Hygiene

A Manual of Personal and Public Health

Arthur Newsholme

Hygiene: A Manual of Personal and Public Health

ISBN: 978-1-64799-356-6

PREFACE

The writing of a preface is perhaps superfluous for a book which has had a large and steady sale for nearly twenty years, and which has evidently met with the approval of a large constituency. A few words of introduction appear, however, desirable in view of the facts that the present edition has been almost entirely re-written; that a large amount of new matter has been introduced; and that, so far as is known, the comments on each subject represent the most recent and authoritative knowledge upon it.

An attempt has been made to meet the requirements of medical students, as well as of science students and general readers, for whom former editions were chiefly intended. A large class of medical students and practitioners do not require the detailed statement of the subject contained in the larger text-books. For them, and, it is hoped, also for a large number of candidates for diplomas in public health and in sanitary science, the present edition will prove to be useful. At the same time, the subject has been treated as non-technically as is consistent with accuracy, in order to retain its suitability for non-medical readers. A large number of new illustrations have been introduced.

The new chapters dealing with Dietetics, Trade Nuisances, Meteorological Observations, Tuberculosis, Disinfection, and Vital Statistics will, it is believed, enhance the value of the book.

Attention is also drawn to the solutions of mathematical problems in the different branches of hygiene, of which a table of contents is given on page viii.

In its new form, it is hoped that this work will be found to have retained its value as a plain and straightforward account of its subject for the general public and for science students; and to have become a practical guide to sanitary inspectors and to medical students, whether preparing for a diploma in public health, or studying hygiene as an important branch of medicine. The use of smaller type for specially technical matter of less general interest will facilitate discriminative reading.

ARTHUR NEWSHOLME

BRIGHTON,
February 28th, 1902

TABLE OF CONTENTS

CHAPTER I

INTRODUCTORY

In classical mythology, Æsculapius was worshipped as the god of Medicine, while his daughter Hygeia had homage done to her as the sweet and smiling goddess of Health. The temples of these two deities were always placed in close contiguity; and statues representing Hygeia were often placed in the temple of Æsculapius. In these statues she is represented as a beautiful maid, holding in her hand a bowl, from which a serpent is drinking—the serpent typifying the art of medicine, then merely an art, now establishing its right more and more to the dignity of a science.

That considerable attention was paid in very early times to matters relating to health, is also shewn by the elaborate directions contained in the Mosaic law as to extreme care in the choice of wholesome foods and drinks, in isolation of the sick, and attention to personal and public cleanliness. It is not surprising, therefore, to find that the Jews, throughout the whole of their history, have apparently enjoyed a high standard of health.

In this country great ignorance of the laws of Health has prior to the last fifty years prevailed, and consequently preventible diseases have been rampant, and have claimed innumerable victims. Each century has been marked by great epidemics, which have swept through the country, scattering disease and death in their course. In the fourteenth century, for instance, there was the Black Death, a disease so fatal that it left scarcely one-fourth part of the people alive; while Europe altogether is supposed to have lost about 40 millions of its inhabitants, and China alone 13 millions. A century and a half later came the Sweating Sickness (though there were a score of minor epidemics in between). This was carried by Henry the Seventh's army throughout the country, and so great was the mortality, that "if half the population in any town escaped, it was thought great favour." Considerable light is thrown on the rapid spread of this disease after its importation, when we remember that there were no means of ventilation in the houses; that the floors were covered with rushes which were constantly put on fresh without removing the old, thus concealing a mass of filth and exhaling a noisome vapour; while clothing was immoderately warm and seldom changed; baths were very seldom indulged in, and soap hardly used.

In the sixteenth and seventeenth centuries there were five or six epidemics of The Plague, and it was only eradicated from London, when all the houses from Temple Bar to the Tower were burned down in the Great Fire of September 2nd, 1666, which destroyed the insanitary and necessitated the building of new and larger houses.

Scurvy, jail-fever, and small-pox, are other diseases which were formerly frightfully prevalent. Jail-fever, the same disease as the modern typhus-fever, has now become practically extinct in its former habitat, owing largely to the noble work of John Howard, "whose life was finally brought to an end by the fever, against the ravages of which his life had been expended." This disease was fostered by overcrowding, ill-ventilation, and filth.

Scurvy formerly produced a very great mortality, especially among sea-faring men. In Admiral Anson's fleet in 1742, out of 961 men, 626 died in nine months, or nearly two out of every three, and this was no solitary case. Captain Cook, on the other hand, conducted an expedition round the world, consisting of 118 men; and although absent over three years, only lost one life. He was practically the first to demonstrate the potency of fresh vegetables in preventing scurvy.

The general death-rate has also greatly declined. Thus while the annual death-rate in London 200 years ago was 80 per 1,000, it only averaged 18.8 in the four years 1896-99; and the death-rate of England and Wales has declined from 22.4 in 1841-50 to 18.7 per 1,000 in 1891-95 and 17.6 in 1896-99.

That much still remains to be done is evident on every hand. There is little doubt that the general death-rate might be reduced to 15 per 1,000 per annum, instead of the present 18, were the laws of health applied in every household and community. It has been estimated that on the average at least 20 cases of sickness occur for every death; therefore nearly half of the population is ill at least once a year. A simple calculation will show how much loss the community annually suffers from this vast mass of preventible sickness. It amounts to many millions of pounds, leaving out of the reckoning the suffering and distress which are always associated with sickness.

In the prevention of this mass of sickness, the knowledge of its causation is half the battle; when once a disease is traced to its source, as a rule, the agency which produces it can be avoided.

The reason why even more progress has not been made in the prevention of disease is not far to seek. In order to prevent a disease it is necessary to remove its causes. The causes of disease can only be ascertained by a careful investigation of its phenomena; and it is only within the last century that these have been studied to any large extent scientifically. Such knowledge of morbid processes not only results in improved measures of treatment, but in more rational and complete measures of prevention. Thus, not only is the number of diseases which are curable becoming gradually augmented, but the number preventible is even more rapidly on the increase.

Inasmuch as the preservation of health involves the prevention of disease, Hygiene, the science of health, is sometimes called Preventive Medicine.

The subject of Hygiene naturally divides itself into two parts, the health of the individual, and that of the community, or Personal and Public Health.

The former treats of the influence of habits, cleanliness, exercise, clothing, and food on health; while the latter is concerned with the interests of the community at large, as affected by a pure supply of air and water, the removal of all excreta, the condition of the soil, and with the administrative measures required to secure the removal of evil conditions. It is obvious, however, that these two divisions are not mutually exclusive. What is important to the health of the community, is equally so to each individual member of it. The purity of air and water, for instance, is of immense importance both personally and collectively.

It will be convenient to study first the three main factors in relation to health—food, water, and air—subsequently considering other matters of importance to health (see pages 4-157).

CHAPTER II

FOOD

PHYSIOLOGICAL CONSIDERATIONS.—All substances are foods which, after undergoing preparatory changes in the digestive organs (rendering them capable of absorption into the circulation), serve to renew the organs of the body, and maintain their functions. Foods have been classified as tissue producers or energy producers, the first class renewing the composition of the organs of the body, and the second class supplying the combustible material, the oxidation (or more correctly the metabolism) of which is the source of the energy manifested in the body. The two main manifestations of energy in the body are heat and mechanical motion, which are to a large extent interchangeable.

All foods come under one of these heads; they are either tissue or energy producers. They may be both, and in many cases are so. Thus, all nitrogenous foods (as meat, legumens, etc.) not only help to form the nitrogenous tissues of the body, but their largest share becomes split up into fats and urea, and so forms a source of heat to the body. Similarly fats may possibly, after assimilation, enter into the composition of the various tissues containing fat (of which the brain is the most important), though they usually supply an immediate source of heat. Proteid foods are, however, the tissue producers par excellence, other foods serving as the immediate sources of energy when metabolised in the body.

Certain foods do not directly serve either as tissue or energy producers, but are useful in aiding the assimilation of food. Such are the various condiments which may be classed as adjuncts to food. Salt is so necessary to the assimilation of food and to the composition of the various tissues, that it may be ranked as an important food. Water, again, though already oxidised, and so not an immediate source of energy, is absolutely necessary to the assimilation of food, to the interchange between the various tissues and the blood, and to the elimination of effete products.

CLASSIFICATION OF FOODS.—Inasmuch as milk supplies all the

food necessary for health and growth during the first year of life, it may reasonably be expected to afford some guidance as to the necessary constituents of a diet for the adult; although the conditions of life being altered in the latter, we can hardly expect the same proportions of the different materials to hold good. In the infant rapid growth and building up of new tissues and organs are going on, involving the necessity for a larger proportional amount of nitrogenous food than in the adult.

The following is the average composition of 100 parts of

	HUMAN MILK.	COW'S MILK.
Casein	2.4	4.0
Albumin	.6	.9
Fat	2.9	3.5
Sugar	5.9	4.0
Salts	.16	.7
	———	———
Total Solids	11.96	13.1
Water	88.04	86.9

It is evident from this analysis of milk that our food must contain (at least) representatives of all the above divisions. We have, therefore:—

1. Nitrogenous Foods.
2. Hydrocarbons or Fats.
3. Carbohydrates or Amyloids.
4. Salts.
5. Water.

Condiments and stimulants (tea, coffee, alcohol) are not foods in the strict sense of the word, and will be discussed in a later chapter.

Nitrogenous Foods include albumin, casein, gluten, legumen, fibrin, and gelatin. They all agree in consisting of a complex molecule containing many atoms of carbon, hydrogen, oxygen, and nitrogen, with the addition of smaller quantities of sulphur, and in some cases phosphorus. The nitrogenous substances used as food may be divided into two groups, (a) those containing gelatin, and (b) numerous bodies which receive the common name of proteids or albuminoids.

The percentage composition of gelatin is:—

CARBON	HYDROGEN	NITROGEN	OXYGEN
50.0	6.6	18.3	25.1

The percentage composition of all proteids lies within the following limits:—

CARBON	HYDROGEN	NITROGEN	OXYGEN	SULPHUR
52.7 to	6.9 to	15.4 to	20.9 to	0.8 to
54.5	7.3	16.5	23.5	1.6

Proteids also contain a small amount of phosphorus, chiefly as phosphate of lime, but also in minute quantity in their essential structure. Various proteids are used in food, e.g. serum-albumin in the blood and tissues of animals; egg-albumin in the white of eggs; myosin in flesh; casein in milk; legumin, or plant-casein, in the seeds of leguminous plants; gluten in wheat-flour, etc.

Proteid foods are pre-eminently important, as they construct and keep in repair the tissues of the body. They are not used solely for this purpose. A large share of the energy of the body is derived from the metabolism of proteids. Meanwhile, it may be said that it is not found to be compatible with efficient health simply to supply an amount of proteid food which will suffice to replace the wear and tear of the tissues, leaving fats and carbohydrates to supply the energy of the body. Deficiency of proteid food always leads to ill-health; and it would appear that in all cases proteid food determines, to a large extent, the metabolism of non-nitrogenous food, and so is favourable to all vital action. The action of nitrogenous food in thus increasing metabolism may make it, when in relative excess, a tissue waster. Banting's cure for corpulence is founded on this principle, lean meat alone being taken, all starchy and saccharine foods being carefully avoided.

By metabolism is meant the changes undergone by food before it reaches the state in which it is finally eliminated from the body. It is commonly spoken of as oxidation, but this word less exactly represents the facts. The complexity of the changes undergone by food in the body may be better appreciated by a glance at the following schematic statement, which only gives an approximation to the truth:-

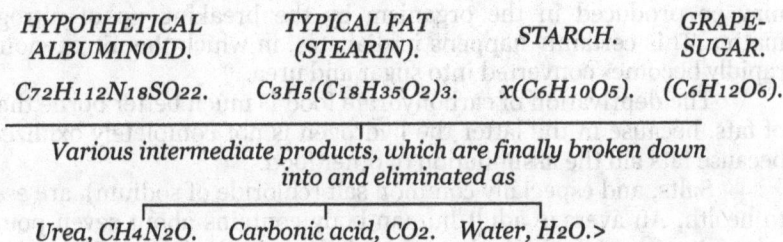

HYPOTHETICAL ALBUMINOID.	TYPICAL FAT (STEARIN).	STARCH.	GRAPE-SUGAR.
$C_{72}H_{112}N_{18}SO_{22}$.	$C_3H_5(C_{18}H_{35}O_2)_3$.	$x(C_6H_{10}O_5)$.	$(C_6H_{12}O_6)$.

Various intermediate products, which are finally broken down into and eliminated as

Urea, CH_4N_2O.   Carbonic acid, CO_2.   Water, H_2O.>

Hydrocarbons, or fats, consist of three elements, carbon, hydrogen, and oxygen, the amount of oxygen present not being sufficient to oxidise completely either the hydrogen or the carbon. Thus the molecule of stearin, which may be taken as a typical fat, has the formula C_3H_5 $(C_{18}H_{35}O_2)_8$.

In respect to their comparatively unoxidised condition fats compare favourably with starch and sugar, $C_6H_{10}O_5$ and $C_6H_{12}O_6$ respectively. It is evident that in starch the $H_{10}O_5 = 5H_2O$, and that in sugar $H_{12}O_6 = 6H_2O$, so that in both cases only carbon remains uncombined with oxygen. Dried fats produce by their oxidation $2\frac{1}{4}$ times as much heat as a corresponding amount of sugar or starch; but the relative advantage of fat is not quite so great as would appear from this comparison, inasmuch as metabolism within the body is not identical with oxidation.

The fat obtained from food is not simply deposited in the body as

5

such, to form a store of combustible matter, and to fill up the interstices between the different tissues. If this were so, the kind of fat deposited would vary with the food, which is not the case. The fat of the body is probably not formed directly from fatty food, but as the result of the metabolism of nitrogenous foods when this metabolism is incomplete. In the formation of milk this can be distinctly proved: the fat cells are formed from the protoplasm of the cells of the mammary gland.

Possibly carbohydrate food may be a source of fat, as well as nitrogenous and fatty food. This appears to be the case in the Strasburg goose, which is kept penned up in a warm room, and fed entirely on barley-meal, in order to produce an enormous fatty liver for the delicacy termed pâté de foie gras. But it may be that the large accumulation of fat in the liver is due to the warmth and inaction of the goose diminishing metabolism, and producing a fatty degeneration of the nitrogenous material of the liver.

Fats and carbohydrates, unlike proteids, do not excite metabolism in the system, and so, if in excess of the requirements of the system, can be stored up with comparative ease. Quiet and warmth, diminishing metabolism, conduce to the accumulation of fat in animals being fed for the market; and the same applies to human beings.

Carbohydrates or amyloids include the various starchy and saccharine foods. They are inferior to fats in nutritive power, but, being very digestible, are in much greater favour. In the process of digestion, starch is converted into grape sugar, and starch and sugar are practically equal in nutritive power.

Even when carbohydrates are entirely absent from the food, they may be produced in the organism by the breaking up of nitrogenous matter. This certainly happens in diabetes, in which the nitrogenous food rapidly becomes converted into sugar and urea.

The deprivation of carbohydrate food is much better borne than that of fats, because in the latter the hydrogen is not completely oxidized, and because fats aid the assimilation of other food.

Salts, and especially common salt (chloride of sodium), are essential to health. An average adult human body contains about seven pounds of mineral matter, of which about five-sixths is in the bones. On analysis the whole body yields about five per cent. of ash.

Chloride of sodium is necessary for the production of the acid (hydrochloric) of gastric juice, and of the salts of bile; half the weight of the ash of blood consists of it. An adult requires 150 to 200 grains of salt per day; a large part of this is taken in meat, bread, etc.; and but little need be taken as a condiment. Potassium salts form an important part of milk, muscle juice, and the blood corpuscles. They are obtained from bread and fresh vegetables and fruits. It has been maintained that deficiency of potassium salts causes scurvy; but this is now discredited, and probably potash is chiefly useful because of the vegetable acids with which it is associated in fruits and vegetables, which when oxidised, help to maintain the alkalinity of the blood, e.g., tartrates, citrates, and malates, which become carbonates in the circulation. Calcium phosphate (bone earth) is essential for the growth of bones, and is very important for the young. The best source for it is milk. There is more lime in a pint of milk than in a pint of lime water. Next to milk, come eggs, and then cereals, especially rice as a source of calcium. Lime salts and phosphates as drugs do not benefit like the same substances taken in natural food, and rickets is not curable by taking such drugs.

Oxide of iron is always present in the ash of blood and muscles, and in smaller quantities in milk. Fish and veal are usually deficient in it, while beef and yolk of egg are foods richest in iron. The amount of iron required in food is minute, and it is amply supplied by ordinary diet.

Phosphorus is an essential building material for the body. It is contained in foods chiefly in organic combination. The foods richest in it are yolk of egg, sweetbread (thymus), fish-roe, calves' brains, and the germ of wheat. Milk and cheese are very rich in phosphates.

Water forms an important article of diet. This is evident from the fact that 80 per cent. of the blood consists of it, and 75 per cent. of the solid tissues; and from the fact that the daily loss of water from the system averages 50 ounces (2½ pints) by the kidneys, and about 40 ounces by the skin and lungs. Water is not simply received into the system as a liquid. It forms a large proportion of the solid food taken. Thus, 87 per cent. of milk, 78 per cent. of fish, 72 per cent. of lean meat, 38 per cent. of bread, 13 per cent. of peas, and 92 per cent. of cabbage, consist of water.

Solid food is dissolved in the alimentary canal by the watery secretions derived from the blood. Water swallowed as food, begins to pass on into the intestine at once. The statement that free consumption of water at meals delays digestion by diluting the gastric juice is therefore not well grounded. In the blood, water serves to carry nutrient materials to all the tissues; and, at the same time being circulated all over the system, equalises the temperature, favours chemical changes, and washes all the tissues. By water again, the effete matters which have been separated by the kidneys are washed out of its tubes.

The Oxygen of the air, in a broad sense, forms one of the foods of the system. This will be considered later.

Besides the above classification, foods have also been classified as follows:—

1. *Inorganic food—Oxygen, salts.*

2. *Organic foods*
   - *Animal* { *Nitrogenous.* / *Non-nitrogenous.*
   - *Vegetable* { *Nitrogenous.* / *Non-nitrogenous.*

Or, as—

1. *Solid foods*
   - *Animal* { *Nitrogenous.* / *Non-nitrogenous.*
   - *Vegetable* { *Nitrogenous.* / *Non-nitrogenous.*

2. Liquid foods
$$\left.\begin{array}{l}\text{Water.}\\ \text{Milk and its products.}\\ \text{Tea and similar beverages.}\\ \text{Alcoholic beverages.}\end{array}\right\}$$

3. Gaseous foods—Air.

CHAPTER III

THE VARIETIES OF FOOD

NITROGENOUS ANIMAL FOODS.—These are divided into two groups, the one containing gelatin, and the other all the proteid or albuminoid substances, which are taken in the flesh of various animals, and in milk and eggs.

Gelatin is obtainable from bones, and from connective tissue wherever found. Being easily digested, and absorbed, it has been very popular as an invalid's food; but the fact that animals cannot sustain life on it without the addition of proteids proves that its value is limited. It is incapable of building tissues, but is a valuable proteid-saver, being able to save from metabolism half its weight of proteid, or twice as much as is spared by an equal weight of carbohydrate. Its utility in this direction is, however, limited, because of the dilute form in which it is taken in ordinary foods. It is useful for invalids, partly because it forms a bulk, and prevents the evil tendency to give their food in too concentrated a form; partly because it forms a source of easily metabolised material, and so prevents tissue-waste; and partly because it commonly contains phosphate of lime, derived from the bones forming the source of gelatin.

Gelatin as prepared for the table contains a considerable proportion of water; as little as one per cent. of gelatin in water will cause it to gelatinise on cooling. Isinglass obtained from the floating bladder of the sturgeon is an example of the purest kind of gelatin; glue is an inferior sort, made from bones, etc.

Gelatin is only a cheap food when obtained, for instance, from bones which cannot otherwise be utilised. When made from veal it is costly out of proportion to its dietetic value.

The Flesh of various animals is one of the main sources of our nitrogenous and fatty food. Meats may be divided into two kinds, viz., red meat and white meat. These gradually merge into one another. As common examples of red meats, we have beef, mutton, pork, game, wild fowl, and salmon.

The common fowl and turkey, most fishes, rabbits, crustaceans, and

8

molluscs, are examples of white meat. As a rule white meats are more digestible than red, having more delicate fibres, and containing a smaller proportion of nitrogenous matter.

Flesh consists almost entirely of muscular tissue, of which there are two kinds, striped and unstriped.

The striped is the variety most commonly used as food. Unstriped muscle has a softer texture, but is not so easily masticated as striped, and for this reason may be indigestible. Tripe is composed of the unstriped muscle and connective tissue of the stomach of the cow, and if well cooked forms a cheap and easily digested dish.

The influence of feeding on the quality of the meat is great. In ill-fed or old animals, connective tissue is more abundant, and the meat is tougher. Well-fed and fattened meat contains for equal weights much more nutritious matter than non-fattened meat, the fat which is deposited in the muscle replacing water and not proteid. Hence the gain in nutritive value is an absolute one, and is not attained at the expense of the proteid part of the meat. Young animals, again, contain more water and fat and a larger proportion of connective tissue than the full-grown, and are consequently not so nourishing.

Meat ought to be eaten either before the onset of rigor mortis, or near its end, before putrefaction has commenced. During rigor mortis it is denser, tougher, and more difficult to digest than after it.

The proportion of fat in meat varies greatly in different individuals of the same species, in different animals, and in different parts of the same animal. According to Dr. Ed. Smith, the proportion of fat in fat oxen is ⅓, in fat sheep ½, in calves ⅙, lambs ⅓, and fat pigs ½.

Good meat, whether beef or mutton, ought to have a marbled appearance, a medium colour, neither pale pink nor deep purple; its texture should be firm, and not leave the impress of the finger; its odour slight and pleasant, the juice reddish and acid, the bundles of fibres not coarse, and free from foreign particles imbedded in them; and lastly, it should not be taken from an animal killed near the time of parturition, nor in consequence of any accident or disease.

Beef is, as a rule, more lean than mutton or pork; it has a closer texture, and more nutritive material in a given bulk. It is also fullest of the red-blood juices, and possesses a richer flavour than the two others.

Liebig's beef extract contains little if any albumin or gelatin. It is a useful stimulant to the gastric secretion, as in soups at the beginning of a meal, but is not a food. Its chief constituents are the various extractives of meat, the most important of which are inosinic acid, kreatin ($C_4H_9N_3O_2, H_2O$), and inosite, or muscle sugar ($C_6H_{12}O_6, 2H_2O$). Even in substances like Bovril, containing powdered meat fibre mixed with Liebig's extract, the amount of nutritive material is very small. The white of one egg contains as much nutritive matter as three teaspoonsful of bovril. None of these substances can be trusted like eggs or milk to keep a patient alive for several weeks.

Mutton is regarded as being more suitable for people of sedentary

9

occupation than beef. Lamb is more watery than mutton, and less nutritious.

Veal, as ordinarily prepared in this country, is difficult of digestion; its shreddy, juiceless fibres eluding the teeth, and consequently not undergoing proper mastication.

Pork is not so digestible as beef or mutton, partly because of the large proportion of fat, and partly because its fibres are hard and difficult to masticate. Its digestibility varies greatly with its age, breeding, and proportion of fat.

The Flesh of Birds contains very little fat, and that found separate from the meat is rarely nice. Most birds are edible, but fish-eating birds are apt to be nasty. As a rule, the flavour of the male bird is richer than that of the female. The chief virtues in poultry are their tenderness, and the large proportion of phosphates they contain. They are deficient in fat and in iron. To compensate for the former, one commonly takes with them melted butter and fat bacon or pork sausages; to compensate for the latter, the addition of Liebig's extract to the gravy is useful. Young, and consequently tender, birds are known by their large feet and leg-joints. When a bird appears at table with violet-tinged thighs and a thin neck, if possible avoid being helped to the leg. Wild fowls are harder and less digestible than tame. In ducks and geese fat is more abundant, and of a stronger flavour; they are, consequently, not so digestible as fowls.

Fish forms an important article of diet. It is easily cooked, and usually very digestible; it possesses a larger bulk in proportion to its nutritive quality, and hence is very valuable for those who habitually take an excess of meat food, which is commonly the case with those leading sedentary lives, and in declining years. There appears to be no foundation for the statement that fish is rich in phosphorus, and is thus a good brain food. Generally, white-fleshed fish is more digestible than red-fleshed (such as salmon), the latter usually containing more fat than the former. When the fat is distributed throughout the flesh, as in the salmon, fish is more satisfying than when it is mainly stored up in the liver, as in the cod-fish. According to Payen, the percentage proportion of fat in soles is only 0.248, in whiting 0.383, conger eel 5.021, mackerel 5.758, eels 23.861. The addition of some fatty food, as melted butter, is very advisable to such meats as poultry, rabbits, soles, whiting, plaice, haddock, cod, turbot, and other fishes; whereas sprats, eels,. herrings, pilchards, salmon, etc., are more or less rich in fat.

A Hen's Egg usually weighs a little under two ounces. It consists of 74 per cent. of water and 26 per cent. of solid matter. The white of the egg is chiefly albumin, the yolk consists of a very digestible oil, rich in phosphorus and iron, each particle of the oil being enveloped in a form of albumin called vitellin. The salts are chiefly contained in the shell. There is no sugar in the egg, the necessity for such oxidisable material for the chick being obviated by the heat produced by incubation. Eggs, when kept for some time, lose weight, owing to evaporation through the porous shell; similarly, air entering from without sets up decomposition. In a solution of brine containing an ounce of common salt to half a pint of water, fresh

10

eggs sink, stale ones float; rotten eggs may even float in fresh water. Eggs may be preserved by keeping them in brine, or, better still in lime water, or by smearing them over with lard or butter, as soon as possible after they are laid.

Cow's Milk has a specific gravity of 1028-34, and on allowing it to stand in a long narrow vessel ought to form ten or twelve per cent of its volume of cream. The legal minimum standard for dairy milk, which is presumably derived from a number of cows, is now 3 per cent. of fat, and 8.5 per cent of "solids not fat." This standard is unfortunately very low, and allows a considerable margin of adulteration, which cannot be prevented by legal means. Thus ordinary milk derived from a herd of cows would probably contain 4.5 per cent. of fat; and it is, therefore, practicable to mix pure new milk with a large proportion of separated milk, and yet keep within the legal standard. This is largely done in towns, and infants suffer much from the deficiency of cream in their sole food. The lactometer determines the specific gravity, which should be taken at a temperature of 60° F. In skimmed or separated milk it will be over 1034; watering on the contrary lowers the specific gravity. If the milk has been both watered and skimmed the specific gravity will give an uncertain indication. Measurement of the cream in a tall narrow glass will enable one to detect the second possible source of fallacy; but the composition of milk can only be certainly determined by analysis. This is done (a) by evaporating a weighed amount of milk to dryness and then re-weighing. (b) From a separate amount of dried milk the fat is extracted by ether, the ether then evaporated, the remaining fat weighed, and its percentage calculated. The weight of fat deducted from the total solids i.e. (b) from (a), gives the "solids not fat." The following example will make the method then followed clear. The sample gives 7.9 per cent. of "solids not fat." Genuine milk contains at least 8.5 per cent. of "solids not fat."

Then the sample contains—

$$100 \times 7.9/8.5 = 92.9 \text{ per cent. of genuine milk,}$$
i.e. 7.1 per cent. of water has been added to it.

Half a pint of milk supplies as much nitrogenous nutriment as two good-sized eggs, and as three and a half ounces of beef. Milk may be deteriorated (1) by skimming or "separating" by machinery, or (2) by the addition of water—the first diminishing the proportion of fats, and the second the total amount of solids.

Skim Milk still contains nearly 1 per cent. of fat, but Separated Milk, in which the cream has been removed by centrifugal apparatus, contains less than 1/8 per cent.

Skim or separated milk forms a cheap source of nitrogenous food; but when it is sold mixed with new or alone as new milk, the public is defrauded, and infants fed on it are robbed of the fat which is so essential for their growth.

Condensed Milk is milk deprived of a large part of its water. It represents three times its volume of fresh milk. There are in the market (a) unsweetened and condensed whole milk, (b) sweetened and condensed

11

whole milk, and (c) sweetened and condensed skim or separated milk. Unfortunately the latter is most largely sold because cheapest; and infants are thus often robbed of fat, a most important element in their food. Always examine the label of each tin carefully, to ascertain whether the milk has been deprived of its cream. The law requires that this fact should be stated on the label. Tins which have bulged should be rejected. Condensed milk is more easily digested by infants than new cow's milk, but it lacks the anti-scorbutic properties of new milk (see page 28). Even the condensed whole milk if diluted beyond 1 part of milk to 3 of water is deficient in fat. Sweetened condensed milk has one-third its weight of extraneous sugar added to it, and on this account it tends in children to produce fatness, and a distaste for simple food; in children fed on it alone ossification (formation of bone) is retarded, and resistance to illness is diminished. The only dietetic advantages it possesses over fresh cow's milk are its freedom from possible disease germs and easier digestibility.

The digestion of milk is preceded by its clotting in the stomach. The same thing happens when junket is formed by the addition of rennet to milk. This is a different process from the curdling of milk, which occurs when milk turns sour. The latter is caused by the splitting up of milk sugar and the formation of lactic acid by certain micro-organisms in the milk. When milk is heated, a skin is formed, consisting of coagulated albumin, in which is also a little casein, fat, and salts of lime. Boiled milk becomes sterilized. Cow's milk should always be boiled, unless it is quite certain that the cows from which it is derived are perfectly healthy, and that the milk has not been exposed to infection before reaching the house. The disadvantages of boiling which are outweighed by its advantages, are that the taste of the milk is altered, some nutritive matter is lost by the formation of the "skin," and the casein is not quite so easily digested. Pasteurization of milk, i.e. keeping it at a temperature of 70° C. (158° F.) for 20 to 30 minutes has been proposed as an alternative to boiling. This appears to destroy the bacilli causing tuberculosis. The typhoid bacilli are killed at 60° C. in five minutes when suspended in emulsion. Pasteurization is not, however, so certainly efficacious for other disease-germs as is boiling, and is not so easily carried out in domestic life as boiling. By boiling milk in a double saucepan, i.e. in a water-bath, very little change occurs in the taste of the milk, especially if it be cooled rapidly and strained.

Cheese is prepared by coagulating milk by "rennet," the mucous membrane of the fourth stomach of the calf, salted and dried before using. By this means the casein is precipitated, carrying down with it the cream, and a large proportion of the salts of milk. The whey, containing the sugar, soluble albumin, and remaining salts, is separated by straining, while the mixed curd and fat are pressed in moulds. Cheese thus consists of casein, fat in varying proportions, water and salts, especially phosphate of lime. It is coloured with annatto, a vegetable colouring matter. When new, cheese is tough; when old, its oils tend to become rancid; the best age is from nine to twenty months. It is probable that cheese in small amount helps the digestion of other foods, though it is itself a highly concentrated and comparatively indigestible food. When toasted it is proverbially indigestible.

There are many different kinds of cheese. The following classification gives the more important varieties:—

(1) Cream cheese is the new curd only slightly pressed, and is more digestible than ordinary cheese.

(2) Next to these are cheeses made with whole milk rich in cream, such as Stilton, Gorgonzola, Cheshire, and Cheddar.

(3) Cheeses made of poor or partially skimmed milk, such as Shropshire, Single Gloucester, and Gruyère.

(4) Cheeses made of skimmed milk, such as Suffolk, Parmesan, and Dutch.

American cheeses may belong to any of these classes; they are generally pure, but occasionally are made from separated milk, margarine being added to take the place of cream. The sale of such cheeses, except under the name of "margarine cheese," is now illegal.

NON-NITROGENOUS ANIMAL FOODS.—These are all fats, and the most important are the various meat fats and butter. They possess a higher food value than carbohydrates in the proportion of $2\frac{1}{4}$; to 1. The composition of the various fats differs somewhat; they usually contain varying proportions of olein, palmitin, and stearin, which are compounds of glycerine with the radicle of a fatty acid (stearin = $C_3H_5 (C_{18}H_{35}O_2)_3$). Thus mutton suet consists of stearin, olein, and palmitin, with a preponderance of stearin. Beef suet contains less stearin and more olein than mutton suet. The more olein a fat contains the less solid it is. Olive oil is composed almost entirely of olein. Palmitin, which melts sooner than stearin, is the chief solid constituent of butter, while olein is its chief liquid constituent. Butter is specially distinguished by containing 7 to 8 per cent. of "volatile fatty acids," such as butyric, caproic, etc., combined with glycerine. The presence and amount of these compounds is an important test for the freedom of butter from adulterating fats.

Cod-liver oil is next to butter the most digestible animal fat known. The best cod-liver oil is frozen at a low temperature, by which means the stearin is frozen out, and nearly pure olein is left. Traces of iodine have been found in it, and more commonly a small amount of bile, which probably increases its digestibility.

The temperature at which a fat becomes hard is a fair guide to its digestibility. Thus we know that beef, and still more, mutton fat, would become solid, under conditions in which bacon dripping is still soft. Where digestion is weak, there may be an instinctive loathing of fat meat; for such persons, especially for children, some other fat should always be substituted. Thus the addition of butter to the potatoes makes up the deficiency.

Butter forms $3\frac{1}{2}$ to $4\frac{1}{2}$ per cent. of cow's milk. It is separated from milk by churning, the oil particles being deprived by this means of their albuminous coats. The more completely the butter-milk is separated the longer the butter keeps. It can be kept longer if salt is added, or in hot weather by keeping it under frequently-changed water. Rancidity indicates the decomposition of traces of the fat of butter into its fatty acid and glycerine.

Cream contains about 30 per cent. of butter fat, Cheshire cheese 25 per cent., and skim milk cheese 7 per cent.

Butter milk differs from skim milk in the presence of lactic acid. It is more digestible than skim milk, the casein being in a more flocculent condition.

The odour and flavour of butter are not due to olein and palmitin, the two chief constituents, but to a smaller quantity of butyrin, caproin, and caprylin fats of a much lower series. Ordinary butter contains a considerable proportion of water, and the presence of about 8 per cent. renders it more palatable; if it is over 15 per cent., the butter is considered adulterated. An excessive amount of salt is sometimes present. The most frequent adulteration is the substitution of foreign fats for butter fat, e.g. lard, palm oil, rape seed oil, or cocoa-nut oil. Margarine is most frequently used for this purpose.

Margarine is prepared from beef-fat by melting, the stearin becoming solid again at a temperature at which olein and margarine still remain liquid. It forms a wholesome and cheap food, being nearly as digestible as butter, for which more expensive food it is often fraudulently sold. When mixed with a small proportion of butter its recognition by smell, etc., is almost impossible, but on careful chemical analysis, it is found to have a higher melting point and a lower specific gravity than butter, and a much smaller percentage of soluble fatty acids than the latter. Thus:—

	MELTING POINT	SPECIFIC GRAVITY	SAPONIFICATION AND FORMATION OF INSOLUBLE FATTY ACID
Butter	32° C.	.913	88 per cent. insoluble fatty acid
Margarine	35° C.[1]	.904-.907	95[2] per cent. insoluble fatty acid

CEREAL FOODS.—Gluten is peculiar to plants, and is chiefly found in plants belonging to the great family of grasses. Gluten is to bread what casein is to milk, and myosin to flesh. If one takes a piece of dough made from wheat flour, and holds it under a stream of water from the tap, a large part of it is washed away, while a sticky adherent mass is left behind. This is gluten, and it is its tenacity which enables bread to be made. If the fluid with which the dough was washed is collected, it will be found to contain a large quantity of starch, a small amount of sugar, of albumin, and certain salts. All cereals possess these constituents in various proportions, as may be seen from the following table:—

---

[1] While the addition of animal fat like margarine raises the melting point, rape-seed oil and other vegetable oils lower it.
[2] The fat to be analysed is saponified with soda or potash, and then the fatty acid set free by hydrochloric acid. If water be now added, 11 or 12 per cent. of the fatty acid will be dissolved, if the fat is butter; less than this if it is a mixture; and not more than 5 per cent. if no butter is present in the fat.

14

	WATR	PROTEID	FAT	CARBO-HYDRATES	CELLULOSE	MINERAL MATTER
Wheatmeal	12.1	12.9	1.9	70.3	1.6	1.2
Fine wheat flour	13.0	9.5	0.8	75.3	0.7	0.7
Oatmeal	7.2	14.2	7.3	65.9	3.5	1.9
Barley meal	11.9	10.0	2.2	71.5	1.8	2.6
Maize meal	11.4	8.5	4.6	72.8	1.4	1.3
Rice (husk removed)	12.0	7.2	2.0	76.8	1.0	1.0

The proteid varies in character in the different cereals; wheat flour has the largest proportion of gluten (8 to 12 per cent.) and therefore makes the best bread.

Good wheat flour ought to be white, not gritty or lumpy, not acid or musty, forming a coherent stringy dough. Examined microscopically, it should show the absence of any fungi, or acarus farinæ, or of foreign starches, such as barley, maize, rice, potato, known by the different shape of their starch granules. (See Fig. 1.) Alum has been occasionally added to flour, to enable the baker to make a white and porous bread from damaged wheat flour. It can be detected as follows:—Pour over the freshly cut surface of a slice of bread some freshly prepared decoction of logwood chips, and then a solution of carbonate of ammonia. If alum is present, the bread turns a marked blue to violet colour; but if the bread is pure, it is only stained pink.

The wheat grain may be used as food in its entirety. Thus boiled in milk, after having been soaked in water, it forms the chief constituent of frumenty. Usually it is converted into flour by grinding or milling. A grain of wheat consists of three parts, an outer envelope, the bran, consisting chiefly of indigestible cellulose, and composing 13½ per cent. of the grain; the kernel, or endosperm, which makes up 85 per cent. of the grain; and the germ, forming 1½ per cent. of the grain. In the old method of stone grinding, the bran was removed, and the germ left along with the endosperm. In the elaborate processes of modern roller milling, the bran is removed as in the old grinding, because it cannot without the greatest difficulty be reduced to powder; and the germ is also removed, because the oil abundantly present in it is apt to become rancid and spoil the flour, and because the soluble proteids in it are apt to change some of the flour into dextrin and sugar, which become brown in baking and spoil the appearance of the bread. The germ is easily removed, because its toughness causes it to be flattened out in the milling, while the endosperm becomes powdery. The central part of the endosperm is the source of 'patents.' It is very rich in starch and is used for making fancy breads and pastry. The outer part of the endosperm is 'households.' 'Households flour' is subdivided into (a) second patents, or 'whites'; (b) first households; (c)

15

second households or 'seconds.' 'Seconds' is richest in gluten, 'whites' in starch. Ordinary bread is normally derived from a blend of these three. Some 'strong' wheats, e.g. Australian, yield a 'patents' which is rich in gluten, and such flour is used for making Vienna bread. 'Strong' wheats take up most water in baking, and so yield most loaves per sack. 'Seconds' flour yields a bread which is richer in proteid than most other kinds; but the dark colour of the loaf makes it unpopular. Various schemes have been devised to utilise the germ and the bran, which are ordinarily discarded. In the preparation of Hovis flour the separated germ is partially cooked by superheated steam. This kills the ferment contained in the soluble proteids, and thus prevents it from changing starch into maltose and dextrin. The action thus prevented is represented by the following formula:—

STARCH.MALTOSE.DEXTRIN.

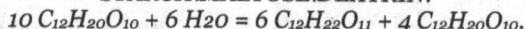

$$10\ C_{12}H_{20}O_{10} + 6\ H_2O = 6\ C_{12}H_{22}O_{11} + 4\ C_{12}H_{20}O_{10}.$$

The germ thus treated is ground to a fine meal, of which one part to three of ordinary flour, forms Hovis flour. Other 'germ breads' are also in the market. In the making of Frame food the bran is boiled with water under high pressure. The watery extract, containing the mineral and part of the nitrogenous constituents of the bran, is evaporated to dryness, and forms the basis of various preparations. It is doubtful if this food possesses any great value.

Brown bread is a somewhat vague expression, meaning either an admixture of bran or of germ or of both with flour, or bread made from whole wheat flour. In each of these cases the loaf would be brown. The bran is rich in fat as well as in phosphates. It acts as a mechanical irritant, ill borne by delicate stomachs, but very useful where a tendency to constipation exists. The excess of nitrogenous matter in brown bread and its richness in fat, do not prove its greater nutritiveness, as it is present in a condition in which only a portion is absorbable from the alimentary canal into the circulation.

The harder wheats, such as Sicilian wheat, contain a larger percentage of gluten; and from them macaroni and vermicelli are obtained, which are nearly pure gluten. They are very nutritious and useful foods. Semolina is prepared from wheat, the millstones being left sufficiently apart to leave the product in a granular condition. In malted breads, a syrupy infusion of malted barley (malt extract) is added to the flour. Malt extract contains in addition to malt sugar (maltose) and dextrins, a ferment (diastase) which, like the saliva, is able to convert starch into the soluble substances, maltose and dextrin (see formulæ above). The action of this ferment is stopped by the temperature of baking. Hence even when the malt extract is allowed a considerable time for its operation on the dough, only about 10 per cent. of the starch in the loaf becomes soluble, as compared with 4 per cent. in an ordinary loaf.

Oatmeal, obtained from the common oat, contains very little gluten, and so cannot be made into vesiculated bread. It contains a large proportion of other nitrogenous material and of fat. As porridge and oatmeal cake it forms a very nutritious diet. The husk ought to be carefully

16

removed from the meal intended for human food, as, although very nitrogenous, it acts as a mechanical irritant. Groats consists of oats from which the husk has been entirely removed. The substitution of rolling for grinding in preparing oats for food and the application of heat during the rolling process, have made oatmeal more digestible, as in Quaker, Provost, and Waverley oats.

Barley contains very little gluten; on this account, like oatmeal, it does not admit of being made easily into bread.

Malt is barley which has been made to germinate by heat and moisture and then dried, "diastase" being formed in the process. Extract of malt, containing diastase in an active condition, is useful in cases of impaired digestion and deficient assimilation of food.

Rye is rarely used in this country for making bread. In Germany it is known as "black bread," but its colour and acid taste make it disagreeable, and it is laxative in its action.

Maize, or Indian Corn, is deficient in gluten, and so not suitable for making vesiculated bread. Like oatmeal, it is made into cakes, called in America "Johnny cake." It contains much fatty matter, and is largely used for fattening poultry and other animals. Oswego flour and corn flour are maize flour deprived by a weak solution of soda, of its proteids and fat; hominy contains all its constituents. Maize is a cheap and nutritious food. When wheat flour is dear, it is occasionally adulterated with maize. The adulteration can be detected by the forms of the starch granules, examined under a low power of the microscope.

Rice contains less proteids and fat than any other cereal. Its chief value as a food depends on the large amount of starch it contains.

LEGUMINOUS FOODS.—The chief seeds belonging to this group are peas, beans, and lentils. They contain a smaller proportion of starch, and a larger proportion of nitrogenous materials than cereals. Thus while flour contains 9.5 and bread 8 per cent. of proteid, lean meat 15.18 per cent., and cheese about 30 per cent., peas and beans contain 21 to 26 per cent. (green peas only 4 per cent., dried peas 21 per cent.) of proteid. The nitrogenous material exists chiefly as legumin, which has been called vegetable casein. Although leguminous seeds contain more nutritive material in a given weight than cereals, dietetically they are inferior, owing to the fact that they are less digestible, often causing flatulence and other dyspeptic symptoms. Cereals, again, are more palatable than leguminous seeds, and are more prolific, and consequently cheaper. In the absence of animal food, legumens form a useful substitute. They are advantageously diluted with oily substances, or with rice. The farm-labourer's dish of broad beans and fat bacon is founded on strict physiological principles. A mixture of lentil and barley flour is sold under the name of Revalenta Arabica. Lentil flour costs 2½d., Revalenta 3s. 6d. per lb. Green peas, French beans, and scarlet runners are much more easily digested than are dried peas or beans. Lentils contain the largest proportion of proteid of any of the pulses. They also contain very little sulphur, and so do not give rise to the same liberation of sulphuretted hydrogen in the intestine, as other pulses. The ash of the Egyptian lentil is particularly rich in iron.

17

AMYLACEOUS FOODS. Amylaceous or starchy substances are contained in many of the preceding foods; but some other foods consist almost entirely of starch. The chief of these are sago, tapioca, and arrowroot.

Sago is obtained from the pith of the stems of various species of palm; a single tree may yield several hundred pounds. Alone it is easy of digestion. Boiled with milk it forms a light, nutritious, and non-irritating food. Fictitious sagos are frequently sold, made from potato starch.

Tapioca and Cassava are derived from the tubers of more than one species of the poisonous family, Euphorbiaceæ. The juices are removed, and the prussic acid removed by heat. Tapioca only differs from cassava in being a purer form of starch; the latter is more nutritious, and among the Indians takes the place of bread.

Arrowroot is obtained from the tubers of Maranta Arundinacea.

Tous-les-mois is a form of starch obtained from the tubers of a West Indian plant, the Canna edulis.

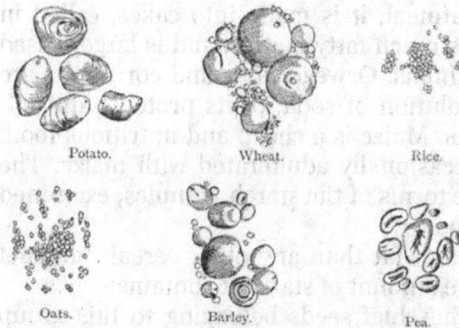

Fig. 1.—Different Forms of Starch Granules.
Potato. Wheat. Rice. Oats. Barley. Pea.

The detection of the varieties of starch is usually possible owing to their fairly characteristic appearance under the microscope. Fig. 1 shows the most important starches. It must be noted that in oats, maize, and rice the contour is completely marked by facets or surfaces, while there are less complete markings in tapioca and sago. In wheat, rye, pea, bean, barley, potato, and arrowroot the contour is even, though there are minor differences of size and shape.

OTHER VEGETABLE FOODS.—Green Vegetables contain comparatively little nutriment, but form valuable additions to other foods. Cellulose, which forms their main constituent, although indigestible, forms a bulk in the alimentary canal, which is necessary to ensure peristalsis. Concentrated nourishment can only be digested in limited quantity, and is very apt to produce digestive disorder. Cabbage contains 92 per cent. of water, and 2½ per cent. nitrogenous matter. Carrots contain 6 per cent. and turnips 2 per cent. of nitrogenous matter; parsnips are intermediate between these. Green vegetables possess valuable anti-scorbutic properties. They may be made an important vehicle for giving fatty food, by adding butter, etc.

Rhubarb and sorrel contain oxalates and tartrates of potash and lime, to which they owe their tartness. Spinach is cooling and laxative, like rhubarb, but not tart. Sea-kale, artichoke, and asparagus are all wholesome vegetables. Asparagus is somewhat diuretic, and gives a peculiar, disagreeable odour to the urine. Salads, such as mustard and cress, water-cress, endive, and the garden lettuce are very useful as anti-scorbutics. Some of them possess a peculiar pungency due to a volatile oil analogous to that contained in horse-radish.

The Potato contains 26 solid parts in 100, of which nearly 20 are starch and 2½ nitrogenous matter. It forms one of our best-appreciated vegetable foods, and as it possesses valuable anti-scorbutic properties, its universal use is, perhaps, the chief cause of the present rarity of scurvy. Alone, it possesses too small a proportion of nitrogenous material to support life, but the addition of butter milk makes up this deficiency; and these two together form a sufficient diet to maintain life and health for a long time.

The Onion, Garlic, Leek, and Shalot, all members of the lily family, are chiefly used as condiments. They contain an acid volatile oil, which gives them a peculiar odour and flavour. By long boiling, this is dissipated (as in the case of the Spanish onion), and the onion is then fairly digestible, as well as nutritious.

Celery possesses a more delicate flavour and odour than the preceding, but even the most tender celery is digested with difficulty; less so, when boiled or stewed, or a constituent of soups.

Only four Fungi are, with us, commonly regarded as safe— mushrooms, champignons, morels, and truffles; but there are many others which are equally edible. The food value of fungi has been exaggerated. They are difficult of digestion and contain little nutritive material. Poisonous fungi usually have an astringent styptic taste and a disagreeable pungent odour. In any doubtful case it is better to abstain.

Oily Seeds contain a considerable amount of fixed oil which renders them unfit for persons of weak digestion. The almond, walnut, hazel-nut, and cocoa-nut are common examples. The sweet almond, when eaten unbleached, occasionally produces nettlerash, and its solid texture and large proportion of fixed oils render it difficult of digestion. The chestnut contains less oil, but a large amount of carbohydrate. It is extensively used as a food in Italy and some other countries. In the uncooked condition it is very difficult of digestion.

Fruits are chiefly used as adjuncts to other foods; but the vegetable salts and the cellulose and sugar which they contain, make them very valuable. Cucurbitaceous fruits are used as vegetables rather than as fruits. Vegetable marrow is wholesome and agreeable, but not very nutritive. Cucumber is most digestible when rapidly grown and freshly gathered.

Stone-fruits or drupes, such as the peach, nectarine, plum, cherry, are rather luxuries than foods, like many other fruits. Before ripening they are unfit for food; when ripening is complete, the acids and astringent matter largely disappear. The date contains chiefly sugar, and forms an important food in the East.

Pomaceous Fruits, as the apple, pear, and quince, are more digestible when cooked; and, speaking generally, all fruit not perfectly ripe should be cooked before eating. The presence of vegetable acids in fruit soon converts the sucrose of cane sugar into dextrose, a less sweet variety of sugar. It is therefore more economical to sweeten after than before cooking.

19

The chief Berries are the grape, currant, gooseberry, cranberry, and elderberry. The grape is the most important, and 1,500 varieties of it have been described. Its juice contains a large amount of grape sugar (dextrose), and small quantities of glutinous material, bitartrate of potash, tartrate of lime, malic acid, etc.

Besides the above fruits, we have strawberries, mulberries, figs, plantains, melons, etc., which are all refreshing and anti-scorbutic. The orange family furnishes us with the orange, lemon, citron, lime, shaddock, and pomelo, of which the orange is by far the most important, and possesses most valuable refreshing qualities.

Sugar exists in two chief forms, viz. sucroses and glucoses. Sucroses, known chemically as disaccharids (Sucrose = $C_{12}H_{22}O_{11}$; compare starch = $C_{12}H_{20}O_{10}$) are exemplified in cane, beet, maple, malt (maltose), and milk sugar (lactose). Cane sugar has been gradually displaced by beet sugar. The two are chemically identical, and equally nutritious. Maltose is given in malt extract as a food, and because of the digestive action of the ferment also contained in the extract on starchy food. Thus:—

STARCH.MALTOSE.
$C_{12}H_{20}O_{10} + H_2O = C_{12}H_{22}O_{11}$.

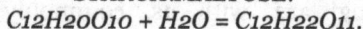

Lactose is comparatively free from sweetness, and is hardly capable of being fermented by yeasts.

Of Glucoses the best example is dextrose = $C_6H_{12}O_6$, H_2O, which can be seen crystallised in dried raisins; it only possesses one-third the sweetening power of sucrose. Starchy food becomes changed into glucose by the action of saliva and pancreatic juice in the alimentary canal. Grapes, cherries, gooseberries, figs, and honey contain lævulose in addition to glucose (glucose = $C_6H_{12}O_6$, H_2O, lævulose = $C_6H_{12}O_6$). Lævulose resembles dextrose except in being uncrystalline, and in its effect on polarised light. Many ripe fruits, such as pineapples, strawberries, peaches, citrons, contain sucrose and lævulose, the latter being not quite so sweet as sucrose.

In the alimentary canal sucroses are inverted into dextrose and lævulose. Thus natural foods containing these sugars are more readily assimilated than those containing sucrose.

The sweetening power of the varieties of sugar depends on their degree of solubility in water. Sucrose is soluble in one-third of its weight of cold, and in rather more of hot water. Dextrose is soluble in its own weight of water; lævulose is more soluble, and therefore sweeter than dextrose. Lactose requires five to six parts of cold and two of hot water, and is therefore not so sweet as the other varieties.

20

CHAPTER IV

DISEASES DUE TO FOOD

Diseases may arise from the noxious character or from deficiency or excess of some particular food, or of the food as a whole.

DISEASES FROM UNWHOLESOME FOOD.—I. The Meat of Diseased Animals.

(1) The flesh of animals which have not been slaughtered should be prohibited from sale, whether death has resulted from accident or disease. The meat from diseased animals is also generally dangerous, sometimes owing to the drugs with which the animals have been dosed before death, e.g. tartar emetic, or opium.

(2) Meat may be unwholesome from the presence of parasites. Of these the most common is—

(a) The cysticercus cellulosæ, which is the undeveloped embryo of the tape-worm; that from the pig becomes the tænia mediocanellata. The cysticercus of the pig is the most common; it forms a cyst about the size of a hemp-seed, commonest on the under surface of the tongue. In hams oval holes are found or opaque white specks, which are the remains of the cysts converted into calcareous matter. When meat containing the cysticercus alive (as in under-cooked or raw meat) is swallowed, it develops into the tape-worm, which consists of a number of flat segments, each capable of producing numerous ova of new cysticerci, with a minute head at the narrow end surrounded by hooklets. A temperature of 174° F. kills the cysticercus. Another kind of tape-worm common on the continent, called bothriocephalus latus, is derived from the cysticercus of fish.

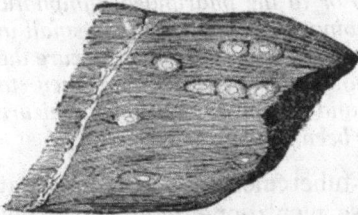

Fig. 2.
Cysticercus ("Measles") in Pork.
(Natural Size.)

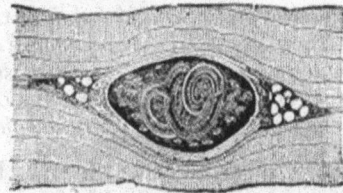

Fig. 3.
Trichinæ Capsulated in Flesh.
Magnified.

(b) The trichina spiralis is not a solid worm like the tænia, but possesses an intestine. In pork it forms a minute white speck, just visible to the naked eye, which forms a nest, and in this one or two coiled up worms can be seen by a magnifying glass in active movement. They are effectually killed by the temperature of boiling water; but no form of drying, salting, or even smoking at a low temperature is sufficient for this purpose. Boiling or roasting does not suffice to destroy all the trichinæ unless the joint is

21

completely cooked in its interior. When trichinous pork is swallowed, the eggs develop in the alimentary canal in about a week into complete worms, and in three or four days more each female produces over a hundred young ones. These burrow into every part of the body, producing great irritation and inflammation. In one case after death upwards of 50,000 worms were estimated to exist in a square inch of muscle. Most of the cases of trichinosis have occurred in Germany, from eating imperfectly cooked sausages. The pig becomes trichinous by eating offal, and man is infected by eating pork. This disease is rare in England.

(3) Tuberculous Meat, from animals suffering from tuberculosis, has been found to cause tuberculosis in small animals experimentally fed on it. Koch has recently thrown doubt on the communicability of bovine tuberculosis to man; but this point must be regarded as still unsettled. Sheep are rarely affected by it, but it is very common in cattle, especially in cows, and it is a serious economical question whether the meat of all such animals should be condemned. The ideal would be to condemn all such animals, as tuberculosis is an infective disease, and the bacillus which causes it (as well as the toxic products of its activity) may be present in meat which shows no actual signs of disease, except in the lungs or other internal organs. In practice, however, the rules laid down by the Royal Commission on Tuberculosis, in 1898, should be followed for the present. These state that:—

"The entire carcase and all the organs may be seized (a) when there is miliary tuberculosis of both lungs, (b) when tuberculous lesions are present on the pleura and peritoneum, or (c) in the muscular system, or in the lymphatic glands embedded in or between the muscles, or (d) when tuberculous lesions exist in any part of an emaciated carcase. The carcase, if otherwise healthy, shall not be condemned, but every part of it containing tuberculous lesions shall be seized (a) when the lesions are confined to the lungs and the thoracic lymphatic glands, (b) when the lesions are confined to the liver, (c) or to the pharyngeal lymphatic glands, or (d) to any combination of the foregoing, but are collectively small in extent." They also add that any degree of tuberculosis in the pig should secure the condemnation of the entire carcase, owing to the greater tendency to generalisation of tuberculosis in this animal; and that in foreign meat, seizure should ensue in every case where the pleura has been "stripped."

(4) Other Infective diseases besides tuberculosis may render meat wholly or partially unfit for food. Of these pleuro-pneumonia may not require condemnation of the entire carcase; but in the following this course should be adopted, cattle-plague, pig typhoid (pneumo-enteritis), anthrax, and quarter ill, as well as in sheep-pox. In puerperal fever, actinomycosis, and sheep-rot (liver flukes) each case must be decided on its merits.

II.—Decomposed Meat.—Putrid meat has often produced diarrhœa and other severe symptoms. Putrid sausages are especially dangerous, and incipient putridity seems to be more dangerous than advanced.

Tinned Meats occasionally produce severe illness, which has been in several cases fatal. It is important to secure a good brand, and to eat the meat as early as possible after the tin is opened. Tins in which any bulging is present, showing the presence of putrefactive gases, must be rejected;

22

and still more tins which have been pricked and resoldered in a second place. All tinned meats and fruits are stated by Hehner to contain compounds of tin in solution. These do not seem to be perceptibly injurious, unlike lead salts, which are now rarely found.

The general subject of Meat Poisoning has had much light thrown on it during the last few years. Brieger, about 1886, showed that during the cultivation of bacteria, alkaloidal bodies known as ptomaines and leucomaines, were formed, which were virulently poisonous. It was commonly supposed that the poisoning occasionally produced by eating meat pies, sausages, hams, brawn, and similar food, was due to these ptomaines. It is now known, however, that there are far more important toxines than the alkaloidal, which result from bacterial life in meat, etc. (see page 286). These are more closely related to substances of an albuminous or proteid nature than the ptomaines. These toxines may be fatal when as small a dose as a fraction of a milligramme (mgm. = about 1/64 grain) is given subcutaneously. The evidence now shows that neither ptomaines nor other toxines (albumoses) or any other bacterial products besides these, cause the outbreaks of acute poisoning occasionally traced to food, but that these are due to bacteria. There is, in other words, actual infection, as well as poisoning. The microbe chiefly found as the cause of these outbreaks is the Bacillus enteritidis of Gaertner, and some allied microbes. In an outbreak at Oldham, 160 pies made on a Thursday, from the veal of a calf killed on the preceding Tuesday, were baked in several batches, and of the persons eating these pies fifty-four became ill. That the contamination was not introduced after cooking was shown by the fact that several persons were made ill who ate pies still warm from baking. The facts indicated that one batch was imperfectly cooked, the time allowed being only twenty minutes, as compared with fifty minutes allowed in corresponding cooking in domestic life. Experimentally it has been found that an exposure for one minute to 70° C. kills the Bacillus enteritidis of Gaertner. That this bacillus was the cause of the outbreak was subsequently shown by the fact that the serum of blood taken from some of the patients showed characteristic clumping with a pure culture of this bacillus, just as happens with the blood of a patient suffering from enteric fever when a cultivation of the microbe of this fever is mixed with it. In this outbreak the symptoms were usually diarrhœa, vomiting, intense thirst, desquamation of the skin, and a slow convalescence, lasting from three to six weeks.

III.—Meat injuries from the food eaten before killing.—Pheasants fed on laurel, hares on rhododendron chrysanthemum, and other animals fed on the lotus, wild cucumber, and wild melon of Australia, have caused dangerous symptoms.

IV.—Fish, especially some kinds, occasionally produce nettlerash and other disorders, especially in warm weather. Leprosy has been ascribed to the eating of decomposing fish, but it occurs in countries where a fish diet is impossible.

Shell-fish and crustaceans (as lobster, crab) are very prone to produce evil results. Shell-fish (mollusca), such as mussels, cockles, and

23

oysters, are dangerous foods. They are generally grown in estuaries, to which the sewage of towns has access; and not infrequently cases of enteric (typhoid) fever, as well as more acute attacks of diarrhœa and vomiting, have been traced to them. Mussels and cockles are seldom sufficiently cooked to render them safe; and oysters are eaten raw. They should never be eaten, unless from personal direct knowledge it is certain that they have been derived from an estuary in which there was no possibility of contamination by sewage.

V.—Milk has been a common carrier of disease. Cows eating the rhus toxicodendron get the "trembles," and their milk produces serious gastric irritation in young children. The milk of goats fed on wild herbs or spurgeworts has produced severe disorders.

The milk of animals suffering from foot-and-mouth disease, although frequently drunk with impunity, occasionally produces inflammation of the mouth (aphthous ulceration). The milk derived from cows fed on grass from sewage farms is, per se, as wholesome as any other, and its butter has no more tendency to become putrid than that derived from any other source.

The great dangers in respect to milk are of its becoming mixed with contaminated water; or of its absorbing foul odours. The absorptive power of milk for any vapour in its neighbourhood, is shewn by exposing it in an atmosphere containing a trace of carbolic acid vapour: the milk speedily tastes of the acid.

Milk also tends to undergo rapid fermentative changes, especially in warm weather, or when tainted by traces of putrefying animal matter. Diarrhœa in children is frequently due to such a condition, or to the rapid decomposition of milk in an imperfectly cleaned bottle. Milk should always be boiled in warm weather; and it should never be stored in ill-ventilated larders, or where there is a possibility of the access of drain effluvia; nor ought it to be kept in lead or zinc vessels.

Epidemic diarrhœa has been ascribed by Klein to a microbe called the Bacillus enteritidis sporogenes. This is not killed by heating the liquid containing it to 80°C. for twelve to fifteen minutes, as is the typhoid bacillus and other non-spore-forming bacilli. In an outbreak of diarrhœa among the patients in St. Bartholomew's Hospital, London, there was strong evidence that this microbe taken in rice pudding had caused the mischief. Eighty-four patients and two nurses were attacked, and the patients who had eaten rice pudding were almost exclusively attacked. A portion of this pudding after being kept twenty-four hours was found sour and acid. The Bac. enteritidis sporog. was found in it. Furthermore it was shewn that the temperature at which the rice puddings were cooked never exceeded 98°C., whereas the spores of this microbe withstand 100°F. a considerable time.

Very many epidemics of enteric fever and scarlet fever, and a smaller number of epidemics of diphtheria have been traced to contaminated milk. Usually in enteric fever the contamination of the milk was traced to the use of water "for washing the milk-cans," derived from specifically polluted sources, and doubtless the water was the real source of the disease. In most of the milk outbreaks of scarlet fever, either there was scarlet fever in the dairy, or persons employed in the dairy were in attendance on patients suffering from the disease; but in an outbreak connected with a supply of milk from Hendon, it was suspected that a certain eruptive disease of the udders of the cow might have been the cause of scarlet fever in man, without infection from a previous case of the disease. This point is still sub judice.

Tubercular disease of the intestines and mesenteric glands may be produced by taking milk derived from tuberculous cows. This was proved in the case of calves, and there are strong reasons for thinking that the same is true for infants, though doubt has been thrown by Koch on the communicability of bovine tuberculosis to the human being. The only safe plan is to sterilise the milk.

VII.—Vegetable Food (especially greens) is indigestible if stale, and all mouldy vegetables are dangerous. Over-ripe and rotten fruit is liable to produce diarrhœa; but the diarrhœa prevalent in summer is due much less to this than to other decomposing foods, particularly milk.

Poisonous symptoms have been produced by the admixture of darnel (lolium temulentum) with flour.

The eating of damaged maize in Italy is the cause of an endemic skin disease, called pellagra, which commonly proves fatal.

Ergotism is due to the growth on cereals (and most commonly on the rye) of a poisonous fungus, the claviceps purpurea, which produces a deep purple deposit on the grain. If bread made from such flour is eaten for prolonged periods, severe symptoms result; in some cases, a dry rotting of the limbs. There have been several epidemics on the continent, due chiefly to eating bad rye bread.

Starvation Diseases.—Simple Starvation causes death in a period varying with the previous state of nutrition. Usually death occurs when the body has lost two-fifths of its weight, whether this be after days, months, or years (Chossat). A supply of water prolongs the duration of life, to as much as three times what it would otherwise be. Good nourishment doubles the power of resisting disease; while deficient food prepares the way for many diseases. A large share of the decline in the English death-rate during the last forty years is due to free trade, and the great cheapening of wholesome food which has resulted from it.

An ill-balanced is more frequent than a deficient diet. Deficiency of fat is more serious than deficiency of carbohydrates, and deficiency of proteid is most serious.

Scurvy is caused by the absence of fresh vegetables. The use of the potato and the orange, as well as of lime juice (the juice of citrus limetta), has led to its extinction among adults in this country. In former times, it caused more deaths among seamen than all other causes put together, including the accidents of war. In infants fed upon tinned foods, whether condensed milk or patent foods, a form of scurvy still occurs. Infants fed on new-milk never suffer in this way. If, therefore, it is necessary to feed an infant on condensed milk for many consecutive months, potato gruel or raw meat juice or fresh milk must occasionally be given.

Rickets is chiefly due to improper feeding in childhood. The substitution of artificial foods (most of them containing starch) for the natural milk is its chief cause. The lower incisor teeth of an infant appear between the sixth and seventh months. Starchy food given before this age is undigested. Such food likewise leads to less fat and proteid being given, which are essential for growth. Deficiency of lime salts in the food does not cause it, and giving them in food or medicine will not cure it. Enrichment of the diet by cream or failing this by cod liver oil is the best means of preventing and curing it. Abundant fresh air and warm clothing are also necessary.

Relapsing fever generally follows epidemics of typhus fever, and is greatly favoured by starvation. Ophthalmia has been chiefly prevalent in charity schools in which the children are underfed, though its essential cause is contagion.

Diseases Connected with Over-Feeding.—A fire may go out for want of fuel, or from becoming choked with ashes; and it is the latter state of things which occurs in Gout and allied diseases. Weakness is commonly complained of, but this is due to excess of food embarrassing vital action; and abstinence and exercise are required to restore the balance. Excess of nitrogenous food—especially if combined with the use of sweet, or strong, or very acid wines, and beer—is particularly prone to produce gout. In these cases, animal food should only be taken once a day, and vegetable food should be allowed to preponderate.

Obesity is favoured by excess of starchy food and sugar, and by copious drinking of water or other beverages. The plan of curing obesity by restricting oneself almost entirely to meat food is only advisable, however, under certain conditions. Gall-stones are favoured by rich foods and excess of sugar; also by alcoholic indulgence. Dyspepsia is commonly due to loading the stomach at too frequent intervals; but on the other hand, it not infrequently leads to the taking of insufficient food, because of the discomfort produced. The result of this is that a chronic starvation results, with impaired vital powers. Dyspeptic patients should abstain from pastry and from tea and coffee, except in small quantities. Alcohol in any form, as a rule, does harm. Not uncommonly mastication is imperfectly performed, and a good dentist may cure the indigestion which has resisted all other treatment.

CHAPTER V

DIET

The importance of a duly proportioned and sufficient dietary is shown by its great influence on health and constitution. An ill-

26

proportioned or deficient diet is certain to lead to failure of health. The anatomy of an animal may be modified in the course of generations by altered diet, as well as its character; thus, the alimentary canal of the cat has increased in length to adapt it to its omnivorous habits. In the case of the bee we have a still more remarkable instance. If by any accident the queen bee dies, or is lost, the working bees (which are sexually undeveloped) select two or three eggs, which they hatch in large cells, and then feed the maggot on a stimulating jelly, different from that supplied to the other maggots, thus producing a queen bee.

The food of mankind varies naturally with—

I.—Climate. A cold climate leads to increased metabolism, and consequently a large amount of fatty matter can be eaten without producing nausea. Witness the difference between a Laplander's and a Hindoo's diet.

The season of the year has likewise some influence. Vital processes are more active in spring than autumn, and more food is consequently required in the former season.

II.—Occupation. Although muscular exercise is not associated with an immediate increase of elimination of urea, yet as a matter of experience more nitrogenous food is required and can be metabolised by hard workers than by idlers. The trappers on the North American prairies can live for weeks together on meat alone, accompanied by copious draughts of tea. They are constantly in the open air, undergoing fatiguing exercises, in a dry and rare atmosphere. For brain workers no special food is required. Foods containing phosphorus have no special value, so far as is known, for mental work. Such work, however, is apt to affect digestion; consequently the digestibility of food is more important for those engaged in sedentary occupations than its chemical composition.

III.—Sex. As a rule, women require about one-tenth less food than men, but probably this rule hardly holds good in the case of women engaged in laborious work.

IV.—Age. Infants require only milk, and the less they have of any other food before a year old the better. Atwater has calculated that——

A child under 2 requires 3/10 the food of a man doing moderate work.
A child of 3 to 5 requires 4/10 the food of a man doing moderate work.
A child of 6 to 9 requires 5/10 the food of a man doing moderate work.
A child of 10 to 13 requires 6/10 the food of a man doing moderate work.
A girl of 14 to 16 requires 7/10 the food of a man doing moderate work.
A boy of 14 to 16 requires 8/10 the food of a man doing moderate work.

Vital processes are more active in early life, and food is required not only to carry on the functions of the body, but also to furnish the materials for growth. Hence, while the proportion of proteids to carbohydrates and fats should be—

As 1:5.3 in adults, it should be about as 1:4.3 in children.

After the age of thirty-five or forty, the tendency is to take too much food. All the tissues of the body are established, and excess of food (especially nitrogenous food) is liable to produce tissue degeneration by loading the system with partially metabolised matter, and may lead to gouty diseases. It is much safer to take what may be regarded as too little than too much food after this period.

Times for Eating.—The best arrangement seems to be to have three meals, each fairly nutritious, and containing all the constituents required. The Romans only had two meals daily, prandium and cœna. This is common among the French at present, but it tends to overloading the digestive organs at these meals.

An ordinary full meal has usually passed from the stomach in four hours. Fresh food ought never to be introduced before this period; it is advisable to allow an interval of five hours between meals for the healthy, so as to give time for the digestive organs to rest, and for the absorption of food. The practice of taking tea with the chief meal, or a "meat tea," is bad. Tea is better taken an hour or two after food.

Regularity in the time of taking meals is important, as the digestive organs acquire habits like other parts of the body. Work ought not, if possible, to be resumed immediately after meals, nor active exercise of any kind. These tend to abstract blood from the digestive organs, and so diminish the efficiency of digestion.

Vegetable and Animal Foods.—The fact that the food we require can be obtained from the vegetable world has led to the proposition that vegetable food should be taken alone. It is urged in favour of this plan, that a large amount of suffering to animals would be prevented. Also that animal food is not so economical as vegetable, land being more economically employed in producing corn than in feeding cattle. Thirdly, there is the indubitable fact that health can be maintained for prolonged periods on vegetable food (including nuts, cereals, fruits, etc.)

On the other hand, the chief objections to a purely vegetable diet are that the undigested refuse is greater than with an equal quantity of animal food; that a longer time and more exertion than for animal foods are required in digesting the most nutritious vegetable foods, such as legumens, while other vegetable foods do not contain a sufficient proportion of nitrogenous material. Also, if one lived entirely on vegetable food, a greater bulk would be required, and owing to the fact that such food is less easily absorbed, satisfaction to the appetite would not so soon be produced. Animal food has a great advantage as regards convenience. Man is not an eating machine; he requires food which is easily converted into the body substance, and this is supplied by the flesh of animals, milk and eggs, with a due proportion of non-nitrogenous food; sheep and oxen work up indigestible vegetable materials into easily assimilable mutton and beef. The greater convenience of animal food as a supply of proteid is shown by the following examples of foods after the removal of water:—

100 parts of rice	contain		7	parts of proteid.
„	wheat	„	16	„
„	pea flour	„	27	„
„	dried lean beef	„	89	„

On the other hand, vegetable foods are a cheaper source, not only of

28

carbohydrates and fats, but also of proteids as well. Thus the approximate cost of—

1 lb.	of proteid in	beef is 2s. 8d.
„	„	milk is 2s. 2d.
„	„	bread is 1s. 6d.
„	„	oatmeal is 7½d.
„	„	peas is 7d.

Under the ordinary conditions of town life, there is considerable danger of indulging in an excess of nitrogenous food, and vegetarians may therefore do good by showing that meat is not absolutely necessary, and can often with advantage be largely replaced by vegetable food.

If we include milk, cheese, and eggs in the vegetarian diet, the objections to it partially disappear; and it would be well if it were much more widely known, especially among the poor, that on these, together with vegetables, health can be maintained with the addition of little or no meat.

The Determination of Diet.—The first principle in making a dietary is that it must be mixed, containing all the necessary constituents, proteids, hydrocarbons, carbohydrates, water, and salts. No one of these alone will support life for any considerable period. Carbohydrates (sugar and starch) can be most easily dispensed with; fats, on the other hand, are essential for the maintenance of health.

The next point is to ascertain the proportion in which these different foods are required. Salts are commonly taken with other foods, common salt being the only one taken alone. The amount required is given on p. 7. The amount of water required varies with the season of the year, the amount of exercise and perspiration, and other factors. As a rule, not more than two pints of water are required per day, and still less if fruit is freely taken. We may therefore confine our attention to the carbonaceous and nitrogenous foods, and try to ascertain the amount of each of these required. Every diet must be subjected to the following tests, to fully ascertain its value:—

1. The Chemical Test.—The metabolism undergone by food in the body being essentially a process of oxidation (though partially modified and incomplete), the amount of heat yielded on complete combustion of a food may be taken as a measure of its value as a source of energy, of which heat and work are convertible forms. The standard of heat production is the calorie, the amount of heat required to raise the temperature of one gramme of water 1° C. This is the small calorie. The kilo-calorie (called the Calorie) is the amount of heat required to raise 1 kilo (1 litre) of water 1° C., or 1 lb. of water 4° F. In calculations on this basis, allowance must be made for foods which are incompletely oxidised in the body. Rubner has shown that the heat value of 1 gramme (=15½ grains) of each of the chief food stuffs is as follows:—

Proteid	4.1	Calories.
Carbohydrates	4.1	„
Fat	9.3	„

29

The method of applying this standard to a food is as follows: the percentage of proteid or carbohydrate given in the following table is multiplied by 4.1, and the percentage of fat by 9.3:—

IN 100 PARTS

	WATER	ALBUMINATES OR PROTEIDS	FATS	CARBO-HYDRATES	SALTS
Uncooked meat with little fat	74.4	20.5	3.5	—	1.6
Cooked meat—without loss	54	27.6	15.45	—	2.95
Salt beef	49.1	29.6	0.2	—	21.0
White fish	78.0	18.1	2.9	—	1.0
Bread, white wheaten	40.	8.	1.5	49.2	1.3
Wheat flour	15.	11.	2.	70.3	1.7
Rice	10	5	.8	83.2	0.5
Oatmeal	15	12.6	5.6	63.0	3.
Peas (dry)	15	22	2.	53.	2.4
Potatoes	74	1.5	.1	23.4	1.
Butter	8	2.	88	—	variable
Eggs (including shell, for which deduct 10 per cent.	73.5	13.5	11.6	—	1
Cheese	36.8	33.5	24.3	—	5.4
Milk	87.0	4.	3.5	4.8	.7

Thus for bread—
Proteid $8 \times 4.1 = 32.8$
Fat $1.5 \times 9.3 =$ 13.95
Carbohydrate $49.2 \times 4.1 =$ 201.72
————
Total Caloric value of 100 grammes of bread =   248.47

The total fuel value in Calories of one pound of certain typical foods is given by Hutchison as follows:—Butter 3,577, peas 1,473, cheese 1,303, bread 1,128, eggs 739, beef 623, potatoes 369, milk 322, fish (cod) 315, apples 238.

2. The Physiological Test.—Not only is a proper proportion of proteid, fat, and carbohydrates required, but these must be capable of digestion and absorption and of oxidation in the body. Cheese is a highly concentrated food, but its value is less than its percentage composition would indicate, because of the difficulty of digesting considerable quantities of it. Green vegetables consist largely of cellulose, which is only imperfectly capable of absorption into the blood, although it can experimentally be oxidised by combustion. The proportion between absorbed food and food rejected in the fæces can be ascertained by analysis. Many experiments made on these lines show that on a purely animal diet (meat, eggs, milk) but little nitrogen is lost, while with vegetable foods (carrots, potatoes, peas, etc.) the waste of nitrogen is

considerable. Fats are very completely absorbed from the alimentary canal. The amount remaining unabsorbed is greatest with mutton fat (10 per cent.), least with butter (2½ per cent.). Experimentally it has been found that an amount up to 150 grammes (about 5½ oz.) of fat can be absorbed without appreciable loss. Carbohydrates are very completely absorbed, even starchy foods rarely escaping digestion. Completeness of absorption from the alimentary canal is not desirable for all foods; a certain amount of unabsorbed residue is required to stimulate peristalsis. With a purely vegetable diet this amount is excessive, and there is physiological waste of effort.

3. In practical dietetics the Economic test is important. Carbohydrate is by far the cheapest food, and generally vegetable are cheaper than animal foods. Thus a shilling's-worth of bread yields 10,764 Calories, while the same sum spent on milk would only yield 1/3, and on beef 1/10 this number of heat units. Similarly a shilling's-worth of peas contains 572 grammes of proteid, about double as much as the same money's-worth of cheese; while to obtain the same amount of proteid from eggs would cost more than eight, and from beef more than five times as much as from peas (Hutchison). The market price of foods is no certain indication of their nutritive value. Thus haddock will supply as much nutriment as sole at a fourth of the cost; Dutch as much nutriment as Stilton cheese at less than half the cost. Similarly the most economical fats are margarine and dripping.

4. An Examination of Actual Dietaries under various conditions has strikingly confirmed the results obtained by other methods. It has been found that (a) the potential energy required by a healthy man weighing 11 stones, and doing a moderate amount of muscular work is 3,000 to 3,500 Calories (=310 grains); and that (b) about 20 grammes of nitrogen and 320 grammes (=4,960 grains) of carbon are excreted by such a man. (c) Expressing the 3,000 Calories required in terms of grammes of food, it is found that 125 grammes of proteid, 500 of carbohydrate and 50 of fat are necessary. These facts are expressed in the following table (Hutchison):—

STANDARD AMOUNT OF FOOD CONSTITUENTS REQUIRED (IN GRAMMES)	SAME AMOUNT OF FOOD FOOD IN TERMS OF		YIELDING ENERGY IN Calories
	CARBON	NITROGEN	
Proteid	125	62	20	512·5
Fat	500	200	——	2050·
Carbohydrate	50	38	——	465·
	675	300	20	3027·5

Three of the best known standard dietaries give the amounts in grammes of each food constituent as follows:

	PLAYFAIR	MOLESCHOTT	ATWATER	AVERAGE
Proteid	119	130	125	125

31

Fat	51	40	125	72
Carbohydrate	531	550	450	510
Calories	3140	3160	3520	3273

Expressing the same facts in English ounces instead of grammes, 42/5 oz. of proteid, 2½ oz. of fat, and 18 oz. of carbohydrate, would represent the ounces of each constituent required according to

	(1) AVERAGE OF ABOVE THREE DIETARIES	(2) HUTCHISON
Proteid	$4/25$	$4/25$
Fat	$2\,1/2$	$1/45$
Carbohydrate	18	$17/35$
Ounces of dry food	$24/910$	$23/45$

The chief point of divergence in the above standard dietaries is in the relative proportion of carbohydrate and fat. Probably the correct proportion between these is as 1 to 10; but it will vary according to climate and other circumstances. Detailed examination of a large number of dietaries shows that the amount of daily proteid should be about 125 grammes, or 4⅖ozs. This is contained in 20 eggs, or in 18 oz. i.e. about 4½ ordinary platesful of cooked meat.

It must be noted that the 23-24 oz. of food given above as the standard daily amount represents dry food. This represents 40 oz. or nearly 3 lbs. of ordinary food.

The following example by Waller, gives a rather liberal standard English diet, for a man doing a moderate amount of muscular work.

		CARBON.	NITROGEN.
Foundation:	1 lb. bread	117	5.5
	½ lb. meat	34	7.5
	¼ lb. meat	84	—
Accessories:	1 lb. potatoes	45	1.3
	½ pint milk	20	1.7
	¼ lb. eggs	15	2.0
	⅛ lb. cheese	20	3.0
		—	——
	Total	335	21 grammes.

This divided up into meals works out roughly as follows (Hutchison):—

Breakfast	Two slices of thick bread and butter.
	Two eggs.
Dinner	One plateful of potato soup.

A large helping of meat with some fat.

Four moderate sized potatoes.

One slice of thick bread and butter.

Tea   *A glass of milk and two slices of thick bread and butter.*

Supper   *Two slices of thick bread and butter and 2 oz. of cheese.*

From the preceding data, practical problems as to dietaries are easily solved. Thus if it be required to find *how much oatmeal, milk, and butter would be required to give a sufficient quantity of albuminoids, fats, and carbohydrates to an adult male,* the calculation may be based on the figures in the table on p. 32, or the following figures may, for the sake of convenient calculation, be taken as representing the percentage amount of each of these chief food principles contained in the foods named:—

	ALBUMINOIDS	FATS	CARBOHYDRATES
Oatmeal	12	6	60
Milk	4	3	5
Butter	2	88	—

Let

o = number of ounces of oatmeal required.

m = number of ounces of milk required.

      b = number of ounces of butter required.

Then

$(120 + 4m + 2b)/100 = 4.5$ ozs. of albuminoid

$(60 + 3m + 88b)/100 = 3$ ozs. of fat

$(600 + 5m)/100 = 14.25$ ozs. of carbohydrate,

according to Moleschott's diet.

When these equations are worked out by substitution and transference—

$o = 19.2$ *ounces.*

$m = 55.4$ *ounces.*

$b = 0.24$ *ounces.*

Similarly if it is required to find how much meat, bread, and butter of the following percentage composition will be required to give a man a sufficient amount of albuminoids, fats, and carbohydrates.

	ALBUMINOIDS.	FATS.	CARBOHYDRATES.
Meat	25	15	0
Bread	8	1.5	50
Butter	2	88	0

Let

m = number of ounces of meat required.

b = number of ounces of bread required.

B = number of ounces of butter required.

Then

$(12m + 8b + 2B)/100 = 4.5$ *ozs. of albuminoid*

$(15m + 1.5b + 88B)100 = 3$ *ozs. of fat*

$$50b/100 = 14.25 \text{ ozs. of carbohydrates}$$

When these equations are worked out—

$$m = 6.28 \text{ ounces.}$$
$$b = 28.5 \text{ ounces.}$$
$$B = 1.15 \text{ ounces.}$$

Relation of Food to Mechanical Work.—In the body the movements of every part are constant sources of heat. It is evident therefore that the potential energy of food can be expressed by (a) the amount of heat obtained by its complete combustion, or (b) by the amount of work capable of being obtained from it. Joule discovered by exact experiment that the mechanical power obtainable from a given amount of fuel is directly proportional to the amount of fuel used, being in fact due to the oxidation of this fuel, the heat produced being transformed into mechanical power. The heat unit or calorie has been already given (p. 32). The gram-metre is the work unit. The heat unit corresponds to 425.5 units of work. Thus the same energy required to heat one gramme of water 1° C. will raise a weight of 425.5 grammes to the height of 1 metre. Conversely a weight of 425 grammes if allowed to fall from a height of 1 metre, will by its concussion produce heat sufficing to raise the temperature of 1 gramme of water 1° C. In England the amount of work done is commonly expressed as foot tons, i.e. tons lifted one foot; while in France it is similarly expressed as kilogrammetres. Gramme-metres can be converted into foot-pounds by multiplying them by .007233, and kilogrammetres into foot-tons by dividing by 311.

Frankland estimated that—

1 oz. dry albumin	yields	174 foot-tons of potential energy.
1 oz. fat	„ 378	„ „
1 oz. starch	„ 135	„ „
1 oz. cane sugar	„ 129	„ „
1 oz. glucose or lactose	„ 122	„ „

In practical dietetics digestibility of food as well as chemical composition is an important factor. Furthermore metabolism in the body is not in every instance so complete as oxidation outside it. Hence estimates of potential energy can only be regarded as theoretically correct. Examination questions like the following are occasionally asked:—

A man does work equal to 176.8 foot-tons in a day. Supposing that he eats only bread, how much will he require to give the amount of energy required, if bread contains 8 per cent. proteid, 1.5 per cent. fat, and 49.2 per cent. carbohydrate?

On the above basis, from 100 ounces of bread the amount of potential energy obtainable is:—

$$8 \times 174 = \quad 1{,}392 \ foot\text{-}tons$$
$$1.5 \times 378 = \quad 567 \quad „$$
$$49.2 \times 135 = \quad 6{,}642 \quad „$$

Total energy = 8,601 „ obtained from 100 ozs. bread.

Let b = number of ounces of bread required to develop 176.8 foot-tons of energy.

Then 8,601: 100:: 176.8: b.

Therefore b = 2.05 ounces.

CHAPTER VI

THE PREPARATION AND PRESERVATION OF FOOD

OBJECTS OF COOKING.—Food may be taken in its crude condition, as directly derived from the animal or vegetable world, or after it has undergone a preparatory process of cooking. Man is the only animal who cooks his food. Many foods, in the uncooked condition are almost entirely incapable of digestion by him—such as the proteid and farinaceous materials contained in the seeds of cereal and leguminous plants. But cooking, as a preparatory help to the digestion of food, is not equally required by all foods. Thus, fruit is commonly taken uncooked, and does not undergo any important alteration on cooking. Salads are taken uncooked, but not for their nutritive properties so much as for a relish to other foods, and for their quasi-medicinal properties. Milk, again, may be taken cooked or uncooked. The oyster is the only animal which is eaten habitually, and by preference, in the uncooked condition; and there is a physiological reason for this universal custom. The large fawn-coloured liver, which constitutes the delicacy of the oyster, is little else than glycogen, associated with its appropriate ferment diastase, so that the oyster is almost self-digestive. When cooked, the ferment is destroyed, and digestion of the oyster becomes more difficult.

Cooking is intended—1. To make the food softer, and in part to mechanically disintegrate it, thus rendering it more easily masticated and digested. In fact, cooking, in the best sense, is an artificial help to digestion; and digestion may well be said to commence in the kitchen.

2. To produce certain chemical changes. Thus, starch is partially converted into dextrine; gelatin is formed from connective tissue, etc.

3. To destroy any noxious parasites present in the food, or obviate any ill effects from putrefactive changes. Diseased meat chiefly produces bad effects when imperfectly cooked.

4. To make the food more pleasant to the eye and agreeable to the palate. The improved savour in cooked meat, for instance, has a very appetising effect, and consequently makes digestion easier.

THE COOKING OF FLESH.—1. Roasting is, perhaps, the most perfect way of cooking meat. It exalts its flavour more than any other method. In roasting, place the meat at first sufficiently near a brisk fire, so that the albumin on its surface may be readily coagulated, and the juices retained in the interior of the joint. After about fifteen minutes, the joint ought to be removed somewhat further from the fire, and allowed to cook slowly. Frequent basting is desirable to obtain a good result. Brown meats, such as beef, mutton, and goose, require a quarter of an hour per pound weight; veal and pork require about ten minutes additional, to ensure the absence of redness. White-fleshed birds require a somewhat shorter time. The time required in roasting will be a little more if the joint is large, or the fire not very clear. To ascertain if the meat is sufficiently cooked, press the fleshy part; if it remains depressed, it is done; if not done, it retains its elasticity. At the first incision, gravy should flow out of a reddish colour.

The changes undergone during roasting are, that the connective tissues uniting the muscular fibres is converted by the gradual heat into gelatin, which is soluble and easily digested; the muscular fibres, consequently, become more separable, and the myosin of which they consist is rendered more digestible. The fat is partly melted out of its fat cells, and partly combines with the alkali from the blood-serum. Empyreumatic oils (i.e. fat partially burnt), developed by charring of the surface of the joint, are carried off when it is roasted in front of the fire; and so, to a large extent, is acrolein. Acrolein (C_3H_4O) is always produced by the destructive distillation of neutral fats containing glycerine, and is the cause of the intolerably pungent odour accompanying the process. Osmazome, a peculiar extractive matter, on which the flavour and odour of meat depend, is developed better by roasting than by any other method of cooking.

It is useful to remember, in buying beef or mutton, that 20 per cent. must be allowed for bone and 20 to 30 per cent. for the loss during cooking.

The following figures are by Johnston:

	IN ROASTING.	IN BAKING.	IN BOILING.
4 lb. of mutton lose in weight	1 lb. 6 oz.	1 lb. 4 oz.	14 oz.
„ beef „	1 lb. 5 oz.	1 lb. 3 oz.	1 lb.

Thus roasting is the least economical method of cooking. The chief loss, however, is of water; the dripping and gravy are recoverable.

2. Baking of meat in a closed oven does not produce so agreeable a result as roasting in front of an open fire. The oven ought always to be very hot before the meat is put in, in order to rapidly coagulate its surface. Baked meat may have an unpleasant flavour, owing to its saturation with empyreumatic oils, which escape in open roasting. The unpleasant flavour can be prevented by covering the meat with a layer of some non-conducting material, as a pie-dish or a crust, no empyreuma being then formed. Baked white of egg, as in the dish of fried ham and eggs, is one of the most indigestible forms of albumin obtainable.

3. Boiling of meat requires the same time as roasting. If the flavour and juices are to be retained, the joint ought first to be plunged into soft boiling water, and then, after three minutes, allowed to stand aside in

water at 170° Fahr. The preliminary boiling forms a coating of coagulated albumin over the joint. Where there is no thermometer to guide the cooking—after the preliminary boiling for three to five minutes, add three pints of cold water to each gallon of boiling water, and retain at the same temperature for the rest of the process, i.e., at about 170° Fahr. If the meat is boiled in an inner vessel surrounded by water (water-bath), the temperature of the inner vessel does not rise above 160°-170° F. Ordinary "simmering" means that the meat is kept all the time at a temperature of 212° F. and is thus spoilt. The boiling of an egg is an example of the same point. If an egg is kept in water at a temperature of 170° F. for 10 to 15 minutes, its contents form a tender jelly, while an egg kept in water at 212° F. for the same length of time is hard and tough. An egg is more digestible when cooked in water at 170° F. for 10 minutes than when boiled in water for 2½ minutes.

The use of soft water for cooking purposes is always advisable; otherwise a longer period must be allowed. A preliminary boiling for a few minutes renders hard water softer, and the addition of a little carbonate of soda has a like effect.

When meat is inserted in water at a temperature below its boiling point, the juices are gradually extracted, while the meat is left a mass of indigestible fibres. A good soup is produced, but the meat is almost valueless. In order that the soups and broths may be nutritious, the less heat is employed in their preparation the better. If a soup is strained to make it clear, much of the most valuable part is removed.

Stewing is a process intermediate between boiling and baking. It possesses the great advantage over dry baking that no empyreumatic gases are produced, and there is no charring. The temperature of the stew-pan ought never to be above 180° Fahr.; at this heat the roughest and coarsest kinds of meat are made tender. The only objection to stewing is that the meat becomes saturated with fat and gravy, and is too rich for weak stomachs. It is advisable to stew lean meats only.

Hashing is a process of stewing applied to meat which has been previously cooked. The consequence of this double cooking, is that the meat becomes tough and leathery. A modified hash in which the meat is simply well warmed throughout is preferable.

Frying, unless carefully done, renders meat difficult of digestion, each fibre becoming coated with fat. The art is to "fry lightly," that is, to burn quickly and evenly, so that no charring is produced. Two methods of frying are described. In the first, the substance to be fried, as an omelette or pancake, is placed with a little fat or oil in a frying-pan. This is really a modified process of roasting, the fat merely serving to prevent the object from adhering to the shallow pan. In the second, the substance to be fried is immersed in fat; for this purpose a frying kettle is required. Olive oil or good cotton seed oil is best for use in the frying-kettle. Lard is a bad material for frying; both it and butter are apt to burn unless heated slowly. Dripping is a good substance for frying. The fat used must be heated to from 350° to 390° F., and then the substance to be fried, e.g. a sole, plunged into it and left for two or three minutes. In this process the substance of the sole is really being steamed by the steam generated in the substance of the sole.

6. Broiling and Grilling are really processes of roasting applied to small portions of meat. In grilling, it is important that the gridiron should be hot before putting anything on it. An external coagulation of albumin is produced, as in good roasting and boiling.

THE COOKING OF MIXED DISHES.—A few instances may be given of common errors in preparing compound dishes. An egg in a custard, or just coagulated in a poached egg, is a light and easily-digested food; baked half an hour in a pudding, it is much less digestible; fried with ham, it is almost as indigestible as leather. Spices, if mixed with a dish before it is boiled, lose nearly all their flavouring power, while they remain irritating. They ought to be added near the end of the cooking process. A soup containing vegetables, as well as meat juices, should be prepared in two parts. The vegetables require prolonged boiling; gravy is spoilt by this. Similarly, the jam in a tartlet, if inserted before baking, loses its proper fruity flavour; and oysters baked in a beef-steak pie are indigestible.

THE COOKING OF VEGETABLE FOODS.—Bread is either vesiculated or unvesiculated; the latter being what is called unleavened bread. Vesiculation of bread has usually been produced by fermentation of some of the sugar of the flour. The starch first becomes sugar (dextrose) and then the growth of the yeast plant in the dough splits this up into alcohol and carbonic acid gas. The carbonic acid percolates the substance of the dough, rendering it porous. When it has "risen" sufficiently, the dough is placed in the oven. The heat of the latter kills the yeast plant, thus preventing any further fermentation, but at the same time expands the carbonic acid gas in the bread, rendering the latter still more porous, and drives off in a gaseous condition the greater part of the alcohol produced by the previous fermentation.

It is objected to this plan of making bread, that a little of the sugar is wasted in producing alcohol and carbonic acid. To remedy this, another plan is sometimes adopted, as first proposed by Dr. Dauglish. In it the dough is charged with carbonic acid dissolved in water under considerable pressure. The gas escapes in the substance of the dough, and on baking expands as in the ordinary method of making bread. Bread made in this manner, is called "aerated bread." Nevill's bread has a solution of carbonate of ammonia incorporated in the dough, which is dissipated by heat, thus causing vesiculation of the bread.

On the continent, a mixture of hydrochloric acid and carbonate of soda is commonly used, carbonic acid and common salt being formed in the dough. Thus $NaHCO_3 + HCl = NaCl + H_2O + CO_2$. The hydrochloric acid employed should be perfectly pure and free from arsenic. Baking powders are also largely used for making cakes. "Self-raising" flour is flour with which baking-powder has already been mixed. Most baking-powders consist of a mixture of carbonate of soda and tartaric acid or bitartrate of potash, diluted with starch. When wetted, carbonic acid gas is evolved. A few contain alum, which is now an illegal material for this purpose.

Ten pounds of flour ought to make thirteen to fourteen of bread. The use of stale bread is much more economical than of newly-made bread;

besides this, it is more digestible. Newly-made bread is more palatable than stale, but it is more cohesive, and does not crumble into separate particles like stale bread. The consequence is, that it is less digestible, being less easily penetrated by the saliva and other digestive juices. The effect of toasting is to render bread more friable, and consequently more digestible. It ought, however, to be thin and eaten soon after it is made; when thick and kept too long, it becomes tough and leathery.

Pastry is less easily digested than ordinary bread. The lard or dripping added renders it more flaky and less easily pulverised; and, in addition, the fat coats over the starch cells; and thus the action of the digestive juices on the pastry is impeded.

Potatoes ought to be boiled in their jackets, or steamed, to avoid loss of nitrogenous material and salts. Moist heat causes the starch granules to swell, and ultimately softens and bursts the cellulose envelopes in which these are contained. Dry heat, as when potatoes are baked, converts starch into a soluble form, and ultimately into dextrine (= $C_6H_{10}O_5$), an intermediate stage towards the formation of dextrose (i.e. glucose = $C_6H_{12}O_6$).

Peas and Beans ought to be boiled slowly and for a long time to render them more digestible. If old, they ought to be soaked in cold water for twenty-four hours, then crushed, and stewed. Hard water must be avoided in the cooking of peas and beans as well as of other vegetables, as the lime-salts form insoluble compounds with legumin.

Green vegetables require thorough and prolonged cooking. This renders their tissues softer and more easily attacked in digestion. The members of the cabbage tribe and carrots can hardly be boiled too long. Soft water ought always to be used; this is one reason why steaming is preferable. Before boiling, all vegetables should be well washed in cold water. A little vinegar will remove any insects present.

COOKING APPARATUS.—The apparatus required in cooking may be divided into kitchen utensils and cooking ranges.

To ensure good cooking, perfect cleanliness of all apparatus is indispensable. The use of the frying-pan, gridiron, spit, and oven has been sufficiently indicated under the description of the different methods of cooking. The form of stove to be used for cooking meat is gradually being settled against the old open stove. Although this secures a somewhat more savoury joint than when meat is baked, it is extravagant in working. The closed kitchener in which coal is employed is less economical than a gas stove at the present price of gas, if the latter is carefully used.

Various appliances for economising fuel have been devised, and at the same time of allowing of the prolonged action of a moderate degree of heat. These are usually constructed on the principle of an ordinary bath, consisting of a double pan, with a layer of water between the two compartments. Warren's cooking-pot belongs to this type. The Aladdin oven consists of an iron box with an opening above to let off superfluous steam. This box is surrounded by another composed of non-conducting material, while a lamp below furnishes the heat. Dr. Atkinson has calculated that in an ordinary oven 2 lbs. of fuel must be expended for every pound of food cooked, while in his Aladdin oven 2½ lbs. of fuel will cook 60 lbs. of food. Time is an important element in cooking. Food is most thoroughly cooked and most digestible when subjected to a temperature below that of boiling water for a prolonged period.

THE PRESERVATION OF FOOD.—All organic foods tend rapidly to decompose and putrefy. Putrefaction only occurs when a warm and moist substance is exposed to the air. The problem of preserving any food, therefore, may be solved (1) by keeping it at a very low temperature, (2) by desiccating it, or (3) by boiling or steaming it so as to destroy any microbes in the food which would otherwise start putrefaction, and then fastening it in an air-tight case.

Milk is commonly preserved as condensed milk, and in this condition is very valuable. A pure condensed milk is now supplied, prepared without the addition of sugar or any antiseptic, but in which, as in other condensed milks, all disease-producing or decomposition-producing microbes have been destroyed during the process of concentration. Milk may also be desiccated; in this condition it is difficult of digestion.

In addition to the household methods of preserving fruits, large quantities of fruits—both moist and dry—are now imported, protected by syrup or sugar, in sealed canisters; and they retain the original flavour almost unchanged.

The preservation of meat is effected by—

1. Drying.—This must be done rapidly. It is a process which is best applicable to fish, but has been applied also to beef. Dried Hamburg beef is used for making sausages. Pemmican, largely used by Arctic voyagers, consists of a mixture of meat and fat, dried and powdered along with some spices; it is generally eaten with some kind of meal.

2. Cold.—Frozen meat now forms a very large part of the food of the English people. If the meat has been frozen before rigor mortis (rigidity after death) has commenced, it keeps well; if frozen later, it rapidly decomposes after being thawed. Freezing arrests putrefaction and tends to conceal its odour. Hence the bad condition of frozen fish may not be detected until it is cooked. In cooking frozen meat, time should be allowed for thawing to occur, before the meat is placed in the oven. Much of the ill-founded prejudice against frozen meat arises from inattention to this point. Frozen meat is equal in nutritive value to and does not lose more in cooking than fresh meat.

3. Salting may be done with brine or saltpetre (nitrate of potassium); the latter does not decolourize the meat like the former. Salted meats have lost much of their nutritive material, in the form of albumin and salts, and the remaining meat is harder and more difficult of digestion than fresh meat.

4. Immersion in antiseptic liquids or gases, as sulphite of soda, is objectionable, on account of the addition of extraneous, and not altogether innocuous, salts. Boric acid powder is largely used for sprinkling on meat, particularly rabbits, etc., and for preserving hams and other meats. Its use

is to be deprecated. All such meats should be thoroughly washed with water, before being cooked.

Solutions of boric acid and borax are frequently added to milk. Their use is objectionable (a) because they tend to conceal incipient decomposition, but do not prevent its possible evil effects, and (b) because they enable the farmer to palm off dirty milk on the public. Were the addition of preservatives to milk forbidden, the farmer could perfectly well keep his milk sweet until it reached the town-consumer by adopting strict measures of cleanliness, and by cooling his milk before it leaves the farm. At the least it should be made obligatory on the milk retailer to declare the presence of preservatives in milk sold by him.

The presence of borax or boric acid can be detected by evaporating the milk to dryness, incinerating and then moistening the ash with a drop of strong sulphuric acid. If a little alcohol be now added, on applying a light, a green flame indicates boric acid. Milk or cream containing boric acid turns blue litmus paper red.

Formalin is also sometimes used as a preservative for milk in very weak solution.

Its presence can be determined by diluting the milk with water in a test-tube, and running strong sulphuric acid down the side of the tube, taking care to prevent mixing. At the junction of the acid and diluted milk a violet ring is seen if formalin is present.

Salicylic acid was formerly used as a milk preservative, but is now seldom used except in beers. All these preservatives are objectionable in milk, although their injurious action may be difficult to prove.

5. Coating with fat or gelatine has only succeeded in conjunction with the exclusion of air. This process is especially applicable to fishes, as tinned sardines. In a modified form, it is useful in coating potted meats, etc.

6. Heating and Air-tight Cases.—Tinned meats prepared according to this method are imported in large quantities. In the process of preparation, the cases are packed with meat and filled up with gravy, and then closed with a cover which is hermetically sealed, except at one point. The case is then heated to 250° Fahr., in order to drive out all air, and destroy any putrefactive germs present. The open point is sealed while the gravy is still boiling, thus making the case completely air-tight. Albumin is coagulated at about 170° Fahr.; the higher temperature, which it is found necessary to employ, overcooks the meat and renders it less digestible (see also p. 40).

CHAPTER VII

CONDIMENTS AND BEVERAGES

CONDIMENTS, ETC.—The name condiment is used in various senses by different writers. In its strictest sense it is a substance containing a volatile oil or ether, which may be taken with salt, and the object of which is to excite the senses of taste and smell, and consequently produce an appetising effect. This definition excludes spices, substances allied to condiments, but usually taken with sugar, as cinnamon, ginger, etc.; also flavouring agents, such as vanilla; and acids, such as vinegar and lemon-juice. If we use the word in its widest sense, to include these various groups of substances, we find that all condiments are taken with the object of improving the taste or flavour of food, or of assisting its digestion; but that they are not foods in the sense of supplying any elements towards building up the body or maintaining its heat. The only partial exception is lemon-juice, the salts of which have a quasi-medicinal use.

Taste is usually a compound sensation, the organs of which are the nerves of taste and smell. True taste is confined to the appreciation of sensations of bitter and sweet; but the flavour of meats is nearly entirely appreciated by the sense of smell. This is shown by the fact that meats appear tasteless and insipid, during "a cold in the head." In the appreciation of acid, astringent, and fiery substances, the sense of touch is also employed. The excitement of these different nerves results in a stimulus which is carried up to the central nervous system, and causes by reflex action an increased flow of the digestive juices. Hot substances, like cayenne and ginger, also cause an increased flow of gastric juice, by directly congesting the mucous membrane. This action is not so desirable as that through the influence of the nervous system. All natural foods are sapid and possessed of flavour, and thus stimulate secretion; but any local irritating effect ought to be avoided.

1. Condiments proper comprise chiefly mustard, pepper, cayenne, garlic, onion, capers, mint, sage, morels, mushrooms, truffles. The last three on the list are also foods, but are more commonly used as condiments.

All these act as stimulants to the digestive organs, and in small quantities aid digestion. The active principle of mustard and horse-radish is sulphocyanide of allyl. Horse-radish is not so wholesome as mustard, the scraped root being apt to adhere to the stomach like the skins of grapes, and produce indigestion. Pepper contains an acrid resin, a volatile oil, and an alkaloidal substance, called piperine. Cayenne contains an analogous substance, called capsicin. Cayenne, unless in extreme moderation, is harmful, as its small particles adhere to the mucous membrane of the stomach, and may set up considerable irritation.

2. Spices are those condiments which contain an aromatic oil, and which harmonize with sugar. They are, as a rule, less irritating to the

42

stomach than those of the pepper group. Cinnamon, cloves, camphor, ginger, and curry powder are the chief of these. Curry powder really belongs to both the first and second divisions. When genuine, it is said to contain turmeric, cardamoms, ginger, allspice, cloves, black pepper, coriander, cayenne, and a few other substances.

3. Flavouring agents, such as vanilla, lemon peel, and fruit essences, are used to give a pleasant flavour to various dishes.

4. Acidulous substances are taken chiefly because of their sharp and agreeable taste. Vinegar is the chief acid employed. It is produced by the action of a fungus (Mycoderma aceti) on alcoholic liquids, as wine, or beer, C_2H_5OH (alcohol) becoming $C_2H_4O_2$ (acetic acid). It is also produced by the destructive distillation of wood. In small quantities it does not stop digestion, but, by exciting the nerves of taste, may be of actual service. It helps to soften the vegetable fibres in a salad; and is also useful for the same purpose with hard meats, as lobster, etc. In large quantities it diminishes the power to assimilate food.

Good vinegar ought not to contain less than 3 per cent. of acetic acid; and sulphuric acid beyond 1 in 1000 in vinegar is to be regarded as an adulteration. A specific gravity below 1015 indicates the addition of water.

Citric acid and lemon-juice are useful for their refreshing properties, and the latter also because of its alkaline salts.

Oils, such as olive oil, have been sometimes classed under condiments, but as they have great nutritive properties, this is hardly accurate. For the same reason, salt is not classed under this head.

BEVERAGES

Water is the universal beverage, and for healthy persons is preferable to any other. All other beverages necessarily contain it as their basis.

It will be convenient to consider first aërated and other natural waters; then tea, coffee, and cocoa; and finally, alcohol.

1. Aerated Waters contain carbonic acid (carbon dioxide) in solution, which gives to them their characteristic sharp taste and sparkling character. Thus distilled water charged with gas is sold as Salutaris or Puralis water. Soda water contains three to five grains, and medicinal soda water fifteen grains of bicarbonate of soda to the bottle. Potash water contains fifteen grains of bicarbonate of potash to the pint, in each case carbonic acid being dissolved under pressure. In lemonade, ginger-beer, etc., the basis is sweetened water, rendered tart by the addition of an acid, and finally charged with carbonic acid. Lemonade frequently contains acetic or phosphoric acid instead of citric or tartaric, and ginger-beer the same constituents with some added tincture of ginger. Home-made lemonade prepared from fresh lemons is a much more wholesome drink. Ginger-beer (stone ginger) is produced by the fermentative action of yeast on a solution containing sugar, bruised ginger, tartaric acid, and oil of lemon. It usually contains at least two per cent. of alcohol.

Natural Mineral Waters usually contain common salt (chloride of sodium) and alkaline salts of soda or lime, and are impregnated with carbonic acid gas. Apollinaris, Rosbach, and Johannis possess these characteristics. The carbonic acid in natural waters is partially combined, and is given off more gradually than that in artificial mineral waters.

In all the preceding waters there is considerable carbonic acid. This acts as a sedative to the mucous membrane of the stomach, and is useful in indigestion. An aërated water added to milk renders it more digestible by diluting it, and by preventing the formation in the stomach of a heavy clot of casein. In the making of artificial aërated waters, it is essential that the water employed should be pure, that the acid used in generating the carbonic acid should be free from arsenic or other impurities, and that the water should not be allowed to come into contact with lead at any stage, as in pewter fittings. One per cent. of proof spirit is allowed in temperance beverages by the Excise.

TEA

Tea is the leaf of an evergreen shrub, the Camellia thea, which is cultivated in China, Japan, British India, Ceylon, Java, and other countries. The tea leaves, as seen in this country, uncurl in hot water. They are lanceolated, with a serrated edge, and the veins do not extend to the edge of each leaf. By these characteristics they may be distinguished from foreign leaves, e.g., the sloe and willow used as adulterants (Fig. 4). The use of old and exhausted leaves can be detected by a determination of the percentage of soluble matter dissolved by boiling water from a given weight of tea. This on evaporation to dryness should be 28 to 30 per cent. of the total weight of the original tea. The presence of clay, iron dust or other forms of dust is detected by igniting a given amount of tea and determining the amount of ash. This should be only about six per cent.

In black tea, the leaves are dried in the sun, rolled and allowed to become soft and to ferment. During this process, some of the tannin appears to be converted into less soluble forms. The leaves are afterwards sun-dried, and these "fired" in a furnace. Green tea leaves are dried in the fresh condition over wood fires. Indian teas have more "body" and astringency than China teas. The smallest and topmost leaves of the tea plant give the finest sort of tea (Orange Pekoe); next to this comes Pekoe; the next largest leaves producing Souchong; after these Congou; while the coarser leaves nearer the base used to yield Bohea, which is now seldom seen.

Tea consists of three important constituents—volatile oil, theine or caffeine, and tannin—and soluble and insoluble extractive matters.

The amount of caffeine varies from 2 to 4 per cent.

" " " tannin " " 10 to 12 " "

" " " volatile oil is about ½ " "

(1) Volatile Oil gives the aroma and flavour to each particular tea. It is this which causes the headache, trembling, wakefulness, and restlessness, occasionally produced by tea, especially by green tea.

44

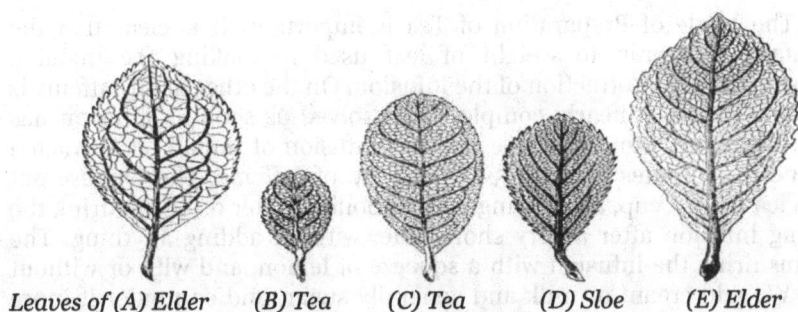

Leaves of (A) Elder   (B) Tea   (C) Tea   (D) Sloe   (E) Elder
Fig. 4.

(2) Theine or caffeine, is an alkaloidal crystalline principle. Its composition is represented by the formula $C_8H_{10}N_4O_2$, H_2O. Ceylon tea, broken leaf contains 4·03 per cent., Assam (Indian) tea, broken leaf 4·02 per cent., while Chinese teas contain from 2·89 (Moyune Gunpowder) to 3·74 (Moning, black leaf) per cent. of caffeine (Allen).

Theine is the most important constituent of tea and coffee. It is a stimulant, but unlike alcohol, acts even more upon the central nervous system than upon the heart. It removes the sense of fatigue, and may, especially if taken in excessive doses, produce sleeplessness. Its stimulant action on the heart is followed by increased flow of urine, and it thus helps in the removal of waste products from the system. The effect on the tissue-changes of the body is somewhat doubtful. It has been stated to arrest or diminish the waste, i.e., the metabolism, constantly going on in the system, and so diminish the amount of food required to repair this waste. This is highly improbable; we cannot conceive the likelihood of the development of energy without a corresponding expenditure of material, and that is what would be the case if theine increased the activity of various organs while retarding their waste. The experiments of Conty and Guimarès on the action of coffee show that this (and tea has the same essential constituent) does not diminish tissue waste. It does not prolong life in starvation, though it may lessen the feeling of hunger. Hence tea and coffee, which owe their value mainly to the caffeine or theine contained in them, are in no sense foods.

(3) The amount of Tannin varies from 12·31 in Ceylon tea (broken leaf, Pekoe) to 11·76 in Moning, black leaf, and 9·9 per cent. in Natal Pekoe Souchong (Allen). The difference in tannin between Chinese and Indian teas is not therefore so great as is usually supposed. Tannin is a powerful astringent, and possesses a bitter styptic taste, and a constipating effect on the bowels. Its amount is increased by long "brewing," as is shown by the following results (Hale White):—

	Three Minutes' Infusion.	Fifteen Minutes' Infusion.
Finest Assam	11·30 per cent.	17·73 per cent.
Finest China	7·77 per cent.	7·97 per cent.
Common Congou	9·37 per cent.	11·15 per cent.

45

The Mode of Preparation of Tea is important. It is clear that the percentage of tannin to weight of leaf used in making the infusion increases with the protraction of the infusion. On the other hand caffeine is so soluble that it is nearly completely dissolved as soon as infusion has begun. Dittmann found that five minutes infusion of Indian tea extracted 3·63 and ten minutes infusion 3·73 per cent. of caffeine. The Chinese put the tea leaves in a cup, and having poured boiling water on them, drink the resulting infusion after a very short time, without adding anything. The Russians drink the infusion with a squeeze of lemon, and with or without sugar. We add cream or milk and generally sugar, and so render it more nutritious, though the delicate flavour is veiled. The Chinese plan of infusion for a short time is the best, as it ensures the extraction of the aromatic and stimulant principles of the tea with only a proportion of the tannin.

In making tea it is important to use a tea-pot which is quite dry, in order to avoid mustiness; to pour a small quantity of boiling water into the tea-pot and then out again, so that the infusion may be made at the temperature of boiling water; and to use water which has only freshly come to the boil, and so has not been rendered flat, and not to infuse longer than five minutes. For persons of weak digestion, the best kind of tea is that obtained by pouring boiling water on the leaves, and then immediately pouring the resulting infusion into another hot tea-pot. In all cases where tea has to be kept a considerable time, it should be poured into a second tea-pot, the leaves being left behind.

Indigestion is not an uncommon consequence of tea-drinking; caused by the excess of tannin in the tea, by the other constituents of the tea, or more commonly by the practice of drinking tea in small sips, with bread and butter. The tea infusion usurps the place of the saliva, the secretion of saliva remaining partially in abeyance. The presence of tannin in tea renders it an undesirable part of a substantial meal. Tannin coagulates albumin, and retards its solution by the digestive juices. Hence "high teas" and "tea-dinners," unless the tea is very weak, are objectionable. The practice of drinking tea with every meal is inexcusable.

For quenching thirst during active exercise, and rendering possible prolonged exertions, tea is unsurpassed.

COFFEE

Coffee is the seed of the berry of the Caffea Arabica. Each berry contains two seeds, or beans as they are sometimes incorrectly called. The coffee is prepared by roasting the seeds until they assume a reddish-brown colour, in which process they lose 15 per cent. in weight and gain 30 per cent. in bulk. During the process of roasting, a volatile oil having a powerful aromatic smell is developed. This is not produced in such large quantities from fresh seeds; the best time for roasting varying, however, for different varieties of coffee.

The amount of Volatile Oil in coffee is much less than in tea. As it is elicited during the process of roasting, this should be done with nicety and care. It is effected in an iron cylinder made to revolve over a fire. After the roasting, the sooner the seeds are ground the better the coffee. When it cannot be immediately used, it should be kept in closed canisters, and not in paper or open jars.

In addition to the volatile oil, which is contained in roasted coffee in the proportion of about 1 part in 50,000, coffee contains caffeine, of which there is ¾ to 1 per cent., and an astringent acid, called caffeo-tannic or caffeic acid, which differs from ordinary tannin in that it does not blacken a solution of an iron salt.

The chief adulteration of coffee is Chicory, which is thought by some to improve the coffee. It is generally harmless, though in some people it produces heartburn and diarrhœa. Chicory is prepared from the root of the wild endive. It contains a volatile oil and a bitter principle, but no caffeine. It is, therefore, of no utility as a stimulant. Its presence can be detected by shaking a little of the suspected coffee on to the surface of the water in a wine-glassful of cold water. Coffee swims on the surface, and gives little or no colouration to the water; while chicory sinks, and gives a deep red tint. The aqueous extract of pure coffee (extracted by boiling water) is, when evaporated, 25 to 30 per cent. of the weight of the original decoction of coffee; while that of chicory is 65 to 70 per cent.; and on this basis, as well as on the fact that a filtered decoction of 10 grammes of coffee in 100 c.c. of distilled water, cooled to 60° F. has a specific gravity of 1009, while that of a similar solution of chicory would be 1021, the proportion of chicory in a mixture of coffee and chicory can be calculated. The microscopical appearances of the two powders differ, coffee showing hexagonal cells and no laticiferous vessels, unlike chicory. There is no law against selling mixed coffee and chicory, if the fact that it is a mixture is stated; and the proportion of the two unfortunately is not required to be stated. As a pound of coffee costs five times as much as a pound of chicory, it is obviously to the purchaser's advantage to make his own mixture in the proportions desired.

The Preparation of Coffee ought to be effected as in the case of tea— by making an infusion and not a decoction, i.e. by pouring boiling water on the coffee and allowing it to stand, but not continuing the boiling. Continuance of boiling dissipates the delicate aroma.

Inasmuch as coffee contains a much smaller percentage of theine than tea, more of the former must be used to obtain a beverage equally refreshing with tea. Two ounces to a pint of boiling water are required. The infusion thus made should be mixed with an equal part of boiled milk. The coffee ought, if possible, to be freshly roasted.

The colour of coffee is no guide to its strength. Many of the black coffees, especially "French coffee," owe their colour to the caramel (burnt sugar) contained in the chicory mixed with them.

Coffee has similar properties to tea, with some minor differences. (1) Like tea, it is restorative and sustaining in its action, but seems to act more quickly than tea. (2) Unlike tea, it does not tend to produce perspiration, but rather a dry hot skin. (3) With some it is decidedly laxative; while tea, especially if badly made, has an opposite effect; but this is not always true.

47

(4) It seems to have a greater power of antagonising the effects of alcohol than tea; and is a valuable antidote, after the action of an emetic, in poisoning by opium or arsenic or alcohol.

As a rule, coffee is not so prone to disorder the digestion as tea, but this is not universally true, and in some persons it always produces "biliousness." When taken in excess, it produces—besides indigestion—palpitation, restlessness, irritability, sleeplessness, and a condition of general nervous prostration; in fact, similar symptoms to those produced by a prolonged over-indulgence in tea.

While the consumption of tea is rapidly on the increase, that of coffee is steadily diminishing. This is partly owing to the greater expense of coffee—a larger quantity being required to form a good beverage; and partly to the greater difficulty in preparing good coffee.

COCOA

Cocoa, or more properly cacao, is obtained from the seeds of the Theobroma Cacao—a native of the West Indies, Mexico, and the central parts of America. Its name Theobroma was given it by Linnæus, and means the "food of gods." The fruit is a large leathery capsule, having nearly the form of a cucumber. It contains from 25 to 30 seeds, each about the size of an almond. Before using, these are roasted like coffee berries, and a peculiar aroma is developed in this process as in the case of coffee. The beans or seeds are then manufactured into three different products. (1) They are simply deprived of their husks and broken to pieces; this forms Cocoa-Nibs. (2) They are ground, husk and all, between hot rollers into a paste, and mixed with starch and sugar; this forms Cocoa. (3) They are shelled and then ground into a paste, as in making cocoa; sugar and some seasoning, usually vanilla, being subsequently thoroughly mixed; this paste is Chocolate.

The purest form is the cocoa-nibs. When these are boiled in water, a brownish decoction is formed, with the fat as a scum at the top; this may be removed, and the decoction flavoured with milk and sugar. In this form, cocoa can be taken by invalids with weak digestion, who would be nauseated by the fat of ordinary cocoa or chocolate.

The best cocoa is prepared as above; but the lowest quality contains the husks of the beans, with hardly any of the beans in it; a somewhat better, though still inferior sort, is made from the smaller fragments of the nibs, and a good deal of husk. In some cases the cacao butter is removed during the process of preparation, and starch or sugar substituted. This form is less likely to disagree with dyspeptics than whole cocoa.

The action of the Volatile Oil (not the cacao-butter) developed during roasting, is probably similar to that of tea and coffee, though it is less in amount. The bitterness is greater than that of coffee, but the astringency less than in either tea or coffee.

The Concrete Oil, or fat of cocoa, forms about half its weight. It is white, and not apt to turn rancid, and possesses an agreeable flavour. Cocoa also contains a certain amount of starch and cellulose.

Theobromine is a white crystalline alkaloid, the exact analogue of caffeine. The latter, in fact, is methyl-theobromine—that is, theobromine plus the theoretical group CH2. Theobromine possesses similar properties to caffeine. It amounts to 1.5 to 2 per cent. of the whole bean. The ordinary preparations of cocoa differ considerably in composition as may be seen from the following table of per centage composition (Ewell). In each instance other nitrogenous and non-nitrogenous constituents go to make up the total 100:

	FAT	FIBRE	CANE-SUGA	ASH	ADDED STARCH
Fry's Cocoa Extract	30·9	3·9	—	4·2	None.
Schweitzer's Cocoatina	31·1	3·7	—	6·3	Do.
Rowntree's Cocoa Extract	27·6	4·4	—	8·5	Do.
Van Houten's Cocoa	29·8	4·4	—	8·6	Do.
Epps's Prepared Cocoa	25·9	1·5	26	3·1	Much arrowroot.

Some of the preparations of cocoa (e.g. Van Houten's) have added to them alkaline salts to increase their solubility. Cocoa is not such a valuable food as might appear from the large amount of fat in it, because only moderate quantities of this can be taken without deranging digestion. In Vi-Cocoa a certain amount of kola is added, which contains a considerable proportion of caffeine. The addition of such a drug to a beverage is distinctly to be deprecated.

Minor Stimulants.—Beverages containing theine, or some analogous principle, appear to be employed in most countries. In moderate doses, they may assist the assimilation of other foods, but their main influence is on the nervous system. Theine-containing substances may be described as both sedative and exciting. They are sedative, in that they allay nervous irritability, and tend to "take the edge off" the disturbance caused by outward circumstances; and they are exciting, inasmuch as they are known to form an admirable antidote to the stupefying effects of opium or alcohol. The wakefulness from tea is an instance of the same thing, while the allaying of sensations of cold and hunger by a cup of tea is an instance of the sedative effect.

In Brazil, Guarana (from Paullinia sorbilis) is used as a drink; it contains theine, the quantity of which is twice as much as in good black tea, and five times as much as in coffee. Like green tea, a cup of guarana infusion is sometimes extremely valuable in nervous headaches.

In Peru, the natives use the leaves of the Coca plant (Erythroxylon coca), which must be carefully distinguished from cocoa. It is chewed somewhat in the same way as the betel-nut. It contains two alkaloids—cocaine and hygrine, as well as tannin. In its stimulant action it resembles tea and coffee. The active principle of this plant, Cocaine, is a valuable local anæsthetic. Internally it has been taken as a stimulant and restorative. Various wines containing Coca, with vaunted restorative powers, are advertised. They are mischievous when taken frequently. Nature's remedy for fatigue, whether mental or body, is rest and recreation. Stimulants of this class, even though they enable work to be continued for awhile, eventually increase the exhaustion for which they are taken.

The Kola-nut is used in some parts of Western Africa as a stimulant. It is about the size of a pigeon's egg, and has a bitter taste. The natives of Guinea generally take a piece of the seeds before each meal, and sometimes nibble it throughout the day.

Kava is prepared from the root of a kind of pepper. The natives of the Fiji islands commonly indulge in it. Its effects resemble those of coffee. In large doses, it destroys the power of walking, and may possibly produce impairment of vision.

The leaves of the Ilex Paraguayense, Ilex Gongorrha, and Ilex Theezans are made into the beverage commonly known as Paraguay tea or maté.

The leaves of the Hydrangea Thunbergii are made into a beverage, which is designated in Japan "the tea of heaven."

Among certain nations of Asia, the Betel-nut (from a palm called Areca Catechu) is chewed, after mixing small fragments with pepper and quicklime, and rolling in a palm leaf. The saliva is tinged blood-red, and a narcotic effect is said to be produced.

The dried flowering tops of the Indian Hemp (Cannabis Indica) are smoked by the Malays and others, or made into a beverage, called haschisch, which produces a kind of intoxication, in which murder has often been committed (hence, assassins equals haschascheens).

The Kamtschatkans drink an infusion made from a fungus, known as the Fly Agaric (Amanita Muscaria), thus producing an intoxication similar to that from haschisch.

Opium in small doses is a stimulant, in large doses narcotic. The crude drug is sometimes taken, and less frequently the active principle, Morphia. It is frequently smoked, as well as taken internally. It is to be feared that secret opium taking is considerably increasing. The taking of morphia, especially hypodermically, is too common. Generally it has been first prescribed for neuralgia or some other complaint causing acute pain; and the patient, having experienced relief by its means, is tempted to revert to the practice apart from medical advice. Such a line of action is most pernicious. Eventually both the physical and the moral nature of the victim are shattered by it; and to break off this insidious habit, when once thoroughly established, is most difficult.

Tobacco may be conveniently mentioned here, though its usual effects are certainly not stimulant. It is smoked, chewed, or taken as snuff; when indulged in to excess it produces serious depression of the heart's action, with frequent intermittence. In moderate doses it is sedative as well as slightly laxative. Prolonged indulgence in tobacco has produced many cases of incomplete blindness (tobacco amblyopia), in some cases it comes on with much smaller doses, and in all cases is only curable by ceasing to smoke. There is no sufficient ground for the statement that cigarette smoking is more injurious than smoking tobacco in a pipe or cigar, unless in the former case the smoke is inhaled into the lungs. The practice of smoking is injurious to growing boys, and should be strictly forbidden.

Other Drugs are now not infrequently taken, apart from medical advice. Of these the most commonly used are Antipyrin and Phenacetin, for headaches. Their use is injurious, and should not be entertained as a frequent practice. Sleeplessness frequently leads to the practice of taking chloral or sulphonal, or occasionally the inhalation of chloroform to induce sleep. Remedies to induce sleep should never be taken except under immediate medical advice. They are only justifiable in extreme conditions, and if frequently taken tend to aggravate the conditions for which they are given.

CHAPTER VIII

FERMENTED DRINKS

Properties of Alcohol.—When a saccharine solution is subjected to the influence of warmth and moisture, and exposed to the air, it rapidly undergoes a process of fermentation. The most favourable temperature is about 70° Fahr. The ferment or agent exciting the change in the sugar is derived from the atmosphere; it is a minute fungus (torula cerevisiæ), the spores of which are constantly floating in the air. When once fermentation has started, exposure in the air is no longer necessary; the process continues in closed vessels. The essential change occurring in the vinous fermentation is that grape sugar ($C_6H_{12}O_6,H_2O$) becomes split up into alcohol (C_2H_5OH) and carbonic acid (CO_2). Thus—

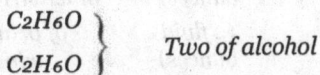

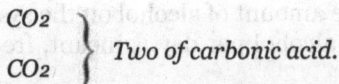

$$C_6C_6H_{12}O_6 = \begin{cases} \left.\begin{array}{l} C_2H_6O \\ C_2H_6O \end{array}\right\} & \text{Two of alcohol} \\[2ex] \left.\begin{array}{l} CO_2 \\ CO_2 \end{array}\right\} & \text{Two of carbonic acid.} \end{cases}$$

There are other fermentations allied to the vinous. Thus the Acetous fermentation results in the conversion of alcohol into vinegar, as in the souring of beer or wine. The Lactic fermentation leads to the conversion of milk-sugar into lactic acid, with consequent souring of the milk.

Alcohol, or more correctly ethylic alcohol, is a colourless liquid, having a pleasant vinous odour, and evaporating rapidly on exposure to air. It burns with a bluish sootless flame, and is a capital solvent for resins and other substances.

Rectified spirit is absolute alcohol mixed with 16 per cent. of water. Proof-spirit is a mixture of 42·7 per cent. by volume of absolute alcohol, and 57·3 per cent. of water. Thus the ratio of alcohol to proof-spirit being as 1: 1·76, the amount of alcohol in any liquid being given, the amount of proof-spirit can readily be calculated. The fermented drinks containing alcohol may be classed as (1) malt liquors, (2) wines, and (3) distilled spirits. The relative properties of these will be considered afterwards; in the next two sections will be considered the effects of diluted alcohol in whatever form it is taken.

Effects of Moderate Doses of Alcohol on the System.—In studying the physiological effects of alcohol, one has to guard against the fallacy that these are the same, only differing in degree, whatever the dose may be. The effects of large doses of alcohol are almost exactly the reverse of those produced by small doses. It will be necessary to define, therefore, what we mean by a moderate dose. By a moderate dose, we understand the amount of alcohol which can be taken without any alcohol being eliminated in the urine. Dr. Anstie found that 1½ ounces, that is three tablespoonsful, of absolute alcohol, taken in twenty-four hours, caused its appearance in the urine; and Dr. Parkes and Count Wollowicz obtained almost precisely the same result. Anything below some quantity between 1 and 1½ fluid ounces per day can be disposed of in the system, and is probably oxidised like ordinary foods.

The amount of alcohol, in the form of alcoholic beverages, corresponding to this maximum dose of absolute alcohol is approximately as follows:—

One imperial pint	(20 fluid ounces)	of bottled beer	(5 per cent. of alcohol).
One tumblerful	(10 fluid ounces)	of claret, hock, and and other weaker wines	(10 „).
2½ glasses	(5 fluid ounces)	of port, sherry, and other strong wines	(20 „).
One glass	(2 fluid ounces)	of brandy or whiskey	(50 „).

It will be understood, therefore, that in describing the effects of a moderate amount of alcohol on the system, an amount below 1½ ounces of absolute alcohol per day is meant, freely diluted, and taken as a rule with meals.

1. Effect on the Stomach.—In very small quantities, alcohol seems to stimulate digestion in the same way as mustard. But like all other artificial helps to digestion, it is best avoided in the healthy condition.

2. The Effect on the Liver is similar to that on the stomach—a temporary redness and congestion being produced; this effect soon disappearing if the dose is small and well diluted. But in all cases where there is a tendency to biliousness, even small doses of alcohol are injurious.

3. The Effect on the Heart and Blood-Vessels is first to increase the force of the heart's action and the rapidity of the pulse. The stimulation of the heart is rapidly followed by a universal dilatation of the small arteries of the body, which diminishes the blood-pressure. Parkes and Wollowicz

found that the daily administration of from 1 to 7½ ounces of rectified spirit raised the pulse rate by ten beats per minute, as compared with other periods; and that this effect was followed by a period of depression in which the beat was both slower and feebler than usual.

4. The Effect on the Nervous System varies. In persons unaccustomed to its effects, even small doses dull the power of thought and the rapidity of perception, owing to the paralyzing effect which it exerts on nerve cells. In most cases, however, it at first produces increased rapidity of thought and excites the imagination, though even here it makes it more difficult to keep to one train of thought. This is clearly owing to the more rapid circulation of blood through the brain. Dr. E. Smith's experiments show that it diminishes the acuteness of the senses. Its influence even in dietetic doses, on the capacity for mental work, is slightly to diminish it.

5. The Effect on the Muscular System is never beneficial. Even when only small quantities are taken, the power of controlling delicate movements is slightly diminished. For persons engaged in laborious occupations, a small quantity does not produce much apparent effect, but where the quantity exceeds two fluid ounces per day the capacity for strong and sustained muscular work is manifestly lessened (Parkes). This effect is probably due partly to the dulling of the nervous system, rendering the muscles less amenable to the will, and partly to the over-excitation of the heart causing palpitation and breathlessness.

6. The Effect on Metabolism is to diminish it, thus favouring the deposit of fat in the tissues. It acts as a poison to the protoplasm of the cells of the body, diminishing their power to break down the floating nutriment, especially fat and carbohydrate.

The Effect on the Temperature is to lower it; but unless the dose is excessive, this effect is hardly appreciable. The resistance to excessive cold is diminished by even moderate doses of alcohol, still more by large doses. In the Arctic regions, this has been abundantly proved. This effect is produced, notwithstanding the fact that alcohol becomes oxidised in the system. The dilatation of the surface blood vessels leads to a greater loss of heat than that produced by the oxidation of the alcohol.

EFFECTS OF IMMODERATE DOSES OF ALCOHOL ON THE SYSTEM.—Bearing in mind the definition given of a moderate dose, one is bound to admit that a large number of individuals exceed this amount daily, apparently without any very serious results. The system becomes habituated to large doses, and if the occupation is a laborious one, they may in part be oxidised in the system. Such, however, are exceptional cases. In the majority of cases evil results are by no means confined to those who indulge in very large quantities of alcohol at varying intervals. In fact these very often escape comparatively free, while others who never take a quantity sufficient to incapacitate them for their work, are sowing the seeds of chronic and oft incurable disease. The labourer who has a drinking bout at intervals is thoroughly nauseated; and the condition of liver and stomach induced, enforces abstinence on him for a time sufficient to bring his organs back to a normal condition; while the city merchant

53

who indulges more moderately, but whose organs are almost continuously impregnated with alcohol, becomes gouty and prematurely old.

The Stomach may become acutely inflamed, when a large dose of alcohol is taken. The chronic irritation of alcohol, especially when taken apart from meals, causes atrophy of the walls of the stomach, and a change analogous to that in the liver.

The Liver, when alcohol is daily taken immoderately, becomes seriously diseased. In some cases it becomes large and fatty; in others the chronic irritation excites an overgrowth of fibrous tissue between the lobules of the liver, which, gradually shrinking, squeezes the liver cells and causes them to atrophy, at the same time obstructing the small branches of the portal vein in the substance of the liver. The consequence of this obstruction to the flow of blood through the liver is that all the organs from which the portal vein brings blood become overloaded with blood, and vomiting of blood and dropsy of the abdomen occur at a later period.

The Lungs are irritated to a less extent by alcohol in large doses. The tendency to chronic bronchitis is increased, followed by emphysema, and sometimes an overgrowth of fibrous tissue (cirrhosis) like that in the liver occurs.

The Heart and Blood-vessels tend to become diseased, owing largely to the gouty condition of system developed.

The powers of Metabolism are diminished. Corpulence is, consequently, a common result of alcoholism. There may also be fatty deposit in the internal organs, such as the heart. This must not, however, be confounded with a much more serious condition, fatty degeneration of the heart, in which the substance of the muscular fibres becomes partially converted into fat, and which also is sometimes due to alcoholism.

The Nervous System is more prone to suffer in chronic alcoholism than any other part of the body, except perhaps the liver. The first effect of a large dose of alcohol is to stimulate the nervous system, as already described. This is followed by a dulling of the nervous faculties, which comes on rapidly in proportion to the amount taken. The phenomena of intoxication are unhappily too familiar to require description, mental incoherence and muscular incoordination (lack of control over the muscles) being the most prominent features.

When the dose of alcohol is still larger, a condition of profound unconsciousness is produced (coma), which may be difficult to distinguish from other forms of unconsciousness.

Delirium Tremens is another nervous condition, which may rarely follow a single debauch, but much more commonly affects the chronic toper. In some cases the immediate exciting cause is a mental shock, or lack of food, or a surgical injury. Alcoholic subjects suffering from any acute disease are liable to this form of delirium, and their chance of recovery is greatly diminished.

Insanity of a more prolonged character than that characterising delirium tremens is an occasional result of alcoholism.

Besides the nervous diseases already named, a chronic thickening of the membranes covering the brain and spinal cord, gradually progressing and finally fatal, is often the consequence of prolonged alcoholic indulgence.

Various Degenerative Diseases are produced by alcohol. It has been well called by Dickinson the very "genius of degeneration." Such degenerations are by no means confined to the intemperate; they are seen in those who are of what would usually be considered moderate habits. The stomach, liver, lungs, and probably the kidneys, are the main organs to suffer in this way. It is probable that the effect on the kidneys only occurs when a gouty condition is developed. In all these cases there is an overgrowth of fibrous tissue, with atrophy of the proper gland structures.

Gout is the common nemesis of those indulging in alcoholic beverages, more especially wine and beer, due to the excessive formation or retention of urate of soda in the body. This produces inflammation of the joints, and other evils—among them the gouty kidney, named above, which is always ultimately fatal. Rigid arteries are likewise commonly due to alcoholism and gout. If one of these bursts in the brain, apoplexy results.

Longevity is diminished by immoderate indulgence in alcohol. The statistics of Temperance Insurance Societies, show much better results among teetotalers than among moderate drinkers. It is only fair to add that although the latter are supposed to consist of moderate drinkers—and particular enquiries are always made on this point before insurance—it is probable that a large proportion of them exceed 1½ ounces of alcohol per day. Making due allowance for this fact, the statistics show a great superiority in the expectation of life of teetotalers.

Factors Modifying the Effects of Alcohol.—1. Age and Sex.—Until adult life is reached, total abstinence from alcohol should be enforced. The delicate nervous system of children is easily disturbed by it, and it appears in some measure to retard growth. Another argument against giving alcohol before adult age is reached, is still more important. It is at this period of life that habits are chiefly formed, and a craving for alcohol may be insidiously produced, destined to have most baneful results.

Old people, if ordered spirits for medical reasons, should drink them well diluted.

Women are much more easily affected by alcohol than men, and if they acquire the habit of excess, the hope of reformation is even less than with men.

2. Exercise has a most important influence in modifying the effects of alcohol. Those of sedentary occupations and living in towns, cannot oxidise as much as those engaged in active out-door work, and are consequently much more prone to suffer. A game-keeper in the Scotch Highlands may possibly live to a good old age, notwithstanding the fact that he consumes an amount of whiskey that would have sent a sedentary man to his grave in the course of a few years.

3. The Condition of the Stomach has also great influence. When the stomach is empty, alcohol produces at once a powerful reflex stimulation of the heart, and becomes quickly absorbed into the circulation. Thus intoxication may be produced by a quantity that would have had little effect if taken with a meal.

4. The State of Concentration or Dilution modifies greatly the action of alcohol, the local action on the stomach and the reflex stimulation being much greater than when it is concentrated, and injurious effects being much more likely to occur.

5. Cold and Heat modify the action of alcohol. A smaller quantity of hot spirits and water will intoxicate than of cold; the heat stimulating the heart, and so making the absorption of the alcohol more rapid. A glass of hot spirits and water will often cause sleep, by drawing the blood towards the abdominal organs. The fact that persons, who have been drinking spirits in a warm room, on going out into the cold air become suddenly intoxicated, seems opposed to what has been already said. But probably this is due to the cold causing contraction of the arteries of the skin, and so driving more of the blood loaded with alcohol to the internal organs and the brain (Brunton).

6. Mental Occupation has some influence in modifying the effects of alcohol. Topers have found that if they try to converse during their debauch—the conversation implying increased functional activity of the brain, and therefore a freer circulation of blood in it—intoxication occurs much more readily, than when the mind is not active.

7. Disease modifies greatly the effects of alcohol. In some diseases, as in inflammation of the lungs and in fevers, it can be given in large quantities without producing intoxication; and in these conditions it lowers the temperature. In other diseases, especially gout and kidney disease, its use is nearly always followed by bad results.

The Advisability of Alcohol as an Article of Diet in Health.—In dealing with this difficult point, two sets of facts require consideration, those obtained as the result of Physiological observations, and those which are the result of Experience. There can be no doubt that the former are much more reliable than the latter. Experience is very prone to give fallacious results, especially when questions of appetite are concerned. In making a trial of abstinence, the mistake has been commonly made of only prolonging the investigation for a few weeks, and then comparing results. Such a method is, however, very unfair, and is certain to lead to an unreliable conclusion.

The records of experience under certain conditions have, however, been so extensive, as to lead to trustworthy results. It has been abundantly proved that prolonged muscular work is best undergone during total abstinence from alcohol; and that the extremes of heat and cold and the exposure and exertions of marching armies, are best borne under similar conditions.

The artificial character of town life is commonly adduced as an argument for the moderate use of alcohol. In the case of healthy workers, this does not hold good; many of our hardest workers and thinkers take no alcohol.

The universality of the habit of taking stimulants is a curious argument on the same side, though if the habit be bad, this can be no more reason for continuing it than can the prevalence of vice be an excuse for indulgence in it.

56

The two chief physiological points bearing on the advisability of alcohol as a part of one's daily diet are—its food properties, and its effect on the appetite and digestion.

It has been already stated that a quantity of alcohol under 1 or 1½ ounces may become oxidised in the system, and may thus form a source of heat. But in all probability, although it may be regarded as a food, it is a most inconvenient one, inasmuch as it diminishes the oxidation of other foods. It has been aptly compared in this respect to sulphur, which is an oxidisable material, but which, when it is burnt in a chimney, in which the soot is on fire, will put an end to the combustion of the latter. Its value as a food, under normal conditions, is practically nil.

Its Effect on the Digestive Organs is three-fold. (a) The contact of alcohol with the mucous membrane of the mouth and stomach, acts as a reflex nervous stimulus, which in moderation excites an increased flow of gastric juice. (b) It also increases the activity of the movements of the stomach. In cases of weak digestion, therefore, small doses of alcohol may, at times, be useful. (c) The effect of alcohol on the food taken varies with its degree of dilution. Concentrated alcohol coagulates albumin, and so stops digestion; largely diluted alcohol has no such effect.

The late Dr. Parkes, the greatest authority on the dietetic use of alcohol, has summarised the argument as to the dietetic use of alcohol as follows:—

"But what, now, should be the conclusion as to the use of alcohol in health after growth is completed? Admitting the impossibility of proving a small quantity to be hurtful, and at the same time acknowledging the dangers of excess, there arises an argument which seems to me somewhat in favour of total abstinence. No man can say when he has passed the boundary which divides safety from harm; he may call himself temperate, and yet may be daily taking a little more than his system can bear, and be gradually causing some tissue to undergo slow degeneration. He may be safe, but he may be on the verge of danger.

"This uncertainty, coupled with the difficulty at present of saying what dietetic advantage is gained by using alcohol, seems to me rather to turn the scale in favour of total abstinence instead of moderate drinking. But if any one honestly tries, and finds he is better in health for a little alcohol, let him take it, but he should keep within the boundary line, viz., that 1½ ounces of pure or absolute alcohol in twenty-four hours form the limit of moderation. I do not then think he can do himself any harm."

The Varieties of Fermented Drinks.—The three chief kinds of alcoholic beverages are malt liquors, wines, and ardent spirits. In addition, we may mention cider and perry, which are the fermented juices of apples and pears respectively; and koumiss, which the Tartars prepare by fermenting mare's milk, though it may also be made from the milk of other animals.

All Beers, Ales, and Porters are prepared from malt, which is the germinating grain of barley. The fermentation of the sugar in the barley produces alcohol, the amount of which varies in different cases. In Pilsener beer it is 3½ per cent. of absolute alcohol; in stout and porter 5 to 6 per cent. The hop which is added to the fermenting barley, gives to beer its characteristic bitterness.

London Porter is coloured with black or roasted malt; stout is only a stronger form of porter. Bottled ales are generally stronger than those on draught, and being slightly effervescent, may agree better.

The effect of alcohol in beer is modified by the hops, which help in producing drowsiness. Beer has a marked tendency to produce obesity, more so than any other alcoholic beverage. Its influence in the production of gout is also very great.

Substitutes for Malt have been largely used. Thus by the action of sulphuric acid on starch, an artificial form of sugar is produced, which is largely used in place of malt for making beer. Many recent cases of poisoning by arsenic have been traced to the use of impure sulphuric acid in manufacturing this form of sugar.

The detection of arsenic in organic liquids requires great care, as so many compounds of arsenic are volatile, especially in the presence of chlorides, as in beer. To detect arsenic in beer a pint of the beer is evaporated to dryness, and treated with 20 c.c. of strong sulphuric acid, heated, and 20 c.c. of strong nitric acid added drop by drop. Violent action occurs: if possible 20 c.c. more of nitric acid are worked in. Transfer the liquid to a small flask, and expel the nitric acid by boiling. By this means all chlorine is expelled, the arsenic is oxidised and the organic matter destroyed. SH_2 gas is now passed into the acid liquid for some hours, the precipitated sulphur and any sulphide filtered off and extracted with ammonia, which dissolves any sulphide of arsenic. The liquid so obtained is subjected to Marsh's test.

In the making of beer from malt, the first stage is to malt the barley, i.e. leave it spread on floors for ten days after soaking. This allows germination to take place, in which process the insoluble starch is converted into starch, dextrine, maltose and glucose. After the dried malt has been screened to break off the sproutings, the brewer places it in the mash-tub, with water, at a temperature of 160° F. This completes the transformation of the starch into glucose. The wort is now boiled to stop the process, and the albumin from the grain is thus coagulated. Hops are added at this stage. The boiled liquid is passed into shallow vessels and cooled. The proper temperature for "top" yeast is 60° F., for "bottom," or Bavarian yeast, a much lower temperature is desirable. When the desired temperature is reached, the liquid is run into the fermenting tun along with yeast. The varieties of beer are due in part to the degree of completeness of fermentation of sugar allowed. If too complete, the beer does not keep well.

Wines are produced by the fermentation of the juice of the grape. The wine produced may be bottled before or after fermentation is complete; in the former case, an effervescing wine is produced, such as the sparkling wines of the Rhine and the Moselle, or champagne. When the sugar is nearly all fermented a dry wine is obtained, of which Bordeaux and Burgundy, Hock and Moselle, are examples.

The difference in colour between red and white wines is produced by allowing the juice in the former to ferment in contact with the skins, from which the colouring matter is extracted by the alcohol. Both red and white wines may be obtained from either red or white grapes. From the skins also are extracted a salt of iron, and a peculiar form of tannin. Tartaric and acetic acids, and tartrate of potass, are present in varying quantities in wines; in old wines the tartrate separates as bitartrate of potass, forming with tannin and colouring matter the "crust" of port and other wines. The "bouquet" of wines is due chiefly to certain volatile bodies, such as pelargonic ether. The proportion of alcohol in wines varies from 6 to 14 per cent. As fermentation is stopped by the presence of 14 per cent. of alcohol, any larger amount of alcohol than this must have been added to the wine.

Wine, like beer, has a strong tendency to produce gout, especially the sweet and strong wines. It has not, however, the same tendency to induce obesity.

Spirits differ from the two last groups, to begin with, in the amount of alcohol they contain. Thus, English beers contain from 3 to 6 per cent., German beers from 2 to 5 per cent., wines from 8 to 20, and all kinds of spirits from 37 to 58 per cent. of alcohol. They differ in the absence of the bitter principle of beer and much of the salts and sugar and ether of wines. They are all prepared by the distillation of some previously fermented liquor. Brandy ought to be made by the distillation of wine; and then contains, besides alcohol and water, small quantities of acetic, œnanthic, butylic, and valerianic ethers. But much of the brandy sold is simply made from potato spirit, by the addition of acetic ether, burnt sugar, etc. The starch of potatoes is converted into dextrin and dextrose by dilute acids, and then fermentation allowed. By the use of patent stills, all bye-products can be separated, a fairly pure alcohol known as silent spirit being produced. This is largely employed in manufacturing spirits and in fortifying wines.

Whiskey is prepared from malted barley, or from a mixture of grains, to which a sufficiency of malt to convert their starch into sugar has been added. In grain whiskey the distillation is effected by steam in a patent (Coffey's) still, which separates most of the bye-products (fusel oil, etc.) from the spirit. In malt whiskey, distilled in the old-fashioned pot-still, these bye-products are not separated.

The improvement of whiskey effected by keeping is not due (Bell) to the diminution of fusel oil. Such a diminution does not occur. The percentage of alcohol diminishes by keeping, 6 to 8 per cent. proof spirit being lost by five years' storage in wood. "Fusel oil" is a mixture of alcohols of higher boiling point than ethylic alcohol (amylic, propylic, etc.). Even in a bad whiskey not more than 1/10 per cent. of fusel oil is present (about one grain in a glassful). Experimentally no marked effects have been produced by fusel oil, when it is less than 1 per cent. Possibly the presence of furfurol, of which there is a trace in malt whiskey, which disappears on keeping, may partially explain the disagreeable flavour of new whiskey. But it is fairly clear that those who argue that it is bad whiskey and not good whiskey which does harm are speaking without knowledge. It is not the quality but the quantity of whiskey which is responsible for so much moral and physical evil.

Gin and Hollands are obtained from barley, and flavoured with juniper berries and other materials. The oil of juniper stimulates the urinary excretion.

Rum is obtained by the distillation of molasses, and is usually kept for a long time in oak barrels. It is said thus to acquire more astringent matters than other spirits contain.

The legal limits of dilution of whiskey, brandy and rum is down to 25 degrees under proof, and of gin down to 35 degrees under proof. The amount of alcohol in an alcoholic liquor is determined by distillation of 100 c.c., making up the distillate to 100 c.c. by the addition of distilled water, and then taking the specific gravity of a portion of this liquid by the aid of the specific gravity bottle. The percentage of alcohol corresponding to a given specific gravity is given in tables prepared for this purpose.

Prolonged indulgence in spirits produces the various organic diseases already described, and unless well diluted they are more harmful than beers or wines. They differ from wines and beers in not tending to produce gout, and from beer in not leading to obesity.

CHAPTER IX

WATER

Uses of Water.—Water is a prime necessity of life. In its absence life can only exist in lowly organised beings, and in them only in a dormant state. From a hygienic point of view, the uses of water are four-fold:—(1) It is an essential part of our food, not only serving to build up the tissues of the body, but also preserving the fluidity of the blood and aiding excretion of effete matters. (2) It is necessary for personal cleanliness, of which the importance can scarcely be exaggerated. (3) In the household it is essential for cooking, as well as for washing the house, the linen, and various utensils. (4) By the community at large it is required for water-closets and sewers, for public baths, for cleansing the streets, and for horses and other domestic animals, as well as in many manufacturing processes. It is obvious that the water to be used for domestic and general purposes, need not be so pure as that for drinking purposes. Hence, a double supply was proposed for London in 1878, by the Metropolitan Board of Works—a less pure river supply for general purposes, and a deep chalk-well supply for drinking purposes. The scheme, however, rightly fell through, because of the expense of a double source of supply, and the danger that the impure water would, through carelessness or ignorance, be often used for drinking purposes, when it happened to be nearest at hand.

Quantity of Water Required.—The quantity of water required for all purposes has been variously stated by different authorities. The quantity required for drinking purposes is found to bear a relation to the weight of the individual, being nearly half an ounce for every pound weight, or 1½ gills for every stone weight. Thus, a man weighing 150 lbs. would require 3¾ pints. Of this water, about one-third is taken in the food; the remainder, averaging 2½ pints, being required as drink. If we add the water required for other purposes, according to De Chaumont, 1 gallon is required for drinking and cooking, 2 gallons (not including a bath) for personal cleanliness, 3 gallons for a share of utensil and house washing, 3 gallons for clothes washing; and if a general bath be taken, 3 gallons more; making a total of about 12 gallons, to which 5 gallons must be added if there is a water closet.

In hot summer weather the consumption is about 20 per cent. above the average of the year; and frost often increases the amount 30—40 per cent. above the average, owing to the bursting of pipes, or the loss from taps foolishly left open to prevent bursting.

Water companies usually reckon 30-60 gallons for each individual, to allow for the water required for scavenging and manufactories and for waste. In large houses and hotels where baths are freely used, often as much as 70 gallons per head is used, and in hospitals the amount averages from 60 to 90 gallons per head. The following is Parkes' estimate of the daily allowance for all purposes:—

GALLONS PER HEAD OF POPULATION

Domestic supply	12
General baths	4
Water-closets	6
Unavoidable waste	3
	—
Total house supply	25
Municipal purposes	5
Trade purposes	5
	—
Total	35

It has been proposed to put a water-meter to each house, so that the rate may be in proportion to the amount of water used. The plan is objectionable for two reasons: 1st—Because it tends to restrict the necessary use of water for purposes of cleanliness. A scant supply of water is always followed by uncleanliness of house and person, with its consequent diseases; at the same time closets may be imperfectly flushed, and may become choked. 2nd—Because of the primary expense of the meter, and of its maintenance.

SOURCES OF WATER SUPPLY.—All our drinking water is obtained in the first instance, by a natural process of distillation on a large scale. The sun is constantly causing evaporation from sea and land. The vapour produced, being condensed by a lower temperature, returns to the earth as snow, dew or rain. All these natural products have been at times utilised as sources of drinking water.

1. Dew has on rare occasions been utilised at sea by hanging out fleeces of wool at night and wringing them out in the morning. A much better plan is—

2. The Distillation of Sea-water. This can easily be managed now that steam power is so largely used. It has even been employed on land, when it was necessary temporarily to continue the use of water derived from an impure source. The first part distilled should always be rejected, as it is always impure. Distilled water is "flat" in taste, owing to its containing no dissolved gases. It can be aërated by letting it drop a considerable distance from one cask into another, through small openings in the upper one, and by filtration through charcoal. Non-aërated water is not easily absorbed into the circulation, and occasionally causes illness.

3. The utility of Melted Snow and Ice is obviously very limited. Moreover, its use is not free from danger if the ice is derived from contaminated water. Outbreaks of enteric fever have been traced in the United States to the taking of ice obtained from impure water.

4. Rain-water is a much more important source of water supply, and after passing through the soil it constitutes the chief part of the water we drink. The term, however, is properly restricted to the water collected immediately after its descent from roofs, etc. Its purity depends on three conditions—the character of the air it passes through, the cleanliness of and absence of lead from the channels through which it runs, and the condition of the water-butts in which it is stored. Rain-water is soft; in fact, too soft to be pleasant to the palate. In passing through the air, it carries with it a certain proportion of its constituents; in towns especially ammonia, soot, etc.; near the sea, it generally contains some salt; and being soft and having dissolved oxygen from the air, it dissolves an appreciable amount of lead from roofs or gutters.

The Rivers Pollution Commissioners found that out of eight samples of stored rain-water only one was fit to drink. They came to the conclusion that rain-water, collected from the roofs of houses and stored in underground tanks, is "often polluted to a dangerous extent by excrementitious matters, and is rarely of sufficiently good quality to be used for domestic purposes with safety." Also, that in Great Britain, and more particularly in England, we shall "look in vain to the atmosphere for a supply of water pure enough for dietetic purposes."

The use of rain-water for drinking purposes is only justified in isolated country houses where no better source is available; and under these circumstances the greatest care should be taken to prevent contamination with lead or organic impurities.

The amount of water falling on any impervious material obtainable from rain can easily be estimated, if the amount of rainfall and the area of the receiving surface are known. The average annual rainfall in this country is 33 inches.

We may assume the amount practically available to be 20 inches per annum, and the area of the receiving surface 500 square feet. Multiply the area by 144, to bring it into square inches, and this by the rainfall, and the product gives the number of cubic inches of rain which fall on the receiving area in a year. One cubic foot, or 1,728 cubic inches, of water being equivalent to 6·23 gallons, the number of gallons of water can be easily calculated. To calculate the receiving surface of the roof of a house, do not take into account the slope of the roof, but merely ascertain the area of the flat space actually covered by the roof. This may be done roughly by calculating the area of all the rooms on the ground floor, and allowing an additional amount for the space occupied by the walls. It has been estimated that, even if a rain-water supply for towns were desirable, the amount collected from the roofs of houses would scarcely average two gallons per person daily—assuming the average rainfall to be 20 inches, and that there was a roof area of 60 square feet for each individual.

The amount practically available from rain falling on different soils varies with their porosity and slope. Thus, according to Professor Rankine, the proportion of the total rainfall available is as follows:—

> Nearly the whole on steep surfaces of granite, gneiss, and slate;
> From three to four-fifths on moorland hilly pastures;
> From two-fifths to half on flat cultivated country; and
> None on chalk.

By available rainfall is meant the amount remaining after allowing for percolation, etc., which can be stored in reservoirs.

5. Upland Surface Water is the water collected in hilly districts, as on moorlands, at the head of a river. By its utilisation for drinking purposes, the sources of water for the river are interfered with, and any water company or local authority using such a source is, therefore, required to run into the stream a quantity of water equal to a third of the available rainfall. The limited and regular supply thus furnished to the stream is found to be advantageous for industrial purposes as its flow is equalised, and the violence of floods mitigated.

In the utilization of upland surface water the water from the surrounding hills is collected at the bottom of a valley, in an artificial, strongly-constructed lake; or in a natural lake, as in Loch Katrine (from which Glasgow is now supplied).

Upland surface water is nearly always soft. Its use is much more economical than that of hard water. It may be brownish, from the presence of peat, but this is not objectionable, so far as health is concerned. Its occasionally solvent action on lead is a more serious objection. The population of many parts of Yorkshire and Lancashire have suffered severely from chronic lead poisoning, due to the action of certain upland surface water on lead service pipes. Only the waters giving an acid reaction possess this plumbo-solvent power.

6. Springs supply water which, originally derived from rain-water, has percolated through the soil until it reaches some impervious stratum, and has then run along this, until it arrives at the point at which the impervious stratum reaches the surface of the soil. A spring is thus the

outcrop of the underground water. Springs are divided into (1) land springs, and (2) main springs. The former flow from beds of drift or gravel lying on an impervious stratum. They are very subject to seasonal variation, and may dry up in certain years; while main springs occurring in chalk, greensand, or other regular geological formation, constantly supply a certain amount of water. Springs often occur in connection with "faults" in geological strata, and then may appear on table-lands and high elevations, unlike springs caused by alternation of strata in valleys of denudation. The two kinds of springs are shewn in Fig. 5 and 6.

In the land spring water crops out at the point where the porous stratum ceases. Deep springs may crop out in the same way as land springs, except that they appear at the bottom of deeper strata. Or they may be formed by faults. Both these are shown in water having percolated through the chalk beneath the superficial clay, is stopped at the "fault" by the lack of continuity of the chalk stratum, and is consequently confined under pressure. It therefore makes its way to the surface, forming a spring. In its passage underground, water (owing partly to the carbonic acid it has obtained from the air and soil), is able to dissolve small quantities of chalk, sulphate of lime and of magnesium, and traces of oxide of iron, aluminium oxide, and silica. Spring-water possesses an equable temperature, generally about 50° Fahr., while impounded or river water is always warm in summer and cold in winter. Spring water is well-aerated, while river water, and still more rain-water, are flat.

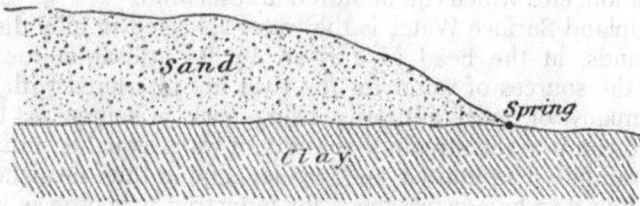

Fig. 5.—Land Spring.

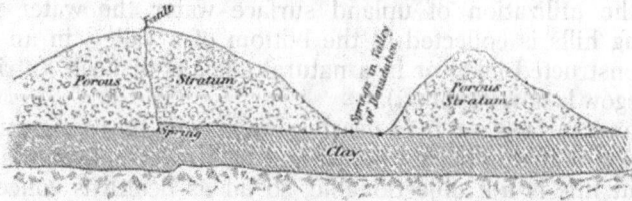

Fig. 6.
Main Springs formed in Valley of Denudation and by a Fault.

7. Wells may form the best or worst sources of water-supply according to their depth and the means of protection against contamination. There are two kinds—Surface wells and deep wells.

Surface Wells do not usually descend further than 15 or 20 feet, and have no impervious stratum between the source of water and the surface of the well. They catch the subsoil or underground-water, which percolates into them from the surrounding soil, and the character of the water they receive will therefore vary with the nature of their surroundings. If there is a cesspool near, this may simply drain into the well. All the soakage from a considerable distance may find its way into the well. In villages and isolated places the water of surface wells is commonly contaminated. One hole may be dug in the garden for a well, and another for a cesspool, while there is possibly a farmyard near at hand—the soakage from the cesspool and farmyard soaking into the well. Danger may also arise from more distant contamination. The ground water which is tapped by the well is an underground stream flowing towards the nearest brook. Heavy rains swelling the ground water may wash impurities from cesspools, leaky drains, etc., at a considerable distance, and carry these into wells lying between these sources of pollution and the brook into the bed of which the underground water ultimately discharges. The danger of contamination of the water in the well by the contents of the cesspool is much greater in the relative position shown in A than in the position shown at B, Fig. 7. After heavy rain, when the underground water is swollen, the danger of contamination is still further increased. The model bye-laws of the Local Government Board state that a cesspool must be at least 40 feet distant from any well, spring, or stream. Probably this is insufficient for safety; cesspools ought to be entirely forbidden. If necessary to retain a surface well, it should be protected nearly to the bottom with brick, lined with an impervious layer of cement so as to prevent water from entering the well except near its bottom. In modern wells iron cylinders are employed to line the upper part of the well; and large glazed earthenware pipes arranged vertically and with water-tight joints are sometimes used for the same purpose.

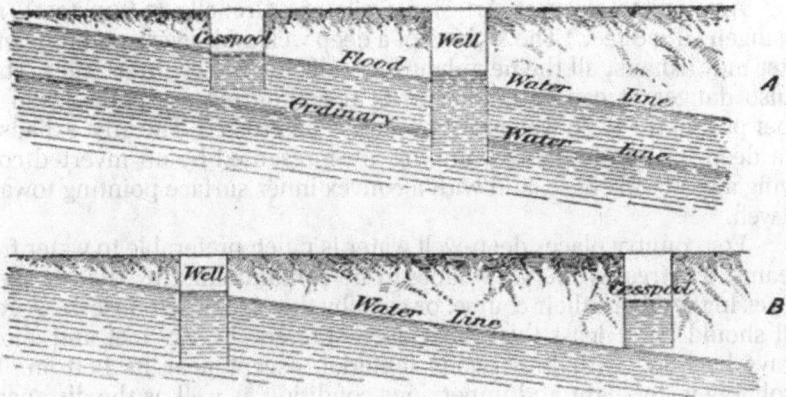

Fig. 7.
Showing Varying Danger of Contamination of a Shallow Well, according to Level of Underground Water and Relative Position of Cesspool and Well (after Galton).

Deep Wells are made by digging a surface well, as above, except that the ground water is prevented from entering the well by means of impervious steining; and then boring from the bottom down through the subjacent impervious stratum until a water-bearing stratum is reached. The difference between a surface well and a deep well is shown in Fig. 8 by A and B. Where the water in this stratum is retained under pressure, deep wells are known as Artesian Wells. Such Artesian wells have been sunk in London. Rain, falling on the chalk hills which lie to the south and north of London, percolates through the chalk downwards, and then laterally, until it lies in the concave London basin. Here the clay stratum above it prevents its escape upwards; and being confined under considerable pressure, it rises to the surface, or into a well in the superficial gravel, when the clay is tapped. In Fig. 8, B is an Artesian well if the pressure is such as to make the water rise through the London clay, when this is cut through and the underlying chalk is reached. C is a well in the chalk, which does not pass through an impervious stratum, and therefore comes within the above definition of a surface well; but as regards depth required to be dug before water is reached it is more like a deep well.

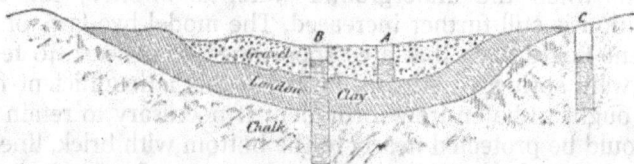

Fig. 8.

Showing Difference between Deep and Superficial Well. A.—Surface Well in Gravel. B.—Deep Well, going through Gravel and Clay to Chalk. C.—Well in Chalk District.

Among the deepest Artesian wells are Grenelle (1,800 feet), and Kissingen (1,878 feet.) The sinking of a deep well and severe pumping of its water may exhaust all the neighbouring wells for two or three miles. There is also danger of contamination from neighbouring cesspools when the upper part of the deep well is not properly constructed. The area exhausted by a deep well undergoing pumping is represented by an inverted cone, having a very wide base, and with a convex inner surface pointing towards the well.

For country places deep-well water is much preferable to water from streams, as streams are very liable to be contaminated by the sewage of houses higher up in their course, or even by that of houses close by. A good well should be at least thirty feet deep—preferably fifty feet and should always be lined with impervious material, except near its bottom. The absolutely water-tight and impervious condition as well as the distance of all drains or cesspools in the vicinity should be ascertained before deciding whether the drinking water from a given well is above suspicion. The direction of flow of the underground water should also be determined. This may be done by measuring the level of all the wells in the neighbourhood. Possible sources of pollution at points from which ground water is flowing towards the well are much more dangerous than those nearer than the well

66

to the river towards which the underground water is flowing (see Fig. 7). Steam pumping greatly increases the area from which contamination may be derived.

An excellent plan to obtain water for villages, in a gravelly soil, is to sink a Norton's Abyssinian tube well for fifty or sixty feet.

In towns it is preferable to trust to the public water supplied, rather than to any private well; and in villages, a general supply from a pure source should also be provided.

The water is obtained from a well by a pump or a draw-well. The former is a safer as well as a less laborious plan. The pump should be fixed some distance from the well, and the aperture through which the pump pipe passes should be rendered water tight. Lead pipes should be avoided, as well water not infrequently has plumbo-solvent properties.

8. Rivers and running streams originate in upland surface water or springs, and their water should be of the same quality as these. Unfortunately, they acquire a large amount of impurities in their course. Towns commonly pour their more or less clarified sewage into them; and the discharge of crude sewage from hamlets and single houses on the banks is still far from uncommon. With the more rigid enforcement of the Rivers Pollution Acts, this pollution of rivers will become less frequent; but river water previously contaminated by even small amounts of sewage cannot be regarded as an ideal source of water-supply.

If no contamination be present in the water of a river, it forms a good source of water-supply; being running water, it is always fairly well aërated, and is not usually so hard as spring-water.

Even if sewage has entered a river, it is asserted that it becomes a safe source of water-supply, after passage through filter beds, the sewage having been got rid of in four ways.

1st.—By subsidence, the organic matter settling to the bottom.

2nd.—By the influence of water-plants, which assimilate ammonia, nitrates, etc., and give out nascent oxygen.

3rd.—Oxidation. Doubtless a large amount of the nitrogenous matter does become oxidised in its course down a river, and in this condition is harmless. The river Seine becomes greatly polluted as it passes through Paris, but so far as chemical analysis can determine its condition, it is purer 30 miles below the city than it was before it received the sewage of the city.

4th.—It is highly probable that the germs (or micro-organisms) of enteric fever and other diseases known to be propagated by polluted water, are practically or wholly destroyed in the struggle for existence with the natural micro-organisms of river-water. When to this is added the fact that river-water supplied to large communities is carefully filtered through sand, after having been stored in reservoirs, in which the chief impurities have time to settle, it is not surprising that the experience of those communities like London, which are supplied with river-water, usually shows no evidence of evil ascribable to drinking this water. For over 30 years the inhabitants of London have been drinking filtered water from the river Lea and from the Thames above Teddington, and this gigantic

67

experiment on a population which has increased from 2½ to 5 millions has not been accompanied by any conclusive evidence of evil effect.

In regard to the comparative merits of the various waters described, it will be useful to give here the classification made by the Rivers Pollution Commissioners in their sixth report:—

Wholesome	1. Spring Water		Very palatable.
	2. Deep-well Water		
	3. Upland Surface Water		Moderately palatable.
Suspicious	4. Stored Rain Water		
	5. Surface Water from Cultivated Land		
Dangerous	6. River Water to which Sewage gains access		Palatable.
	7. Shallow-well Water		

Passage through certain geological strata has a great influence in rendering water palatable, colourless, and wholesome by percolation.

The following strata are said by the Commissioners to be the most efficient:—(1) Chalk, (2) oolite, (3) greensand, (4) Hastings sand, (5) new red and conglomerate sandstone. Fissures or cracks in these strata may cause the water to pass through them unpurified by filtration.

CHAPTER X

THE STORAGE AND DELIVERY OF WATER

The methods of storing and delivering water will vary with its source. In rural districts, deep wells and springs are the best sources of supply; but in large towns they are found to be insufficient for the wants of a rapidly-increasing population; and they can only be multiplied in a given district within certain limits, as every well drains a large surrounding area. The supply from surface wells in gravel or sand beds or in chalk districts is liable to fail in seasons of drought; but deep wells in oolite or chalk formations, and in the new red sandstone, generally yield a constant and abundant supply.

When the water is supplied from upland surfaces, springs, or small streams, a collecting reservoir is required. This is generally a natural valley below the level of the source of supply, but of sufficient elevation above the place supplied to allow the water to be distributed by gravity, without any pumping apparatus. The reservoir should be large enough to hold five or six months' supply, and its embankment should be perfectly water-tight, and of great strength.

When water is collected from upland surfaces, it is important to know the amount of rainfall to be reckoned on. If we know the area of the surface which drains towards the reservoir, and the average rainfall, the total rainfall is easily calculated. This will, however, differ greatly from the available rainfall, owing to the losses from penetration into the ground, evaporation, and other causes. The amount lost will vary, according to the season, from one-half to seven-eighths of the total rainfall; and according to the soil. The proportion of percolation in the chief water-bearing strata surrounding London varies from 48 to 60 per cent. (Prestwich). It is less when the ground is steep and the rainfall rapid, and usually less in winter than in summer.

Water collected near its actual place of fall, and from uncultivated districts, is always purer than that collected further from its source, and from cultivated land.

From the collecting or impounding reservoir, water is carried by the aqueduct or conduit either directly into the service-pipes, or when the pressure is too great, into a second service-reservoir, resembling the impounding reservoir in general structure, and capable of holding a few days' supply.

This must be high ground, above the level of the highest houses to which water has to be supplied, as water cannot rise above its own level. When this cannot be arranged, the water is pumped into tanks at a higher level, and distributed from them.

The greatest hourly demand for water being double the average hourly demand, the water-mains supplying a town must have double the discharging power that would be required, supposing the demand was uniform. The first requisite of a supply of water is that it should be abundant, and sufficient in amount for any extra strain on its capacities. Water ought to be laid on to every house, and to at least two floors of the house. Anything preventing free access to water, militates against cleanliness.

Cast-iron is the most serviceable material used in the construction of the main water-pipes; it is coated with pitch, or Dr. Angus Smith's varnish, or with magnetic oxide of iron (Barff). The service-pipes to each house are generally made of lead, and the ease with which this material can be bent and curved, and carried to the different floors of a house, makes its use very convenient. Lead pipes, furthermore, can be easily obliterated in case of bursting, and so any waste of water and flooding of the house minimised. Some kinds of water, unfortunately, act on and dissolve lead; this is especially true of soft waters and those containing organic matter. Shallow wells, being very liable to organic pollution, ought never to have the supply-pipe of their pumps made of lead. With hard waters, lead pipes may generally be used safely. When the quality of the water renders lead pipes objectionable, the use of iron, tin, zinc, tinned copper, earthenware, gutta-percha, and other materials, has been suggested. Of these, cast and wrought-iron pipes are the most serviceable, or pipes composed of an inner lining of block-tin and an outer of lead, a layer of asbestos intervening to prevent galvanic action between the metals. According to Rawlinson, "supply-pipes of wrought-iron are cheaper, stronger, and more easily fitted than service-pipes of lead;" but it is urged against them by Perry, that with soft water they become choked by rust in a few years. If galvanized they are more durable. Cast-iron pipes are rusted less easily than wrought-iron.

When the water-supply is from a river, filtering beds are needed, in addition to the parts of a water-service hitherto described. Moreover, since the river is usually at a low level, the water, after passing through the filtering beds, requires to be pumped into raised tanks, from which it is delivered.

In laying down water-pipes, in the streets and to houses, it is very important to make the distance between them and all drains and gas-pipes as great as possible. Suction of gases or liquids may occur into leaky pipes, even though these contain water, and still more when they are empty; and disease has occasionally been traced to this source. Thus if sewers and water-mains are laid in the same trench, foul matters which have escaped into the soil from the former may be sucked into the latter. This may happen if the water-mains are leaky, even when they are running full. Experiments have shewn that the flow of water causes a partial vacuum and insuction at the defective points. During intermissions of supply when the mains are partially or entirely empty, the danger of leakage into them is still greater. Coal-gas has been similarly sucked into water-mains.

The pipes bringing the water to a house may be kept constantly filled with water, or only for a limited time once or twice a day. The intermittent system of supply necessitates the provision of cisterns or water-tanks, in which water can be stored in the intervals of flow of water. With a sufficient and properly-distributed public supply of water, no cistern ought to be required.

Cisterns.—Cisterns for the supply of potable water may be made of iron, slate, stone, glass, glazed earthenware, or brick lined with Portland cement. Other materials have been used, as timber, lead, and zinc. Timber is inadvisable, as it easily rots; lead is very objectionable, owing to the possible solvent action of the water on it. Zinc or galvanized iron cisterns are also acted on by soft water; but they may be used with most waters. Galvanized iron is iron coated with a thin layer of zinc. Iron cisterns soon rust; but this may be prevented by giving them a coating of boiled linseed oil before they leave the foundry. Stone cisterns are too heavy for use, except in basements. Slate cisterns are good, but are apt to leak; the points of leakage have occasionally been stopped with red lead, which is attacked by the water, and thus lead poisoning results. If the slate is set in good cement (not mortar, as this makes the water hard), it is a good material for a cistern.

Every cistern should have a well-fitting lid, always kept closed, to avoid the entrance of dust of various kinds, or even dead cats, birds, etc. Noxious gases may be absorbed by the stagnant water.

The cistern should be easy of access. If it is indoors, the cistern room should be well ventilated; and in any case the cistern should be periodically visited and cleaned out. When the cistern is full, a ball-tap prevents any further flow of water; and if this does not act properly, an overflow pipe carries off the excess of water.

Cisterns badly arranged or neglected have been in the past a common source of disease. (1) The overflow pipe should not pass into any part of the water-closet apparatus or the soil-pipe, or into the supply pipe to the water-closet.

Where the overflow-pipe discharges into the soil-pipe or closet pan, foul gases or even solid particles may find their way into the cistern.

(2) No water-closet ought to be supplied from the same cistern as supplies drinking water, as the pipe leading down to the closet may when the cistern is accidentally empty carry noxious effluvia into the cistern. A separate flushing cistern capable of discharging two to three gallons of water should be provided for each closet.

With a constant supply of water, cisterns are only required for water-closets and for hot-water apparatus (see pages 168 and 164).

Constant and Intermittent Services.—With an intermittent service of water, during the intervals of supply, water is only obtainable from cisterns, water-butts, etc. The objections against this system are that—(1) The cisterns required are expensive, and liable to get out of order and become foul. (2) Their overflow pipes may improperly communicate with the soil pipe or with some other part of the drainage, instead of opening into the external air. (3) Putrid gases, from neighbouring ventilating-pipes or other parts of the drainage system, are liable to be absorbed by the stagnant water in the cistern. (4) The chief objection to an intermittent supply is that, during the intervals in which the water-mains are empty, foul air and liquids from the contiguous soil and drains are liable to be sucked through imperfect joints into the pipes. (5) In case of fire, the supply of water in the system is insufficient. In certain towns rates of insurance against fire have been reduced on replacing an intermittent by a constant service of water.

On the other hand it is urged that more expensive fittings are required for a constant service; and that, when taps are left open or pipes burst, the waste of water is much greater than with a cistern supply. The balance is decidedly in favour of a constant supply without storage cisterns. Where storage cisterns are in use, the taps for drinking-water should be connected with the "rising-main," before it supplies the cistern.

The Advantages of the Constant Service may be thus summarised:—

(1) Owing to the absence of cisterns, the risks connected with stagnant water, and with improper arrangement of overflow pipes, are obviated.

(2) The risk of suction into supply mains of external contaminations is reduced to a minimum, since the pipes are never empty.

(3) The pipes are less liable to rust. Air in the presence of a little moisture, causes rapid corrosion.

71

(4) There is an abundant supply of water in case of fire.

Of course, when there is a temporary stoppage of supply, as for repairs, some of the dangers incurred by an intermittent supply will arise.

CHAPTER XI

IMPURITIES OF WATER

Properties of Water.—When pure, water is colourless, or bluish when seen in large quantity. It should be quite inodorous. If, after keeping it for some time in a perfectly clean vessel, or if on heating it a smell is developed, the water is bad. Its taste should be pleasant and sparkling from the atmospheric gases dissolved in it. Bitterness generally indicates the presence of sulphate of magnesium (Epsom salts). Saltness is always a suspicious property, except in water obtained in the neighbourhood of salt mines or brine springs, or near the sea. It should be soft to the touch, and should dissolve soap easily. It should be bright and clear, and contain no suspended matters. Clear water is not necessarily pure, but turbid water is always to be rejected; the only exception being the brownish-tinged water from moors, which is not hurtful. In all other cases, printed matter should be legible through at least 18 inches of water in a clear glass cylinder. Thoroughly dissolved organic matter is less dangerous than suspended; the turbidity of water is therefore of great importance. But water may be bright and sparkling and apparently perfectly clear, and yet highly dangerous. The most important of the physical properties of water in regard to health are the absence of smell and turbidity, and these can be ascertained by even the most inexperienced. The chemical tests for the more important impurities are given.

The impurities of water may be classed under four heads—gaseous, mineral, vegetable, and animal.

The gases ordinarily present in water cannot properly be regarded as impurities, inasmuch as they are always present, and greatly increase its palatableness. The dissolved nitrogen and oxygen bear to each other the proportion 1·42 to 1; where sewage contamination occurs, the oxygen will be diminished or disappear, owing to oxidation of the organic matter.

The amount of carbonic acid gas in water varies greatly. It may be considerable in chalk waters, and in contaminated well-water.

Mineral Impurities.—Mineral impurities are dissolved by water in its course through the soil, and so will vary with the character of the latter. 1. The water obtained from granitic formations contains very little mineral matter, often not more than two to six grains per gallon. Clay slate water is also generally very pure, as is the water from hard trap rocks. 2. The water from millstone grit and hard oolite is very pure, often containing only four to eight grains per gallon, chiefly calcium and magnesium sulphate and carbonate. 3. Soft sand-rock waters usually contain thirty to eighty grains per gallon of sodium salts, with a little lime and magnesia. 4. Loose sand and gravel waters vary greatly. They may be almost free from mineral matter, or the solids may be more than seventy grains per gallon, including much organic matter. 5. Waters from the lias clays vary somewhat, but commonly contain a large quantity of calcium and magnesium sulphates. 6. Chalk waters generally contain from seven to twenty grains of calcium carbonate, with smaller quantities of other salts. 7. Limestone and magnesian limestone waters differ from the last, in containing more calcium sulphate and less calcium carbonate, as well as much magnesium sulphate and carbonate in the dolomite districts. 8. Selenitic waters contain calcium sulphate in considerable quantities. 9. Clay waters usually possess the characters of water from surface wells, and are objectionable. 10. Alluvial waters generally contain a large amount of various salts, including the various calcium, magnesium, and sodium salts. 11. Artesian well water varies greatly in composition. It may contain a large amount of sodium and potassium salts, or a small quantity of iron, or calcium salts.

The commonest and most important mineral constituent of water is calcium carbonate, next to this calcium sulphate. These two salts are the chief causes of hardness of water. For practical purposes as regards use in domestic matters and in manufactures, the most important classification of waters is into hard and soft. The degree of hardness varies within wide limits—from rain-water, which has no hardness at all, to the water from new red sandstone rocks which sometimes possesses a hardness of 90 degrees; or wells in the gravel, in which it may be as much as 152 degrees.

The following classification of waters, according to the degree of hardness, beginning with the least hard and gradually increasing in hardness, is from the sixth report of the Rivers Pollution Commissioners:— 1. Rain-water. 2. Upland surface. 3. Surface from cultivated land. 4. River. 5. Spring. 6. Deep-well. 7. Shallow-well water.

Calcium carbonate is the most common cause of hardness, and the hardness produced by it is remediable by boiling or chemical means. Calcium carbonate (chalk) is rendered soluble in water, by the carbonic acid contained in the latter, a double bicarbonate being thus formed. The air contained in the interstices of the soil through which water passes, often contains 250 times as much carbonic acid as ordinary air. The water, in percolating through the soil, dissolves this carbonic acid, and thus is able to take up a considerable amount of chalk.

The amount of hardness in any given water is expressed in degrees, one degree being equivalent to a grain of calcium carbonate in a gallon of water. Clarke's soap test is employed to detect the amount of hardness. It consists of a solution of soap of a known strength. Soft water will form a lather at once with this; hard water will only form a lather after all the calcium salt is neutralised. The amount of Clarke's solution required before a lather is produced, will give an estimate of the amount of hardness.

To Determine the Total Hardness take 70 c.c. of the water and place

73

in a stoppered bottle. From a burette run in a sufficient quantity of the standard soap solution (of which 1 c.c. equals 1° of hardness), to produce a lather on shaking the water, which remains unbroken after standing five minutes. Thus, if 7.5 c.c. of the soap solution were required, the hardness is 6°·5, as 1 c.c. of the solution is required to produce a lather in soft water. The 6°·5 means 6·5 milligrammes of calcium carbonate in 70 c.c. or 6·5 grains in a gallon of the water.

To Determine the Permanent Hardness boil 70 c.c. of the water in a flask for half-an-hour; allow the precipitated carbonates of calcium and magnesium to settle. Some of the latter will be re-dissolved. Carefully decant, and make up the liquid to the original 70 c.c. with distilled water. Filter through fine filter paper and estimate hardness as above.

The amount of soap wasted in consequence of the hardness of water is very great. Thus, in the case of water of one degree of hardness, as every gallon contains one grain of chalk, 7,000 gallons would contain 7,000 grains—that is, a pound. But every grain of chalk wastes 8 or 9 grains of soap; therefore, a pound of chalk, contained in 7,000 gallons, would waste about 8½ pounds of soap. But nearly all waters are harder than this, and they not uncommonly possess a hardness of 20° or more. If the hardness be 20°, the waste would be 170 pounds of soap. This quantity would be easily used annually in a family of seven or eight persons, if we include the washing of clothes. The amount of money thus wasted can be easily estimated.

Not only does soft water require less soap, but it is much more suitable for making tea and soup, and for boiling meat and vegetables— both time and fuel being saved. The reason why better tea is made when a little carbonate of soda is added to the water is that the chalk is by this means precipitated.

Carbonate of calcium is precipitated from water by boiling it; carbonic acid being driven off, the neutral salt falls to the bottom of the vessel. This is the origin of the "fur" inside kettles, which lessens their conductivity to heat, and renders necessary a greater consumption of fuel.

The chalk may also be removed by adding to the water, while still in the reservoir, some milk of lime—that is, quicklime made into a milky solution with water. This is done on a large scale at various waterworks. The reaction may be expressed thus:—

Calcium bicarbonate + calcium oxide = calcium carbonate + calcium carbonate.

The calcium carbonate, as it is precipitated, carries down with it organic and other matters, thus clearing and purifying the water.

The hardness due to calcium sulphate is not removable by boiling. It is, therefore, called permanent hardness, to distinguish it from the temporary hardness of chalk waters, which is removable by boiling. It may, however, be partially removed by the addition of washing soda to the water, as well as the nitrate and chloride of calcium which are also present. The magnesium salts are not removable by boiling or soda. This is shown by the fact that the "fur" inside kettles does not usually contain magnesium salts.

The amount of hardness varies greatly in different waters. In the deep wells in magnesium limestone, it varies from 14°-57°; in the deep wells from chalk beds, it varies from 13° to 27° and may be higher. In the water from Bala Lake, Wales, the temporary hardness is 0°·1, the permanent hardness 0°·3; in the Loch Katrine water there is no temporary hardness, 0°·9 permanent hardness; in the water from the new red sandstone (Nottingham), the temporary hardness is 9°·6, permanent 10°·2; in a chalk spring at Ryde, temporary hardness 16°·7, permanent 3°·9 (Wanklyn). The total hardness in the metropolitan water supplies from the rivers Thames and Lea, varies from 13°·2 (Southwark Company) to 14°·6 (New River Company); in the Kent Deep Wells 20°·1; in deep wells from the chalk at Brighton it varies from 12° to 13°. In all these, the hardness is chiefly temporary.

The amount of permanent hardness is always great in water from clays, as the London, Oxford, Kimmeridge, and Lower Lias clays; or in places where there are large deposits of calcium sulphate, as at Montmartre, near Paris (hence the name Plaster of Paris, given to desiccated calcium sulphate). Water from fissures in the clay often contains, also, a large amount of organic matter.

Chlorides are always present in small quantities in water. As a rule the presence of more than 1 grain per gallon, i.e. ·7 parts per 100,000 of water, indicates contamination with some animal refuse, unless the water is derived from new red sandstone, or brine springs, or from the neighbourhood of the sea. This rule does not, however, hold universally good. The absence or the presence of only a minute quantity of chlorides indicates the probable absence of animal contamination; but in exceptional cases waters of the highest organic purity may contain more chlorides than the same bulk of sewage.

To determine the amount of Chlorine take 70 c.c. of the water, add a few drops of solution of potassium monochromate ($KCrO_4$). From a burette run in gradually a standard solution of silver nitrate (of such a strength that 1 c.c. of the solution is equivalent to 1 milligramme of chlorine). The silver solution forms milky chloride of silver ($AgCl$) by combination with the chlorine of the chlorides in the water. When all the chlorine is thus combined, the next drop of the silver solution forms a deep red tint with the chromate. The number of c.c.'s of the silver solution required to produce this effect, equals the number of milligrammes of chlorine in 70 c.c. of water, or the number of grains of chlorine in a gallon of water. To convert this into parts per 100,000, divide by 7 and multiply by 10.

To express the amount of chlorine in terms of common salt ($NaCl$), multiply the parts per 100,000 of chlorine by 1·65.

Nitrates in any water are suspicious; but their import varies with the circumstances under which they occur. A minute quantity of ammonium nitrate is present in nearly all waters; and the water of deep wells, especially of wells in the chalk, which, as a rule is perfectly free from sewage, may be highly charged with nitrates. Nitrates, when derived from sewage, represent a completely oxidised condition of its nitrogenous

75

matter. Crude sewage generally contains no nitrates. Nitrites as a rule indicate more recent contamination, and therefore greater danger than nitrates. The presence of more than a trace of phosphates is a strong indication of contamination with sewage matter.

To determine the amount of Nitrites and Nitrates the best known methods are by the indigo, the phenol-sulphuric, the aluminium, or the zinc-copper couple tests. For nitrites the metaphenylene-diamine test is employed. The following qualitative tests will suffice for elementary work.

Nitrates. An equal amount of a solution of brucine is added to the suspected water in a test-tube, then a little pure sulphuric acid is poured down the side of the tube. A pink zone is produced if nitrates are present in considerable amount.

Nitrites. A few drops of each of diluted sulphuric acid and of metaphenylene-diamine solution give a red colour with water after standing for a few minutes, if nitrites are present.

Lead is an occasional contamination of slightly acid waters. The purest and most oxygenated waters act most readily on lead; as also those containing organic matter, nitrates or nitrites. Waters containing chlorides also act on lead, the chloride of lead being sufficiently soluble to produce poisonous symptoms. Upland surface waters derived from moorlands in certain districts, e.g. around Sheffield, have been found to be capable of dissolving considerable lead from lead service-pipes. The water taken first from the tap in the early morning is the most heavily charged with lead. Such waters are very soft; but other moorland soft waters do not dissolve lead. It is the water having a slightly acid reaction which possesses this property. The source of this acid, whether sulphuric acid from the products of combustion in a neighbouring town, or an organic acid, is uncertain. The plumbo-solvent action of such water is greatest in autumn, when the amount of acid is at its maximum. The property of dissolving lead is removed by passing the water on a large scale over filters of sand, spongy iron, chalk, or limestone. The addition of a small quantity of carbonate of soda has the same effect. In such districts the use of tin-lined iron pipes for domestic services has been recommended, but these are liable to fracture when bent. Pipes consisting of an outer case of lead and an inner pipe of tin with a layers of asbestos between have also been placed on the market.

Hard waters have the least action on lead; a coating of insoluble carbonate of lead being formed on the interior of the pipe, which prevents any further action. Thus the use of lead pipes for water containing carbonates or sulphate, or calcium phosphate, is comparatively safe. Hard water containing carbonic acid gas under pressure will dissolve a small amount of carbonate of lead; this explains the cases of lead poisoning from soda water which was formerly supplied in syphon bottles with lead tubes.

Lead is dissolved much more easily by water if other metals are in contact with it, as iron, zinc, or tin, galvanic action being thus set up. Zinc pipes containing some lead are very dangerous, especially with the distilled water used on board ships.

To determine the presence of lead in water, place a given quantity, say 100 c.c. in a white dish, and stir with a rod dipped in a solution of ammonium sulphide; if the water becomes coloured, this is generally due to the presence of iron or lead. If the colour remains after adding a drop or two of hydrochloric acid, lead is present.

To determine the amount of lead, a standard solution of lead acetate containing 1/10 milligrammes of lead in 1 c.c., is made by dissolving ·183 gramme of crystallised lead acetate in a litre of distilled water. Place 100 c.c. of the water to be examined in a Nessler glass, acidify by a few drops of acetic acid; now add ½ c.c. of a saturated solution of ammonium sulphide. A brownish-black discoloration is produced if lead is present. To a second Nessler glass, containing 100 c.c. of distilled water, the same amounts of acetic acid and ammonium sulphide are added, and then a sufficient quantity of the standard lead solution is added, until the tints of the contents of the two Nessler glasses are identical. The amount of the standard solution added being known, we know the amount of lead in 100 c.c., and the amount per litre (1,000 c.c.) will be tenfold. Thus if 2 c.c. of the solution were required for matching colours, there were ·2 parts of lead per 100,000 of water, or ·14 grains per gallon.

Traces of Iron are sometimes present in water, giving it an astringent taste. Such water is apt to turn brown; and tea made from it is very dark.

Organic Impurities.—Organic impurities may be either vegetable or animal, the latter being by far the most dangerous. The water from moorlands is often brown, but this is not noxious. Growing plants, again, may be beneficial to water, by absorbing dissolved organic matter, and aiding its oxidation. Decaying vegetable matter is objectionable in water, and may set up diarrhœa.

The most important organic impurity of water has an animal origin—from sewage; the liquid or solid excreta (i.e. the urine or fæces) gaining accidental access to the water. Besides sewage, the eggs of various intestinal worms have been swallowed with water; and in a few cases, even leeches. But whatever the source of the organic matter contained in water, it contains nitrogen as an essential constituent; and tends under the influence of warmth, and therefore especially in summer, to undergo putrefactive changes, owing to the action of bacteria. These split up the more complex molecules of organic matter into simpler matter; ammoniacal compounds and salts, of which the most important are nitrites and nitrates, being final products of their activity. The detection of nitrates, and still more of nitrites, is important, as they may indicate the occurrence of previous sewage contamination. These products are quite harmless in water, except as an indication that the water has been polluted, and that possibly a certain proportion of the nitrogenous matter in the form of the complex organic matter forming the germs of such diseases as enteric fever, may still be present. Organic matter may be suspended or dissolved, the former being most dangerous to health. The germs or microbes causing disease consist of suspended, i.e. particulate matter. The amount of organic matter is determined by the amount of free ammonia and albuminoid ammonia which are present (Wanklyn's process), by Frankland's combustion process, or by Forschammer's oxygen process; all of which give indications, rather than an exact estimate of its amount.

METHODS OF WATER ANALYSIS

The following scheme of qualitative examination may be followed, when an immediate opinion is required as to a water. It can only be trusted when the examination shows pollution. The following results will be obtained, for instance, when a minute quantity of urine is added to a gallon of water.

(1) The water has a faint odour.

(2) Its colour is greenish yellow in bulk.

(3) On adding a few drops of Nessler's solution, a deep yellow colour appears.

(4) A few drops of an acid solution of permanganate of potassium become yellow when added to it.

(5) Acidify some of the water in a test-tube with nitric acid, then add silver nitrate solution. Distinct cloudiness is produced, much greater than with pure tap water.

(6) Addition of hydrochloric acid and barium chloride solution shows a much greater quantity of sulphates than the same quantity of tap water.

(7) A quantity of the water evaporated in a porcelain dish over a Bunsen's flame gives a white residue, which speedily turns brown, with a urinous odour.

(8) Ignite the ash and add some nitric acid to oxidise it more completely. Then dissolve in distilled water, and add acid molybdate solution. A yellow colour, followed by a precipitate, indicates high phosphates and sewage pollution.

The Complete Systematic Examination is (a) physical, (b) bacteriological, and (c) chemical. Of the physical tests, colour, which should never be yellow or brown except for peaty water, is important. Taste is a somewhat uncertain guide, but any badly-tasting water should be rejected. The odour on heating to 80° F. in a closed flask may indicate pollution. The degree of hardness can be roughly tested by rubbing between the hands. The absence of turbidity is most important, as suspended impurities are more dangerous than all others. Printed matter should be legible through a column of 18 inches of water.

Microscopally the suspended matter in water which has been allowed to settle should be examined. Particles of vegetable matter, e.g. fibres of cotton, linen, cells of potato, or spiral cells of cabbage, are important as indicating domestic impurities. Bits of wool, hair, wings and legs of insects and epithelium may be discovered. The presence of algæ, diatoms and desmids, or of water-fleas, cannot be held to indicate pollution, as these are found in all running streams and in many wells. The eggs and embryos of worms are much more serious.

Bacteria are almost invariably present in water. The majority of these micro-organisms are harmless. But as they may number among them the germs producing diseases like enteric fever and cholera, the estimation of their number and particularly of any deviation from the number usually present in a given water, and if possible the detection of special disease-producing bacteria, are very important. This method has been made more practicable since Koch's method of "plate cultivation" of bacteria was discovered. A small quantity of the water to be examined (kept surrounded by ice until this test is applied, to prevent multiplication of bacteria in the bottle), is mixed with sterilised gelatine which has been melted over a water bath. Then the mixture is spread in a thin layer on a glass plate and allowed to solidify, having been covered to prevent atmospheric germs from settling on the gelatine. The bacteria in the water thus become fixed, each growing and forming "colonies" dotted over the plate. These colonies can be recognised by their size and appearance, and by sub-culturing according to recognised methods. The number of such colonies, and the number of bacteria, from which, presumably, such colonies sprang in 1 c.c. of filtered Thames water is usually much below 100; in the water before filtration many thousands are present. It has been suggested that no water should be regarded as wholesome which contains more than 100 bacteria in each c.c.

This standard is, however, obviously arbitrary. Chalk water ought to have a smaller number than this; river waters may have more, and yet be wholesome. Everything depends on the character of the bacteria found. The detection of the Bacillus coli communis, which is present in sewage, and normally in the human intestine, is very suggestive of contamination by sewage. The bacteriological method of examination of water is still in its infancy.

CHEMICAL ANALYSIS

(1) The total solids are ascertained by evaporating a given quantity of the water to dryness, and weighing.

(2) Determination of Chlorine.

(3) Determination of Hardness.

(4) The Determination of Nitrites is based on the reddish-brown colouration produced when an acid solution of metaphenylene diamine is brought into contact with a weak solution of nitrous acid. 100 c.c. of the water under examination are placed in a clean glass cylinder. Add 1 c.c. of H_2SO_4 solution (1 in 3), then 2 c.c. of metaphenylene diamine solution (5 grains in 1 litre of water with a little H_2SO_4 added). Stir well with a glass rod. If a colouration is produced at once, a smaller quantity of water must be taken, and made up to 100 c.c. with pure distilled water. The quantity of nitrous acid present is measured by introducing different fractions of a c.c. of the standard sodium nitrate solution[3] into similar glass cylinders. Each is then made up to 100 c.c. with distilled water, and the metaphenylene diamine solution and acid added as before. The colour develops slowly; time must, therefore, be allowed in matching.

(5) The Determination of Nitrates can be conveniently made by the following method. When phenyl-hydrogen sulphate solution is poured upon a nitrate, and sulphuric acid is formed, picric acid is formed:—

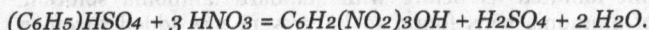

$$(C_6H_5)HSO_4 + 3\ HNO_3 = C_6H_2(NO_2)_3OH + H_2SO_4 + 2\ H_2O.$$

The addition of free ammonia in excess forms yellow ammonium picrate, the intensity of the colour of which is an index of the picrate, and of the nitrate from which it was produced. (a) Evaporate 25 c.c. of the water under examination, and (b) 5 c.c. of standard KNO_3 solution (containing 1 part N in 100,000) to dryness in two porcelain dishes over the water bath. Add 1 c.c. of phenyl-sulphate solution to each of these as soon as cool, stir well with a glass rod, then add 1 c.c. distilled water to each dish and 3 drops of strong H_2SO_4. Next add 25 c.c. of water to each dish, and after heating for five minutes over the water bath, add solution of ammonia to each dish in excess. A yellow colour is produced in proportion to the amount of nitrate present. Transfer the liquids to glass cylinders, and dilute each to 100 c.c. Take 50 c.c. of the solution showing the least colour, and dilute the other with distilled water, until it has the same tint.

Supposing the 100 c.c. of the sample required to be diluted to 150 c.c.—

Then the amount of N will be $150/100 \times 5/25 = \cdot3$ parts per 100,000.

---

[3] Freshly made; of which 1 c.c. = $\cdot00001$ grm. of N_2O_3

If the two solutions (a) and (b) when diluted have the same tint, then the Amount of N in the sample = 5/25 = ·2 parts per 100,000.

(6) Determination of Organic Matter. Frankland's combustion process involves the use of delicate and costly apparatus, and is seldom employed. In this process the organic carbon is evolved as carbonic acid, and the nitrogen as such.

Wanklyn's ammonia process is based on the reduction of organic matter to ammonia. Part of this ammonia, free or saline ammonia, is simply combined with carbonic, nitric, or other acids, or is easily derived from the urea of urine, $CH_4N_2O + 2H_2O = 2(NH_4)_2CO_3$. Another part is only set free when the water is boiled with a strongly alkaline solution of permanganate of potassium. This is called the albuminoid ammonia.

In carrying out this method, a retort is taken, and after having been washed out, first with a little sulphuric acid, and then with some of the water to be analysed, 500 c.c. of the latter is put in, and the retort is connected with a condenser, and distillation begun; 50 c.c. of the distilled water is collected in a cylindrical glass tube called a Nessler glass. To this 1½ c.c. of Nessler's reagent (mercuric iodide dissolved in a solution of potassic iodide and made alkaline by potass) are added. A rich brown colour is produced, if any ammonia is present in the distillate. The amount of ammonia in the distillate is determined by exactly imitating its colour by adding a known quantity of a standard solution of ammonium-chloride to 50 c.c. of ammonia-free distilled water, and then Nesslerising as before. Each c.c. of the dilute standard ammonium chloride solution is equivalent to ·00001 gramme of ammonia (NH_3).

If the first 50 c.c. of water distilled over gives only a slight colouration with the Nessler solution, no more water needs to be distilled over for free ammonia. If more is present, two more 50 c.c.'s must be distilled over, and the amounts of the standard solution required for imitating the test in each Nesslerised 50 c.c. added together. Thus, if 2 c.c. were needed. This

= ·00002 grm. NH_3, which is contained in 500 c.c. of the water

= ·00002 × 200 = ·004 parts saline NH_3 in 100,000 of water.

The free ammonia having been distilled over, 50 c.c. of an alkaline permanganate solution (containing 8 grammes $KMnO_4$ and 200 grammes of NaOH in 1100 c.c. of distilled water, boiled until the bulk is reduced to 1,000 c.c.) is poured into the retort, and distillation is begun again. Three successive 50 c.c.'s of water are collected, and then the distillation stopped. Each of these is Nesslerised, and the tint imitated as before with standard ammonia solution. The three amounts of ammonia thus found to be present are added together; and when multiplied by 200, we obtain the amount of albuminoid ammonia in 100,000 parts of water. This test is universally employed by water analysts along with the next test.

The amount of Oxygen Absorbed from permanganate of potassium is regarded as an approximate test of the amount of organic matter in water. Qualitatively this forms a favourite method of testing the purity of water. Two glass cylinders are taken, one filled with distilled water, one with the water to be tested. To each is added a given small amount of an acid solution of permanganate of potassium. The distilled water to which permanganate has been added will retain its pink colour; while, if the water being tested is very impure, it will speedily become decolourised. The rapidity and degree of decolourisation are a rough test of the amount of impurity. A rapid decolourisation proves the presence of organic matter having an animal origin, or of sulphuretted hydrogen, iron, or nitrites. Sulphuretted hydrogen is rarely present, and can be easily recognised by its smell; iron or nitrites are readily distinguished by their appropriate tests. In the absence of these, the rapid discolouration is an indication of animal contamination.

To Determine the Amount of Oxygen Absorbed, two glass-stoppered bottles, each holding about 350 c.c. are required. Into one, 250 c.c. distilled water, and into the other the same amount of the water under examination are placed. To each are then added 10 c.c. of standard permanganate of potassium solution[4] and 10 c.c. of a standard pure 25 per cent sulphuric acid solution. The two bottles, after being shaken, are placed in a water-bath at 27°C for four hours. At the end of this time add a few drops of potassium iodide solution to each bottle. The pink is now replaced by a yellow colour.[5] A standard thiosulphate solution ($Na_2S_2O_3$, $5H_2O$)[6] is placed in a burette. From this the thiosulphate solution is run into the control bottle until the yellow colour almost disappears. Now a few drops of starch solution are added, and a blue colour is produced. The thiosulphate is then added cautiously until all the blue colour disappears. The amount of thiosulphate necessary for this is read off on the burette. The same process is repeated with the bottle containing the sample of water. The starch acts as an indicator. The amount of iodine liberated is an index of the amount of permanganate in the water, which has not been used up by its impurities. The amount of iodine liberated is measured by the amount of thiosulphate required to decolourise the solution. Thus—

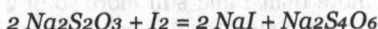

$$2\ Na_2S_2O_3 + I_2 = 2\ NaI + Na_2S_4O_6$$

Suppose that 20 c.c. of thiosulphate solution were required to decolourise the iodine liberated in 250 c.c. of a sample of water, while the distilled water required 25 c.c. Then 25 c.c. thiosulphate represents 10 c.c. of the permanganate solution = ·001 grains of available oxygen.

$$25-20 = 5$$
As 25 c.c. = ·001 grm. O, 5 c.c. = 5/25 of ·001 = ·0002 grm.

This is the amount of O absorbed by 250 c.c. of the sample.
Therefore the amount of O absorbed by 100,000 c.c. of the sample. = ·08 grm.

It is usual to make a similar determination of the amount of oxygen absorbed in fifteen minutes.

The Interpretation of Results of analysis is more difficult than the analysis. A single analysis may be misleading, unless the source of the water is known. Constancy in composition or analysis is almost as important a criterion of purity as the actual character of the constituents. A knowledge of the source is essential in interpreting results of analysis, as the chemical composition of water varies with its source. The following rules are only approximately correct, and are subject to the above general considerations. The total dissolved solids in river-water are usually 10 to 30 parts in 100,000. Shallow well-water may contain from 30 to 200 parts or even more, and deep well-water from 20 to 70 parts.

Saline Ammonia in water is commonly of animal origin, ammonia (NH_3) being one of the first products of decomposition of nitrogenous animal refuse. Upland surface water usually contains about ·002 parts per 100,000, but it may reach ·008 or more if the land over which the water passes has been manured. Shallow well-water may be free from ammonia, or this may be very excessive in amount. Deep well-water may contain no ammonia or any amount up to ·1 per 100,000. Its presence is suspicious if the albuminoid ammonia is above a trace, or if the oxygen absorbed is appreciable in amount. Generally water is suspicious if

---

[4] Made by dissolving ·395 grm. of $KMnO_4$ in 1,000 c.c. of water. Each c.c. of this solution =·0001 grm. of oxygen available for oxidation.
[5] Caused by the liberation of iodine. Thus—
$K_2Mn_2O_8 + 8\ H_2SO_4 + 10\ KI = 6\ K_2SO_4 + 2\ MnSO_4 + 8\ H_2O + 5\ I_2$.
[6] Of the strength of 1 grm. of crystalline sodium thiosulphate to 1 litre of water.

saline ammonia is up to ·01 per 100,000. Albuminoid Ammonia indicates the amount of organic nitrogenous matter present in the water. It should not exceed ·005 parts per 100,000, while at the same time the saline ammonia should not usually exceed ·01 per 100,000. For Oxygen consumed the following table of the weight of oxygen required for 100,000 parts of water is given by Clowes and Coleman:—

	UPLAND SURFACE WATER.	WATER FROM OTHER SOURCES.
Water of Great purity	Not exceeding ·1	Not exceeding ·05
Medium purity	From ·1 to ·3	From ·05 to ·15
Doubtful purity	From ·3 to ·4	From ·15 to ·20
Impure	Exceeding ·4	Exceeding ·20

The presence of more than 1 and still more so of 2 grains of Chlorine per 100,000 of water is most suspicious, except in saline districts. Nitrites if present in an appreciable quantity indicate comparatively recent contamination by sewage. In deep well-water they may be produced by deoxidation of nitrates. Nitrates in upland surface waters should not be equivalent to more than ·03 of N. per 100,000; in shallow well-waters the amount varies greatly; in deep well-waters it may be excessive. As a rule it ought not to be equivalent to more than 5 parts of N. per 100,000 of water; but the significance of nitrates depends greatly on the source of the water and on the amount of the other constituents present.

Chemical analysis alone cannot ascertain the safety of a given drinking water. A minute amount of impurity inappreciable to analysis may be competent to produce disease; while another water may be drunk with impunity, which contains considerable organic matter. Chemical analysis "can tell us of impurity and hazard, but not of purity or safety" (Buchanan). An accurate opinion as to the character of a drinking water can only be expressed when one knows the amount of each chief constituent (as above), and whether these amounts deviate from the same water at other times or from other waters in the vicinity.

CHAPTER XII

ORIGIN AND EFFECTS OF THE IMPURITIES OF WATER

Origin of Impurities of Water.—Parkes classifies impurities of water as:

1. Those Received at the Source.—The character of water varies with the geological structures through which it has passed; with its origin from the subsoil or cultivated land, or deep wells, or graveyards, or near the sea, etc. It is a mistaken policy to commence with an impure water and proceed

to purify it; though communities supplied from rivers may be compelled to submit to this. They must then insist on the most stringent measures of purification. Inorganic impurities are of much smaller consequence as regards health than organic; hence the great advantage of deep well-water over river water. It has been suggested, however, that when deep well-water becomes polluted, it is more dangerous than equally polluted river-water, because in the latter the normal bacteria of water are more abundant, and possibly interfere with the continued life in water of disease-producing bacteria. This statement is unproved; and if correct, is rather an indication for further precautions being taken to prevent access of pollution to deep wells, than in favour of the continued use of river-water.

2. Impurities of Transit from Source to Reservoir, acquired during the flow in rivers, canals, or other conduits. These impurities have been broadly divided by the Rivers Pollution Commissioners into "sewage" and "manufacturing;" the former including the solid and liquid excreta, the house and waste water, etc.; the latter including the refuse from manufacturing processes, as from dye and bleaching works, tanneries, etc.

3. Impurities of Storage, whether in wells, reservoirs, or cisterns. Organic impurities are commonly received at this stage. A well, for instance, drains the soil around it in the shape of an inverted cone, with a very broad base, unless the entrance of water from its sides is prevented.

4. Impurities of Distribution. Lead, and occasionally other metals, are dissolved by certain waters. If the pipes are left empty, as with an intermittent supply, sewage may be drawn into them; in a few cases coal-gas has found its way into the water pipes.

Effects of Impure Water.—1. Effects of Mineral Impurities. Suspended Mineral matters in unfiltered water occasionally produce diarrhœa. The hill diarrhœa of some parts of India has been traced to water containing fine mica particles in suspension.

Hard water is said by some to be hurtful, but the salts causing hardness are probably innocuous when not amounting to more than 12 or 16 grains per gallon. Persons in the habit of drinking hard water find soft water unpalatable. Hard water has been thought to favour gout and calculus (stone), but this is not so. The salts producing permanent hardness are said to be injurious, producing indigestion, but this is doubtful in the amounts ordinarily drunk.

Goitre, a swelling of the thyroid gland in the neck, is often associated with the use of drinking water from magnesian limestone formations; but that any kind of excessively hard water causes goitre is very doubtful.

Lead dissolved in water may produce serious and lasting ailments, and they are often present for a long time before their cause is detected. The amount of lead capable of producing poisonous symptoms has been as little as 1/100 grain per gallon of water (Dr. Angus Smith). According to De Chaumont, 1/10 grain per gallon, that is 1 part in 700,000 is usually required to produce such symptoms. In the well-known case of the poisoning of Louis Phillippe's family at Claremount, there was 7/10 grain

83

of lead in a gallon of water; and this affected 34 per cent. of those who drank it. The symptoms produced by lead poisoning are those of indigestion, accompanied by colic; a blue line at the junction of the gums with the teeth; "wrist drop," a paralysis of the muscles of the forearm, or some other paralysis; and if the poisoning is continued, attacks of gout, followed by its usual consequences, chronic kidney disease. The latter affections chiefly occur when the poisoning is continued for a long time, as in the case of painters or type-setters: poisoning from water is generally discovered before any other than dyspeptic symptoms and colic are produced.

The presence of traces of iron in water may give it a slightly astringent taste; and such water is liable to cause headache and constipation.

2. Effects of Vegetable Impurities.—Living plants are unobjectionable, but decomposing vegetable matter may produce diarrhœa and other severe symptoms.

3. Effects of Animal Impurities.—Animal impurities of water are by far the most important from a sanitary point of view. They are most commonly derived from leaky drains or cesspools, or from surface accumulations of filth. The quality of the contamination is more important than its quantity; and this will explain why water containing a large amount of sewage may be drunk for a prolonged period with impunity, while at another time the least trace, if it contain the active germs of disease, will lead to serious mischief.

Suspended animal impurities are much more dangerous than those completely dissolved. Hence the examination of the colour and turbidity of drinking water is very important. Fæcal contamination is by far the most dangerous of all, and chiefly so when it is derived from a patient suffering from some communicable disease, like enteric fever or cholera.

Certain Parasites occasionally are swallowed with water in the form of embryo or egg. The liver fluke, round worm, and less frequently other kinds of entozoa have been introduced in this way. The occasional swallowing of small leeches has occasionally given rise to hæmorrhage.

Diarrhœa may be caused by animal contamination of water. It most often occurs in summer, when all the circumstances are favourable to active fermentative changes. The summer diarrhœa of infants is caused by similar changes in milk or other foods. The presence of fœtid gases in water may lead to diarrhœa. This may occur when the overflow pipe of a cistern opens into the soil pipe or into the trap of the W.C.

Dysentery, like cholera and enteric fever, may be propagated by water contaminated with the stools of a patient suffering from the same disease.

Malaria or Ague has been stated to be caused by the water of malarious marshes. The evidence on this point requires revision, in view of the part which the mosquito is now known to play in the propagation of this disease.

Enteric (otherwise called Typhoid) fever is most often due to the drinking of water contaminated with sewage.

The balance of evidence is in favour of the view that in order to produce enteric fever water must be contaminated with the stools or urine of a patient who has suffered from this disease. Numerous instances are on record in which villages, the inhabitants of which drink sewage-contaminated water, have remained free from enteric fever, until a patient suffering from it has come to the village, when the spread by water has been very rapid. Occasionally no known contamination from a case of enteric fever has preceded the outbreak of this disease which has been caused by sewage-contaminated water. It must be remembered on this point that the urine of an enteric fever patient may occasionally contain large numbers of the bacillus causing this disease for several months after the patient is well.

The contamination of water with sewage may occur in various ways. In country places surface wells and small streams commonly supply the drinking water, and these are frequently contaminated. The illustration shows the percolation of excretory matters from an out-door closet through the porous gravel, into a neighbouring well; the result being an epidemic of enteric fever among those who drank the water of the well. Alterations in the level of the subsoil water are sometimes followed by an outbreak of enteric fever. A sudden fall of rain occurs, and the excess of water in the soil absorbs the soakings from country privies or cesspools, and carries them into the nearest well. The percolation of tainted water through a considerable tract of land, possibly along fissures, is sometimes insufficient to purify it, as proved by a remarkable epidemic in the small village of Lausen, in Switzerland.

In other cases sewage gains access into leaky water-pipes. Formerly contamination was occasionally due to improper connection between the overflow pipe of the cistern and the soil-pipe, or to the water-closet being flushed by a pipe directly connected with a water-main (as in the Caius College outbreak at Cambridge), or connected with the drinking-water cistern.

Milk may, by the admixture of water, become contaminated with enteric matter, and produce widespread epidemics. Where the water is very impure, the small amount used in washing cans may suffice to cause infection.

Cholera was first proved by Dr. Snow, in 1849, to be due to the specific contagium of cholera gaining an entrance into drinking water. This contagium is derived as in enteric fever from the intestinal evacuations, the urine, and the vomit of patients suffering from the same disease.

85

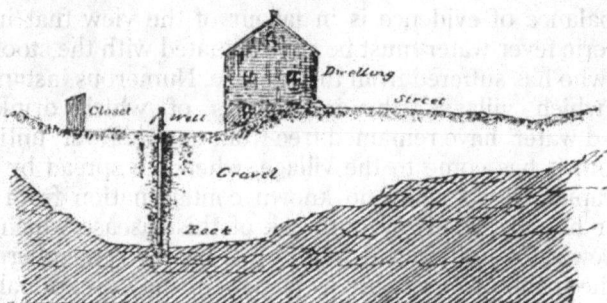

Fig. 9.

The close connection of the spread of cholera with an impure water supply has been repeatedly shown in this country. The cholera epidemic of 1854 was very severe in the southern districts of London. At that period these districts were supplied with water by the Southwark and Vauxhall Company, deriving its water from the Thames at Battersea, and by the Lambeth Company, having its intake at Thames Ditton, where the water was purer. The two companies were acting in rivalry, so that in many streets their mains ran side by side; and houses in the same street similar in all other respects, received a different water supply. An investigation of the distribution of cholera in these districts gave the following results:—

	POPULATION IN 1851.	CHOLERA DEATHS IN 14 WEEKS.	CHOLERA DEATHS PER 10,000 OF POPULATION.
Houses supplied by Southwark Co.	266,516	4,093	153
Houses supplied by Lambeth Co.	173,748	461	26

The facts, when examined in detail, brought out still more strikingly the exemption of the houses supplied by the Lambeth Company; the infection picking out in a given street the houses supplied by the Southwark Company. The great epidemic of cholera at Hamburg in 1892 proves the same point. Hamburg, Wandsbeck and Altona are three towns adjoining each other, and really forming one large community; but while Hamburg suffered terribly, the two other towns had no cases of cholera, except the few that were brought into them. In all respects except water-supply the conditions were alike; but Wandsbeck obtained filtered water from a lake, Altona obtained filtered water from the Elbe below the town, while Hamburg was supplied, previous to the epidemic, by unfiltered water from the Elbe just above the town.

Diphtheria and scarlet fever have never been traced to polluted water.

Effects of an Insufficient Supply of Water.—The influence on personal health is most baneful. Water is used sparingly for purposes of

86

cleanliness, with the necessary results that cutaneous diseases become more common, and the whole body suffers; the linen is imperfectly and infrequently washed; the house becomes dirty; drains are imperfectly flushed; the streets are not cleaned; and the whole atmosphere becomes loaded with impurities. According to Parkes, it is probable that the almost complete disappearance of typhus fever from civilized and cleanly nations, is not merely owing to better ventilation, but also to more frequent and thorough washing of clothes.

Insufficient cleansing of the surfaces of streets and of sewers, owing to a deficient supply of water, has a very important influence on the spread of enteric fever and epidemic diarrhœa. A heavy fall of rain often causes a rapid diminution in the prevalence of the latter disease.

CHAPTER XIII

THE PURIFICATION OF WATER

When a public water-supply is provided, it may reasonably be expected to be furnished pure and fit for use; but this, occasionally is not so. The reports, for instance, of the condition of the London Water Supply, occasionally show that it is turbid and contains a slight excess of organic matter. This is especially the case when, after heavy rainfall, storm-water is brought into the reservoirs, and owing to deficient storage, sufficient time is not allowed for deposit. Rain-water always and other waters frequently require to be purified before use.

Methods of Purification.—The only certain way of obtaining pure water is by Distillation; but this plan is scarcely applicable to water on a large scale. Furthermore distilled water is not so palatable as ordinary water. The distillation of water is more especially required on board ship, during long voyages. It should be followed by the use of some measure to secure efficient aeration.

2. Boiling water serves to remove the temporary hardness, and the chalk carries down with it a large proportion of any organic matter that may be present. Boiling deprives the water of its dissolved gases, and renders it flat; it is desirable, therefore, to aerate it by filtration or from a gazogene after boiling. All the microbes which are known to produce disease are destroyed by efficient boiling. Certain putrefactive microbes are more persistent of life, owing to the fact that they form spores, which are not killed at the temperature of boiling water. Tyndall showed that by boiling the liquid containing these spore-forming microbes on three successive days, thus giving time for the spores to develop into less resistant microbes, they could be effectually destroyed. Boiled water will not cause enteric fever or cholera, the two chief water-borne diseases.

3. The exposure of water in divided currents to the air by passing it through a sieve has been proposed as a means of purifying water, but it is inefficient when trusted to alone. Plants in reservoirs help to absorb organic matter; and fish, by destroying small crustaceans, have been found useful. Hard waters do not bear exposure to light, as a thick green growth of chara occurs, which may block pipes, and give a bitter taste to the water.

4. The Addition of Chemical Substances.—(1) Clarke's process consists in adding milk of lime, i.e. an emulsion of quicklime with water, to the water in the reservoir on a large scale. By this means calcium carbonate is precipitated, but no effect is produced on calcium and magnesium sulphates and chlorides. The hardness of the Thames water can thus be reduced from 16° to 3° or 4° (Clarke's scale). The calcium carbonate carries down with it suspended and possibly dissolved organic matter. In the Porter-Clarke process lime-water, i.e. milk of lime diluted, and the excess of lime separated by settlement or filtration, is mixed with the water to be purified, the water being freed from the precipitated calcium carbonate either by subsidence or by being forced through a filter of stretched canvas.

(2) Carbonate of Soda added to boiling water throws down calcium carbonate, and possibly lead if present. Much less is required when added to boiling than to cold water. Maignen's process consists in adding anti-calcaire powder, containing chiefly carbonate of soda, lime, and alum.

(3) Aluminous salts are very effectual in removing suspended organic matter, if the water contains calcium carbonate. On the addition of alum, calcium sulphate and aluminium hydrate are formed, both of which fall to the bottom, carrying with them other impurities. The amount of alum required is about 6 grains per gallon of water. If the water is not hard, a little calcium chloride and carbonate of soda should be put in before the alum is added, in order that a precipitable substance may be formed.

(4) Potassium permanganate readily removes the offensive smell of stagnant water, but it gives a yellow tint to the water. The addition of a little alum will help to carry down the decomposed permanganate.

(5) Perchloride of Iron, in the proportion of $2\frac{1}{2}$ grains to a gallon of water, has been found to completely purify water from finely suspended organic matters and clay.

(6) More recently, other substances, such as iodine and hyposulphite of soda, have been recommended. These are supposed to act by sterilizing the water, and iodine in suitable quantities undoubtedly effects this.

Chemical processes for the purification of water, with the exception of the softening process, are not to be recommended for general use. Efficient filtration, or boiling, is safer than chemical treatment; and it would only be justifiable to trust to the latter, when, as in a military campaign, an attempt at purification was necessary, and no means were available for filtering or boiling water.

7. Filtration.—The object of filtration is to remove the impurities of water. The most dangerous impurities are suspended in it, especially the microbes causing infectious diseases. Hence the most perfect filter is the one which most completely prevents the passage through it of microbes. If

88

the water supply is pure, domestic filtration is not only useless, but likely to do more harm than good. This is true for such upland surface waters as those supplied to Liverpool, Glasgow, and Manchester; for such deep well-water supplies as those of Brighton (deep chalk), of Nottingham (new red sandstone), and others, when pumped from wells remote from inhabited houses. For upland surface waters known to attack lead pipes, filtration through charcoal or spongy iron may be advisable; for river water, filtration through a germ-proof filter is best.

Filtration on a large scale is generally carried on as follows:—A preliminary step consists in collecting the water into settling reservoirs, wherein the more bulky substances subside. The water is then filtered through beds of gravel and sand, containing perforated tubular drains below, into which the filtered water flows. The drains are covered by a bed of gravel about 3 feet deep, over which is spread a layer of sand about 1½ to 2 feet deep. Sharp angular particles of sand are the best; and the gravel should gradually increase in its coarseness as it descends.

The effect of this filtration is chiefly mechanical; it separates any suspended matter, whether organic or inorganic. A certain amount of biological action possibly also takes place. Piefke found that a perfectly cleaned and sterilised filter when first used, increases the microbes in water, instead of decreasing them. Gradually a gelatinous layer of slimy matter is formed on the top of the sand; the water now filters through much more slowly, but it gradually becomes freer from microbes, these being intercepted by the slimy layer. It is important that this layer should not be disturbed by too rapid or forced filtration, and that when the surface layer requires to be removed, because the filter has become impervious, time should be allowed for another thin film to form before the filtered water is again utilised. Koch concluded that the rapidity of filtration should never be allowed to exceed 100 millimetres (about 4 inches) per hour; and that the number of microbes per c.c. in the filtered water should never exceed 100. Some oxidation of organic matter, as well as detention of microbes, may take place during the filtration of water, nitrates being formed by the vital activity of certain "nitrifying" microbes in the filter. (On nitrification, see pages 195 and 274.) P. Frankland's observations show that the number of microbes in Thames water is reduced by filtration through sand and gravel beds, as practised by the London Water Companies, so that only 3·4 per cent. of those originally present remained. He also concludes that the majority of the microbes present in filtered water are derived from post-filtration sources. Thus the number is greater in tap-water than in water derived from near the reservoirs.

Other materials besides sand have been used for filtration on a large scale, but none with proved success.

Domestic Filtration ought, as already explained, not to be needed, but circumstances often arise in which the public supply is open to suspicion, and a second domestic line of defence against infection through the water supply is desirable. When this is so, the form of filter which will best protect the household is one attached to the house-tap, so that all drinking-water is perforce filtered. When filtering involves the transfer of water from the tap to the interior of the filter, opportunity is left for carelessness or forgetfulness. The one essential point of a domestic filter is that it will prevent the passage through it of microbes. Every filter must be tested from this standpoint.

On this point the experiments of Woodhead and Cartwright Wood are conclusive. They first of all experimented on various filters with fine artificial ultramarine containing particles 16 μ to 0·6 μ or even less in diameter in suspension; and milk containing granules and globules of fat 0·5 μ to 30 μ or more in diameter, freely diluted with water.

	TIME IN MINUTES REQUIRED FOR FILTRATION OF 1 PINT OF WATER	PRESENCE OR ABSENCE OF ULTRAMARINE IN FILTRATE	PRESENCE OR ABSENCE OF MILK IN FILTRATE
Silicated carbon filter	68	++	+++
Carbon filter	18	+	+++
Maignen's Filtre Rapide	4	0	++
Spongy iron filter	14	0	+++
Pasteur-Chamberland filter	420	0	0
Berkefeld filter	140	0	0

The number + indicates the relative amount of the experimental substances that made their way through the filtering medium.

Experiments were then made with the actual microbes of certain infectious diseases, and it was found that certain filters allow these to pass. Thus a silicated carbon filter allowed 1,000 out of 15,000 typhoid bacilli suspended in water to pass through its substance; a manganous carbon filter allowed 600 to 800 out of 10,000 cholera vibrios to pass through; Maignen's filter on the second day of experiment allowed 150 out of 5,000 cholera vibrios to pass through; Lipscombe's charcoal filter experimentally only reduced typhoid bacilli from 20,000 to 5,000; the magnetic carbide filter only reduced them from 20,000 to 10,000; the spongy iron filter from 20,000 to 3,000; while, on the contrary, the Pasteur-Chamberland and the Berkefeld filter completely stopped all microbes and produced a sterile water.

Of the materials enumerated animal charcoal was formerly regarded as an excellent filtering medium. It is capable of oxidising organic matter dissolved in water, but so far from sterilizing water, it favours the growth of microbes in it. Water filtered through charcoal, after the first few days of use of the charcoal, deteriorates, as the charcoal yields up impurities to it.

Manganous Carbon consists of animal charcoal and black oxide of manganese mixed with oil, and heated strongly together out of contact with the air. The oxidising power of the carbon is said to be thus greatly increased. It shares the objections to carbon.

90

Silicated Carbon consists of 75 per cent. of charcoal and 22 per cent. of silica, with a little oxide of iron and alumina. It is not an efficient filtering medium.

Spongy iron is prepared by the reduction of hæmatite ore with fusion, so that the iron is obtained in a porous and finely-divided condition. The Rivers Pollution Commissioners found spongy iron to be "a very active agent, not only in removing organic matter from water, but also in materially reducing its hardness, and otherwise altering its character." It is a powerful oxidising agent, some of the water being decomposed, and hydrogen set free, and the oxygen acting upon any organic matter present. It also removes lead from water. As already seen, it does not, however, fulfil the primary object of water, by depriving it of any microbes contained in it.

Magnetic carbide of iron is obtained by heating hæmatite ore with sawdust. Its action is similar to that of spongy iron.

The Pasteur-Chamberland filter consists of a cylinder of unglazed fine porcelain made from a well-baked Kaolin of a certain degree of porosity and hardness. (Fig. 10.)

The water passes through the porcelain from without inwards, and with the pressure of 1½ to 2½ atmospheres which is usually present in the pipes of a water-service, passes through at the rate of about three quarts per hour. The filter can easily be cleaned by brushing it in a stream of hot water, or by subjecting to the heat of a Bunsen burner. The filtration is entirely mechanical, the filtered water being quite freed of microbes. No chemical action takes place.

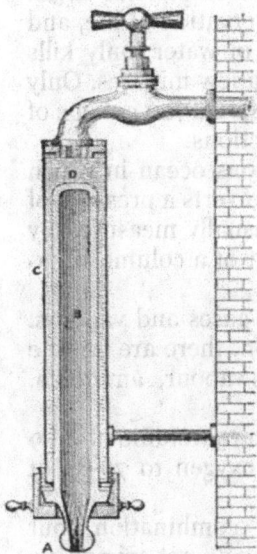

Fig. 10.
Pasteur-Chamberland Filter.
A.—Outlet of filtered water. B.—Pasteur tube.
C.—Metal tube containing unfiltered water.
D.—Unfiltered water delivered through tap.

The Berkefeld filter is cylindrical like the Pasteur-Chamberland filter, and is used in the same way. It is made of infusorial earth, which is soft and friable and liable to break. The cylinder becomes gradually worn thin by cleaning, and it then ceases to filter efficiently. Its sole advantage over the Pasteur-Chamberland filter is the more rapid rate of filtration; and against this is to be set the greater liability to fracture and the lack of continuance of efficient filtration. Woodhead and Wood in the report already quoted, state: "The Berkefeld filter appears to have the largest pores among the efficient filters, as is evidenced by the fact that the water organisms were not apparently weakened, that more species of organisms appeared in its filtrate, and that lowering the temperature to 11° C. did not prevent their appearance. The Pasteur-Chamberland filter, on the other hand, at 11° C. was able to give an

91

apparently sterile filtrate for a prolonged period." More recent experiments have shewn that pathogenic (disease-producing) microbes contained in water after awhile grow through the substance of a Berkefeld filter, and that this does not happen with a Pasteur-Chamberland filter. The latter is therefore preferable.

In determining the number of bougies required for any filter to secure a given amount of pure water, it is necessary to calculate on the basis of the output after several weeks' use, not on the original output. If this is done, pure water will be secured without disappointment as to the amount supplied.

CHAPTER XIV

COMPOSITION AND PROPERTIES OF AIR

An abundant supply of fresh air is necessary at all times. And yet its importance is commonly ignored in practical life. Strenuous efforts are made to ensure a supply of food, and water is commonly filtered or otherwise purified before drinking; but many are content to live in an impure atmosphere, which hardly suffices for the preservation of life, and certainly not of health. Deprivation of food, or even of water, only kills after several days or weeks; deprivation of air kills in a few minutes. Only about three pints of water are required daily, while at least 1,500 gallons of air are necessary every day for carrying on the vital functions.

Composition of Air.—The air constitutes a gaseous ocean in which we live, as fishes live in water. In virtue of its weight, it exerts a pressure of about 15 lbs. on every square inch. This pressure is usually measured by the barometer, and is equivalent on an average to that of a column of 30 inches of quicksilver.

Chemically, air consists of a mixture of various gases and vapours. These are chiefly Oxygen and Nitrogen; but in addition, there are minute quantities of carbonic acid, argon, hydrogen, water vapour, ammonia, ozone, and suspended matters.

The oxygen and nitrogen exist, in the proportion by volume of 20·9 of oxygen to 79·1 of nitrogen, or of 23·16 grains of oxygen to 76·84 of nitrogen, by weight.

These two gases do not exist in chemical combination, but mechanically mixed. This is proved by the fact, that they do not exist in air in the proportion of their combining weights, or any multiple of these; that the proportion varies slightly at different parts; and that the air which is dissolved in water does not contain the nitrogen and oxygen in the proportion 4 to 1 (as in the atmosphere), but in the proportion 1·87 to 1.

This means that oxygen, being more soluble in water than nitrogen, has dissolved in a larger proportion; as it certainly would not have done, had the oxygen and nitrogen been chemically combined. The oxygen dissolved in water supplies fishes with the necessary oxygen for their respiratory processes. Similarly the oxygen in the atmosphere is its most essential constituent, being required in all processes of oxidation (i.e., combustion), whether in living organisms or in the inanimate world. Nitrogen serves as a diluting agent. It is incapable of supporting life alone; and many of the fatal accidents which have occurred through men descending deep wells without first testing, by means of a lit candle held well below them, the quality of the air near the bottom, have been due to an accumulation of nitrogen in the well.

Ozone is a condensed form of oxygen, which is present in minute quantities in pure air, and especially during a thunder-storm or after a fall of snow, and in the air near the sea. In it three volumes of oxygen are condensed so as to occupy two volumes. In this condensed condition it has powerful chemical affinities; often oxidising substances which oxygen cannot attack. It is generally absent from the close air of towns and dwelling houses, having been used up to oxidise the organic matter present in these places. Air without it is said to be "devitalised"; and ozone has been described as the scavenger of the air.

Ozone can be produced by hanging a piece of moist phosphorus in a room; and it is stated by Dr. Daubeny, that part of the oxygen given out by plants, especially by scented flowering plants, is in the condition of ozone. A small quantity is produced when an electrical machine is worked; its presence is evidenced by a peculiar smell (the name ozone is derived from the Greek word for smell).

Test of Ozone in Air.—Traces of ozone in air are detected by exposing strips of blotting paper moistened with a mixture of a solution of potassic iodide and starch. If ozone is present, the paper assumes a blue tint, due to the liberation of iodine, and its combination with the starch. Other acid gases may, however, produce the same effect. A second test should, therefore, be tried. Soak red litmus paper with a very dilute solution of potassic iodide, and expose as before. Potassic oxide is produced if ozone is present, and this turns the litmus blue.

Aqueous Vapour is always present in air, though the amount varies greatly. It is invisible in the ordinary condition, but by condensation becomes cloud or fog, rain, snow, or hail. The quantity of moisture present varies with the temperature of the air; the higher the temperature, the more water can be vaporised, without the point of saturation being reached. An increase of 27° Fahr. doubles the capacity of air for moisture. The amount of moisture that would saturate air at 50° Fahr. only gives 71 per cent. of the saturation amount at 60° Fahr. The amount of moisture is estimated by the hygrometer.

Air saturated with moisture at 32° Fahr., holds vapour equal to 1/160 of its weight; at 59° it holds 1/80, at 86° 1/40, at 113° 1/20, and at 140° 1/10.

Ammonia in normal air does not exceed one part in a million of air;

93

but it is always present—either as free ammonia or as sulphate, chloride, carbonate, or sulphide of ammonia. From this source, plants derive some of the nitrogen they require as food; some also from the free nitrogen, which is fixed by certain microbes, growing in the nodules connected with the roots of peas, lentils, and other plants.

Traces of nitrous and nitric acid are also present in the air, produced by the direct combination of nitrogen and oxygen occurring as the result of the electric spark during lightning.

Carbonic Acid or carbon dioxide is always present in air, in the proportion of 3·36 to 4 parts in 10,000; but in impure air may be present in much larger amount. It is a heavy gas, incapable of supporting combustion, and therefore of supporting animal life. Being a heavy gas, it tends to accumulate where it is produced, as about lime-kilns by the heating of chalk. Thus $CaCO_3$ (chalk) (heated) = CaO (lime) + CO_2 (carbonic acid). Tramps have occasionally died of carbonic acid poisoning through sleeping near lime-kilns.

It is produced by the oxidation of carbonaceous matters, hence in all ordinary combustion, in many cases of putrefaction and fermentation, and in the respiratory processes of all animals.

Plants diminish the amount of carbonic acid in the atmosphere. Two processes occur in most plants: a process of respiration, as in animals; and a process of assimilation, by which the leaves and all other green parts of a plant under the influence of sunlight decompose the carbonic acid of the atmosphere, fixing its carbon and liberating its oxygen. Plants such as fungi, which are destitute of green colouring matter, cannot decompose carbonic acid; nor can any plants during the night. During the day green plants are air purifiers; during the night all plants vitiate the air to a slight extent.

The Air in Relation to Respiration.—The oxygen of air is absolutely essential for the continuance of life. In every organised animal, lungs or analogous organs are provided, in order to supply the necessary oxygen to the system, and to remove the impure air from it.

The act of breathing occurs in man about seventeen times per minute. While the inspired air is in contact with the interior of the lungs, it undergoes important alterations. It comes into contact with the five or six millions air-vesicles which form the minute dilated terminations of the windpipe, and have an aggregate area of ten to twenty square feet. Each of the air-vesicles has extremely thin walls; and outside these delicate walls lie capillary blood-vessels, full of impure blood. An active interchange now occurs between the air and the gases dissolved in the blood. Oxygen passes through the intervening membrane into the blood, while carbonic acid and other impurities of the blood pass into the air-vesicle. The consequence of this is that the impure dark-coloured blood becomes bright scarlet and pure. This purification is not confined to any one portion of the blood; for the heart contracting 60 or 70 times per minute, pours successive portions of blood into the capillaries surrounding the air-vesicles; while at the same time, pure air is brought into the air-vesicles seventeen times per minute, and so the interchange is constantly kept up.

94

In view of the incessant character of respiration and circulation, it is clear that all the blood will be purified if the external air is pure; and that if there is any detrimental matter in the air, it probably will come into contact with the blood in the lungs.

The amount of air taken in with each inspiration is about thirty cubic inches. This is called the tidal air, as it is constantly ebbing and flowing from and to the lungs. By means of a very forced inspiration, about 100 cubic inches of additional air can be inspired; and similarly after an ordinary inspiration, one can expire forcibly an additional 100 cubic inches, though there will still be left in the lungs another 100 cubic inches of air. Thus:—

Tidal air	30	cub. in.
Complemental air	100	„
Supplemental air	100	„
Residual air	100	„
	——	
Total capacity of lungs	330	„

Corresponding to the respiratory changes in the lungs, there are changes in the tissues throughout the body. The pure and oxygenated blood leaving the lungs, is carried to all parts of the system. Oxidation and allied processes are actively carried on, the result of which is the formation of urea, carbonic acid, and smaller quantities of other effete matters. These are then carried by the blood to the excretory organs, urea being chiefly eliminated by the kidneys, and carbonic acid by the lungs.

Examination of Expired Air shows that—1. It is heated; in its passage through the nose and deeper respiratory passages it has acquired a temperature approaching that of the blood.

2. Its moisture is increased. By the skin and lungs from 25 to 40 ounces of water pass off in the twenty-four hours; the relative amount varies somewhat.

3. It contains 4 to 5 per cent. less oxygen, and 4 per cent. more carbonic acid than inspired air. The carbonic acid, instead of being 4 parts in 10,000 of air, becomes over 400 in 10,000, while the oxygen is diminished in a somewhat larger proportion. Thus:—

	OXYGEN	NITROGEN	CARBONIC ACID
Inspired air contains	20·81	79·15	·04
Expired air contains	16·033	79·557	4·38

The amount of carbonic acid expired varies under different circumstances. It is increased by active work, by an increase of food, by a diminution of the external temperature; it is greater when the surrounding air is pure, and when it is moist; and it varies with the season, being greatest in spring, and least in autumn.

Children require more oxygen, and expire more carbonic acid than adults, weight for weight. A child six or seven years old requires nearly as much oxygen as one twice that age. Boys usually require more air than girls, as they are more active and exhale a larger amount of carbonic acid and other impurities.

The average amount of carbonic acid eliminated by a healthy adult is at least 0·6 cubic foot per hour, or 14·4 cubic feet per day. This reckoned as carbon is equivalent to 160 grains per hour, or half a pound of carbon in the twenty-four hours. Liebig gives the amount of carbonic acid expired as 0·79 cubic foot per hour, or 19 cubic feet per day.

4. It contains organic impurities. These are chiefly gaseous, solid particles only being expired during coughing, or possibly during conversation. The danger from the "breath" of patients in infectious diseases is really associated rather with the dried discharges on handkerchiefs, etc., than from the "breath" itself; unless droplets of saliva discharged during speaking, or mucus during coughing, are directly inhaled.

CHAPTER XV

SUSPENDED IMPURITIES OF AIR

Pure air being essential to life and health, it is important to ascertain the character and origin of the impurities of air. Innumerable substance—in the condition of gases, vapours, or solid particles—constantly pass into it, and deteriorate its quality. To counteract this, certain purifying agencies are at work, the mechanism of which will be considered hereafter.

Impurities are much commoner and more abundant in the air of enclosed spaces than in the external air, as the natural processes of purification cannot be brought to bear so efficiently in the former case. In sick rooms, hospitals, etc., impurities arise, which are not present where only healthy people are collected. The most important impurities are derived from the respiration of animals, and the combustion of gases, candles, or lamps in rooms, from sewage emanations, from various occupations, and the air of marshes, mines, church-yards, etc. These may be classed under two heads—solid and gaseous; the solid being simply suspended in the air in a finely divided condition, or floated about in a coarser condition by currents of air. They are revealed in an atmosphere in which one did not previously suspect their existence, by the passage of a beam of sunlight. Light itself is invisible, but its course is rendered visible by the particles from which its rays are reflected. Tyndall demonstrated the presence of minute particulate matter in the air of all ordinary situations, and showed that a large proportion of this matter consists of germs (microbes). In his experiments with vapours in closed tubes, floating matter was always revealed by a concentrated beam of light, even though the air entering the tube had been first drawn through sulphuric acid and through a strong solution of caustic potash. If this air was then passed through a red-hot platinum tube and across folds of red-hot platinum gauze, it became optically empty; the floating matter had been burnt, and disappeared. It was therefore organic. In subsequent experiments, he took organic solutions, as of meat, turnip, and the like, and rendered them sterile by repeated boiling. They remained sterile when kept in air-tight vessels or in vessels covered with a thick layer of cotton-wool, which would efficiently filter any entering air; but when exposed to the air, they invariably became turbid, owing to an enormous multiplication of germs. Clearly, therefore, air contains organic, matter, and much of this organic matter consists of living germs. Most of these germs are comparatively harmless under ordinary conditions. They are, however, the causes of fermentation, putrefaction, and all the processes of decomposition which occur in organic substances. The importance of the exclusion of the dust of air has received an important application in Lister's antiseptic and in the aseptic system of treatment of wounds. Formerly accidents and operations were frequently fatal; now vast numbers of lives are saved by improved surgical methods. The original antiseptic method acted on the supposition that some germicidal application to the wounds was necessary; now it is realized that if, during the operation, germs are not allowed to remain in the wound, all that is afterwards necessary to insure rapid recovery is that they shall be prevented from entering the wound from the external air during its process of recovery. By the adoption of such means, large wounds can be made to heal, without the formation of a drop of "pus" or "matter."

Suspended Matters are mineral or organic, the two being commonly associated together. The mineral matters consist largely of fine particles of common salt, silica, clay, iron rust, dried mud, chalk, coal, soot, and similar substances. Not uncommonly the mineral particles are coated by, or mixed with, organic matter, the comparative lightness of the organic matter enabling the mineral matter to float about more easily. The objection to dust is thus intensified, for not only is it irritating to the respiratory passages and generally disagreeable, but it carries with it putrescent and possibly morbific particles. The prevention of infectious diseases resolves itself largely into means for preventing the inhalation of dust.

Organic Suspended Matters in the open air are, most commonly, minute fragments of wood and straw, dried horse litter, fragments of insects, the spores and pollen of plants, and microscopic plants and animals. In addition, there is the putrescent organic matter resulting from respiration and other organic functions.

Indoors, the air commonly contains, in addition, fragments of cotton, linen, silk, or other fibres, fragments of vegetables, starch cells, soot, charred wood, splinters from floors, etc.

In Sick Rooms, products of the morbid conditions may be evolved; thus, pus-cells, particles from the expectoration, blood cells, fat particles,

97

epithelium, or the special germs or microbes to which infectious diseases are due. These are disturbed by the movements of persons, causing the dust to rise; and thus the infection of consumption, and of the acute infectious diseases, is frequently spread.

Flies and other winged insects are important auxiliaries in the diffusion of disease-carrying particles. Receiving some morbid secretions on their limbs, or other parts of their bodies, they have occasionally been the means of spreading erysipelas in hospitals, and glanders in veterinary stables. The specific contagia of cholera, enteric fever, and summer diarrhœa are occasionally conveyed to food by flies which have previously alighted on latrines or privies or other places where the stools of such patients have been deposited. The excreta of flies, which are not uncommonly deposited on food, or on articles of furniture, have occasionally being found to contain the minute ova of intestinal worms.

Effects of Suspended Matters.—The inhalation of dust is followed by deleterious effects. We may divide the solid substances inhaled as dust into three kinds:—dead substances, living substances, and the contagia (microbes or germs) of various diseases.

1. Dead Substances inhaled for a prolonged period in various occupations are a common cause of premature death. The potter draws into his lungs a fine silicious dust, which irritates his lungs, and finally produces a fatal disease, known as potter's asthma.

Mill-stone Cutters and Stone Masons inhale the fine particles of stone given off from the material which is being chiselled. These produce serious disease of the lungs.

Pearl Cutters inhale fine particles of pearl-dust, and as they generally work in close rooms, and the dust is light and tasteless, serious disease of the lungs results.

Sand-paper Makers inhale minute portions of glass and sand; and needle and knife grinders are exposed to similar dangers, and at one time the mortality among them was frightful. It has greatly diminished since the introduction of wet grinding, the use of steam fans, and wearing of respirators.

Hemp and Flax Dressers inhale a dust which is peculiarly irritating. Workers in rags and in wool suffer in like manner from dust. The dust from fleeces of wool, and especially from the alpaca fleece, has produced in many cases (in the neighbourhood of Bradford and elsewhere) an acute disease (anthrax) proving fatal in a few days. The spores of this disease are very persistent of life, and remain active for mischief for months after the death of the animal which had suffered from it. The fleece can be disinfected by steam; and the use of fans for diverting the dust created during "sorting" minimises the danger from it.

The miller commonly suffers from a form of asthma, not so severe as potter's asthma, as the particles in this case are not equally irritating. The hairdresser is liable to inhale the short fragments of hair cut by the scissors, and the mortality of this class of workers is high. Miners in coal have a surprisingly low mortality, when accidents are excluded from the calculation; except in South Wales, where it is slightly higher than for all males in the same district. Coal dust is relatively free from sharp angles, and is therefore not so irritating to the lungs as metallic dust. Consumption is relatively rare among miners.

The Fur-dyer is very prone to suffer from the dust of the dyed furs, great irritation and disease resulting in many cases.

Artificial Flower-makers, and those engaged in colouring arsenical wall-papers, suffer from the inhalation of arsenical vapours, as well as from the irritating effects of its absorption by the skin. These are now seldom seen, owing to the almost complete abandonment of the use of arsenic for wall-pigments.

Cigar-makers are liable to have their lungs irritated by inhalation of the dust of the tobacco-leaf; and may suffer from tobacco-poisoning.

Workers in Lead are very liable to be poisoned by the metal, e.g., house painters, potters engaged in the glazing process, in which the ware is dipped into a solution containing lead, manufacturers of white lead, and others. The lead is partly absorbed by the skin; in some cases it is inhaled as dust; and more often it is swallowed, when the workman eats his meals with unwashed hands. Of the symptoms "painter's colic" and "drop-wrist" are the two most important, though, in some cases, lead shews its effects more insidiously, leading to gout and chronic renal disease. It is now compulsory on employers to provide in the workshop, complete washing arrangements for the use of workers in lead. Every doctor called to attend a case of lead or phosphorus or arsenic poisoning or anthrax, which has been acquired in an industrial occupation, must notify the same to H.M. Inspector of Factories. This implies inspection of the factory or workshop and the subsequent adoption of further measures of precaution.

Brass-founders occasionally inhale the fumes of oxide of zinc; and diarrhœa, cramp, waterbrash, and other troubles are the result. Those engaged in the manufacture of bichromate of potass, are liable to partial destruction of the mucous membrane of the nose, and to irritation of the skin, with the formation, in some cases, of small ulcers.

Workers with Phosphorus, as those engaged in the making of phosphorus matches, not uncommonly suffer from a gradual necrosis (death) of the jaw-bone. Those having carious teeth are especially attacked by this disease, which is due to the fumes of oxide of phosphorus, attacking the jaw. Improved ventilation of workshops, careful attention to the teeth, and other measures, have greatly diminished this disease; and it has disappeared where safety matches made from red non-volatile phosphorus, have replaced matches made from the yellow variety.

Chimney Sweeps occasionally suffer from irritative skin diseases, as well as bronchitis. In some cases the chronic irritation of the soot has produced cancer of the skin.

The effect of dust on workers can be seen in the mortality returns: Among men aged 25 to 65 years in 1881-90, the comparative mortality figure in England and Wales was as follows, all males throughout the country being taken as a standard and given as 1,000:—

Comparative Mortality Figures.

All males   1000

OCCUPATIONS WITH NO DUST.		DUSTY OCCUPATIONS.	
Clergyman	533	Coal miner (Derby and Notts.)	727
Gardener	553	Carpenter	783
Farmer	563	Bricklayer, mason	1,001
Teacher	604	Coal miner (Lanc.)	1,069
		Tool and scissors maker	1,412
		Potter	1,706
		File-maker	1,810

Remedial Measures.—Means have been taken to diminish the prevalence of the above dust diseases, in several cases with remarkable success. In the case of steel-grinding, for instance, the mortality is greatest with dry grinding, and least with wet grinding. Wet processes have been applied to others of the industries named, with a like success. Where the dust cannot be avoided, the use of steam or electric fans, to deflect the dust away from the workman, has been found successful; and in many cases, free ventilation of the workshops has greatly diminished the mortality. Where none of the above measures suffice, the use of respirators ought to be insisted on. Breathing through the nostrils ought to be carefully maintained, as thus the dust is to a large extent stopped before reaching the lungs.

The dangers of lead poisoning may be avoided by absolute cleanliness, the hands being always washed before taking meals, and the nail-brush used to secure complete cleanliness beneath the nails.

2. Living Substances.—The pollen of plants in some persons produces a distressing form of disease, called hay-asthma, which is apt to recur each year, and is sometimes only curable by living in a town or removing to the sea-coast. The amount of pollen floating about in the atmosphere is considerable; 95 per cent. of it is grass-pollen, and this form and the pollen from pine-trees appear to be the most powerful in inducing hay-asthma. According to some authorities, hay-asthma is rather due to the minute particles constituting the scent of various flowers, than to the pollen; but that is probably not the usual mode of origin of the disease, though it may be in some cases. In some cases, true asthma results from smelling particular plants. Here as in the case of hay-asthma a peculiar idiosyncrasy is involved, only a very small proportion of those exposed to the minute particles suffering from asthma.

The spores of many fungi and of other living organisms are constantly being floated about in the air, until they find a suitable resting place, when they settle and proceed to grow and multiply. The souring of milk, the fermentation of a saccharine solution, the moulding of bread, the presence of mildew, the blighting of corn, and numerous other phenomena are due to the growth of organisms carried by the atmosphere from one part to another.

3. The Contagia (microbes or germs) of the acute infectious diseases are minute living organisms, known as bacteria. Hence these diseases may be carried about by currents of air, some much more easily than others.

Some of the contagia have a persistent vitality. Thus the contagia of scarlet fever, diphtheria, or small-pox may infect a room for months, causing the disease in question, when infected articles in the room are disturbed. The contagia of typhus fever and of measles, on the other hand, are short-lived, and do not usually resist free ventilation and exposure to sunlight.

Besides the contagia of the acute fevers, septic organisms may be carried by the atmosphere. Formerly, blood-poisoning from operation and other wounds was common; but Lister, by insisting on absolute cleanliness of wounds, and only allowing air to have access to the wound which had been filtered through layers of gauze and deprived of its septic germs, has secured that wounds can now be kept perfectly "sweet," the suppuration in them reduced to a minimum, and the danger of blood-poisoning almost annihilated. It had often been noticed that recovery from even very severe injuries was common, if only the skin remained unbroken; while the same injuries, with the addition of a rupture of the skin, and consequent access of air, were rapidly fatal. But to Lister is due the great honour of proving that it was not the air which produced the mischief, but the germs it contained, and that filtered air might be admitted with impunity.

Erysipelas and hospital gangrene have occasionally been carried about in hospital wards by dirty sponges and dressings; and if the ventilation is not perfect, particles of epithelium and pus from diseased persons may be carried to other patients at a distance. Some forms of purulent disease of the eyes are transferable from patient to patient, and in children some forms of eczema are also contagious.

CHAPTER XVI

GASEOUS AND OTHER IMPURITIES OF AIR

Gaseous impurities of the air are very commonly associated with suspended matters, and it is often difficult to separate the effects of the two.

Different gases are also often associated, and so produce modified results. It will be convenient to consider, first of all, certain well-marked gaseous impurities, and then others in which there is a mixture of several gases, or of these with suspended solid particles.

Under the first head the most important impurity is—

(1) Carbonic Acid.—This is reckoned an impurity if amounting to more than 5 parts in 10,000 of air. Owing to the large amount produced in the respiration of animals, in the combustion of fires, gas, lamps, etc., and

in other natural processes, it would be much greater in populous parts, were it not for the rapid diffusion occurring in the air, and the purifying action of plants. The following analyses (Angus Smith) illustrate the facts that in towns the amount rises, and is greatest in the most populous parts, while during fogs it is greatly increased.

VOLUMES OF CARBONIC ACID IN 10,000 VOLUMES OF AIR

On the mountains and moors of Scotland—mean of 57 analyses	3·36
In the streets of Glasgow—mean of 42 analyses	5·02
London, N., N.E., and N.W. postal districts—mean of 30 analyses	4·384
London, E. and E.C.—mean of 12 analyses	4·745
Manchester streets, ordinary weather	4·03
During fogs in Manchester	6·79

The effects of carbonic acid gas alone must be carefully distinguished from those of the same gas plus the organic impurities from respiration, with which it is commonly associated. Dr. Angus Smith found that air containing 3 per cent. of carbonic acid produced difficulty of breathing, but he was able to breathe comfortably an atmosphere containing 0·2 per cent. carbonic acid. Other observers have found they could breathe without discomfort air containing 1 per cent. carbonic acid. When the carbonic acid is derived from respiration, headache and giddiness are produced in many persons when the carbonic acid amounts to 0·15 per cent. A fatal result has occasionally occurred from the inhalation of the carbonic acid at the bottom of brewing vats, or about lime-kilns. The gaseous impurity at the bottom of wells is more commonly nitrogen than carbonic acid.

The presence of an excess of carbonic acid diminishes the elimination of carbonic acid from the lungs, nutrition and muscular energy being consequently impaired. This is seen in workshops where the air is confined and gaslight is commonly employed; though the air here also contains carbonic oxide, sulphurous acid, and organic impurities, and these probably have a large share in producing the evil results.

(2) Carbonic Oxide in the proportion of more than 1 per cent. is rapidly fatal, and has poisoned when under ½ per cent. Poisoning by its means occurs where charcoal stoves are used, and especially when the charcoal is burnt in rooms with no chimney flue. This is an occasional mode of suicide on the continent. Carbonic oxide is a much more deadly poison than the dioxide (carbonic acid); it forms a stable compound with the hæmoglobin of the red blood-corpuscles, displacing oxygen from them, and is got rid of with great difficulty. Lace-frame makers place a coke stove under their work, and thus inhale the invisible gas. Headache, giddiness, irregular action of the heart, and depression of the general health result.

Carbonic oxide is the most poisonous constituent of coal-gas, and is present in much larger quantity in carburetted water-gas with which coal-gas is now commonly mixed, than in pure coal-gas.

(3) The inhalation of Sulphuretted Hydrogen produces headache, nausea, and diarrhœa; but in manufactures involving the inhalation of a small proportion of this gas the symptoms are much slighter.

(4) Sulphurous Acid is always present in small quantities in the air of towns, derived from the combustion of coal and coal-gas. Straw-bleachers and the bleachers in cotton and worsted manufactories, often suffer from severe cough and bronchitis due to inhaling its irritating vapours.

(5) Carbon Disulphide when vaporised and inhaled produces headache, general muscular pains, and nervous depression. It is used in the manufacture of waterproof coats, toy balloons, etc.

(6) Ammonia produces irritation of the eyes and bronchial irritation. Hat-makers commonly suffer from its effects, being generally pale and feeble. It is difficult to say how much is due to the ammonia, and how much to the high temperature at which they work.

(7) Acid Fumes are very irritating to the lungs, and in the case of alkali manufactures, they destroy all vegetation for considerable distances. Hydrochloric acid produces great irritation, and chlorine even more so. The fur-dyer is not only subject to the dangers of dust, but also of the fumes of nitric acid, used to remove fat and give certain shades of colour to the fur.

(8) Other Vapours evolved in various processes produce special symptoms. House-painters suffer from the inhalation of turpentine vapour, headache and loss of appetite commonly resulting. The symptoms from the commonly coexistent lead-poisoning are distinct. Brush-makers have a persistent cough, due to the inhalation of resinous fumes, evolved in making brushes.

Workers in paraffin are liable to an irritative disease of the hair-follicles of the body, followed by the formation of scars, almost like small-pox marks.

Workers in quicksilver, as those engaged in making mirrors or thermometers, are prone to suffer from mercurial poisoning. The gums become spongy, and there is profuse salivation, also generally alimentary disturbance; and in some cases nervous affections, resulting in persistent muscular tremblings, etc.

Under the second head—cases of inhalation of mixed gaseous and particulate contamination—we must consider

(1) The Effects of Air Rendered Impure by Respiration.—It has been already stated that an amount of carbonic acid which could easily be borne alone, is intolerable when other products of respiration are mixed with it. These are chiefly organic gases and solids, which (unless removed quickly) render the atmosphere close and "stuffy"—an effect which is readily perceptible by the sense of smell of those entering an occupied room immediately from the outer air. When such a room is inhabited for a few hours, headache, langour, drowsiness, and yawning (which is really a cry

103

for purer air) result. The soporific effects so commonly produced in churches, etc., are commonly due to the vitiated atmosphere, rather than as is supposed to the soothing effects of the sermon.

When the exposure to foul air is more chronic, and occurs day after day, there results a general lowering of strength and vigour—both bodily and mental—even where no actual disease is set up. Oxidation processes are retarded; the consequence is an anæmic sallow complexion, which compares badly with the ruddy complexion of those spending a great part of the day out of doors.

The prolonged breathing of air, foul from the products of respiration, is perhaps more common in workshops and schools than in private houses; but in both, a faint smell is commonly perceptible on entering from the open air, indicating imperfect ventilation and accumulation of organic putrescible matter. The preceding remarks are left as in the last edition. It must be noted, however, that recent research attaches more importance to the particulate matter (dust) in the atmosphere than to the amount of gaseous impurity, though the latter remains a convenient index of impurity. Experiments made by Drs. Haldane and L. Smith on themselves negative the older conclusion that a special organic poison exists in expired air. They were able without any appreciable effect on themselves to breathe air which was vitiated to such an extent as to completely prevent a match from burning; and they conclude that excess of carbonic acid and deficiency of oxygen are the sole cause of danger from breathing air highly vitiated by respiration. This conclusion may be accepted under the conditions of these experiments. Under ordinary conditions, however, the evil effects produced by breathing the air of crowded rooms, are due not only to the excess of carbonic acid and deficiency of oxygen, but also to the dust which is usually associated with them. This dust, which may be derived from handkerchiefs of patients suffering from influenza, consumption, sore throat, &c., or from other sources, is apt to be inhaled by the persons occupying such rooms.

The tendency to catarrhs is greatly increased by living in a vitiated atmosphere. In the causation of "colds" two elements are concerned, the infective agent, and the condition of the patients. "Colds" are caused primarily by infection from previous patients. The nasal discharge of a "cold in the head" contains the contagium. This is dried on handkerchiefs, and is subsequently scattered as dust, and thus conveyed to others. Ordinarily there is considerable resisting power against such catarrhs. When, however, the general vitality or the local vitality of the mucous membrane of the nose, throat, and lungs is impaired by the breathing of impure air or by sitting in wet clothes after exposure to wet and cold, a catarrh is produced.

The close connection of phthisis (consumption) with overcrowding and the breathing of a vitiated atmosphere will be discussed hereafter. The polluted air acts in producing consumption by depressing vital functions, and diminishing the powers of resistance against the actual contagium of the disease, which is inhaled as dust, produced by the drying of the expectoration of consumptive patients.

The germs of infectious diseases are propagated very rapidly in an impure atmosphere; and typhus fever occurs almost solely in conditions of overcrowding.

In the cattle-plague of 1866, it was found that nearly all the cows died when crowded together in unventilated sheds, while only a third died when there was free ventilation.

The effects of air containing the products of respiration in a concentrated condition, and of a deficient supply of air, have been shown only too well in the oft-quoted case of the Black Hole of Calcutta. In this case, persons were confined in a space eighteen feet every way, with two small windows on one side. Next morning 123 were found dead, and the remaining 23 were very ill.

In the experience of this country, the highest death-rates are in the most densely populated districts. The death-rate from phthisis, childbirth, and typhus fever for instance, is far higher in cities than in country-places. The fact may be explained in various ways. Density of population commonly implies insufficient or unwholesome food, unhealthy work, and poverty; but especially impurity of the air, uncleanliness, and imperfect removal of excreta. Of these factors, the vitiated air is probably the most powerful for evil. Children suffer more than adults from close aggregation of population, largely owing to the greater ease with which infectious diseases spread in towns.

(2) Coal-gas is obtained by the destructive distillation of coal, free from access of air. The average composition of London coal-gas is hydrogen 50 to 53, saturated hydrocarbons 33 to 66, unsaturated hydrocarbons 3·5 to 3·6, carbonic oxide 5·7 to 7·1, carbonic acid 0 to 0·6, nitrogen 2·5 to 4·1, and oxygen 0·2 to 0·3 per cent. Of these the illuminants are olefiant gas (C_2H_4) and the higher hydrocarbons. Sulphuretted hydrogen and other sulphur compounds are present in small quantities, averaging 12 grains of sulphur per 100 cubic feet of London gas.

The inhalation of coal-gas, even in small quantities, is liable to produce headache, and may lead to chronic poisoning if allowed to continue. Where the escape of gas is more extensive, as when a tap is left turned on accidentally during the night, two dangers may arise. If a light is struck in the room an explosion occurs; or persons may be poisoned in their sleep by inhalation of the gas. The most poisonous gas in coal-gas is the carbonic oxide. The chief product of the combustion of coal-gas is carbonic acid. Some sulphurous acid is also produced, which is irritating to breathe, and injurious to bookbindings, picture-frames, etc. If the flame is imperfect, as when the pressure of gas is too great, some carbonic oxide may also escape.

In recent years Carburetted water-gas has been largely mixed with coal-gas in certain districts. This is made by passing steam over heated coke. Thus

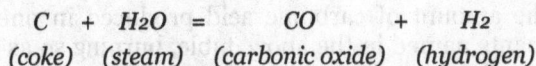

$$C \ + \ H_2O \ = \ CO \ + \ H_2$$
$$(coke) \ (steam) \ (carbonic \ oxide) \ (hydrogen)$$

The product is water-gas which burns with a non-luminous flame and has no smell. For illuminating purposes it is enriched with vaporised paraffin oil, which gives it a high illuminating power, and a smell rather like that of coal-gas. In some towns as much as 60 per cent. of this carburetted water-gas is mixed with 40 per cent. of coal-gas. Now as the former contains about 30 per cent. of carbonic oxide, and the latter only 7 per cent., a mixture of equal parts of the two gases would contain 18·5 per cent. of carbonic oxide, and would therefore be much more dangerous than coal-gas. This has been found to be so in actual experience of escapes of gas.

In speaking of these products of different illuminants, it is necessary to adopt a standard of light. In this country the standard has hitherto been a light known as "one-candle power" which is given by a sperm candle burning 120 grains per hour, or in V. Harcourt's standard flame by a mixture of air and pentane (C_5H_{12}). A good fish-tail or bat's wing burner for coal-gas gives an illuminating power equal to 16 candles, and burns from 4 to 5 cubic feet of gas per hour. Most flat flame burners known as 4 or 5, and supposed to burn that number of cubic feet of gas per hour, really consume nearly double this amount of gas. In the following table the amount of various products produced and of vitiation of air caused by various forms of illuminants is compared, when an illumination equal to 16 candles is produced in each instance:—

	AMOUNT BURNT	CARBONIC ACID PRODUCED	MOISTURE PRODUCED	OXYGEN REMOVED	AMOUNT OF VITIATION PRODUCED STATED IN TERMS OF THE NUMBER OF ADULTS WHO WOULD CAUSE AN EQUAL VITIATION
Sperm candles	1740 grains	6·6 c.ft.	6·6 c.ft.	9·6 c.ft.	11
Paraffin oil	992 „	4·5 „	3·5 „	6·2 „	7
Coal gas burned in Argand burner	4·8 c.ft.	2·5 „	6·4 „	5·8 „	4
Flat-flame burner	5·5 „	3·5 „	7·4 „	6·5 „	6

Thus as an adult expires 0·6 cubic feet of carbonic acid per hour, it follows that the amount of carbonic acid produced in one hour by the various illuminants named in the above table, burning so as to give a light equal to 16 standard candles, varies from 4 to 11 times the amount produced by the adult. Candle and oils possess the advantage over coal-gas

106

that no sulphurous acid is produced in combustion. If the pressure in the mains is excessive, some gas may escape through the burner unburnt or carbonic oxide may escape.

In England the flashing-point of mineral oils has been fixed at 73° Fahr. The material of which the reservoirs of lamps are composed should not be glass or other breakable material, and the wick should be contained in a small wick chamber extending nearly to the bottom of the reservoir. Only a tight fitting wick must be used.

The best illuminant for domestic purposes is incandescent electricity, in which no products of combustion are formed, and only a comparative small amount of heat is produced. Electrical illumination possesses the further advantages that there is no blackening of ceilings and no damaging of other decorations as in illumination by gas.

(3) Air Rendered Impure by Exhalations from the Sick. In addition to the ordinary impurities of occupied rooms, special impurities are produced, varying with the character of the disease. They may include infectious particles from the sick. In wards for consumptives and for diphtheria, dust in the room has been found to contain the special microbes of these diseases. Making beds, sweeping floors, &c. may help to scatter infectious dust; hence the importance of adopting means of cleansing which will not scatter dust, and of keeping sick-rooms spotlessly clean. In many diseases e.g. consumption, a patient may re-infect himself with such infectious dust, and thus diminish his own chance of recovery. Hospital wards can scarcely be too freely ventilated; but even more important than ventilation is the strictest cleanliness in every minute detail.

(4) The Air of Sewers, Cesspools, etc., may contain the products of decomposition of sewage, such as volatile fœtid organic matter, carbo-ammoniacal substances, sulphuretted hydrogen, carbonic acid, etc. The amount of these various products varies greatly under different circumstances, such as dilution of the sewage, ventilation of sewers, temperature, etc. The effluvia from cesspools are usually more concentrated than those from sewers. It appears fairly certain that the emanations from sewers or drains may give rise to diarrhœa and gastric disturbances, and to certain forms of sore throat, which favour the production of diphtheria. On the other hand, there is much evidence showing that the danger from sewer-emanations has been exaggerated. Carnelley and Haldane found that the air of the sewers of the Houses of Parliament and of certain sewers of Dundee was not very impure, containing a smaller number of bacteria than external air. There is reason to believe that the emanations from well-ventilated sewers, possessing a good gradient, so that the contents of the sewers are hurried away to the outfall, are free from danger. The chief source of possible danger would be the escape of the bacteria of such diseases as enteric fever or diphtheria, which had been discharged into the sewer from patients suffering from these diseases. But, in the absence of splashing, these bacteria could not escape from a liquid medium. Their escape could only occur when the sewer became dry, and the dust was carried up by rapid currents of air, a

107

very improbable occurrence in sewers. Hence in the majority of instances sewer emanations must be freed from the accusation of producing infectious diseases. Sewer-men usually enjoy good health, and there is no excess of infectious diseases among them.

The emanations from obstructed drains or sewers may cause serious mischief, similarly to that occasionally produced by the emanations from cesspools. Under such conditions, sulphuretted hydrogen, carburetted hydrogen, and other gases are evolved, and fatal asphyxia has been caused by these. In other instances acute sewer-gas poisoning, without pneumonia, has followed.

The exhalations from cesspools or privies while cleaning them out, may produce severe disorders, which are sometimes fatal. When a drain is newly opened or sewer gas gets into a house, a less marked form of poisoning sometimes occurs, chiefly characterised by languor, headache, vomiting, and diarrhœa. In some cases there may be febrile attacks lasting a few days. Children are especially sensitive to such conditions and quickly fall into ill health.

The direct origin of acute infectious diseases from the effluvia from drains or cesspools has occasionally occurred. Leaky and choked drains under a house are especially dangerous. The subsoil becomes contaminated more and more as time goes on; foul gases are aspirated into the house, owing to its interior being warmer than the subsoil; and finally infectious matter may find its way into the house, or carried by insects or vermin, through cracks in the earth.

Diphtheria has been ascribed to emanations from drains and sewers. There is reason to believe that a non-specific form of sore throat may originate in this way; but diphtheria is generally, if not always, spread by personal infection. Diarrhœa has been occasionally ascribed to sewer-emanations. It chiefly occurs in hot weather, and is usually associated with a foul condition of the surface soil, and speedily ceases after this has been scoured by copious rain.

Enteric or typhoid fever, has been frequently ascribed to drain and sewer effluvia. It was formerly thought that putrefactive changes alone, under certain conditions of temperature, etc., would produce it, and Dr. Murchison, one of the greatest authorities on the subject, who adopted this view, proposed for enteric fever the name "pythogenic fever" (i.e. filth-produced). Isolated cases of enteric fever, occurring where there is no system of drainage, support the same view, as does also the fact that, with the adoption of drainage, the enteric mortality has steadily diminished. On the other hand, numerous cases can be quoted to show that emanations from excreta have been breathed, and sewage-contaminated water drunk, for years, without the production of a single case of enteric fever—until a case is accidentally imported. The weight of evidence is clearly on the side of the view that only emanations from the liquid or solid dejecta of previous enteric patients will produce enteric fever, and that it is the solid particles of the urine or fæces, either inhaled as dust or carried on to food by flies, &c., or mixed with food by contaminated water, &c., which cause infection. Furthermore, modern investigation shows that infection by dust

108

is the exception in England; and that the enteric infection is usually swallowed and not inhaled, being taken in infected water or milk or other food.

(5) Effluvia from Decomposing Organic Matter.—(a) The air of marshes contains an excess of carbonic acid, marsh gas, etc., in addition to other organic matters. Malarial diseases are commonly ascribed to the inhalation of the marsh effluvia under certain conditions, though the recent proof of the part played by the mosquito in spreading malaria, puts the inhalation of such effluvia in the background as cause of this disease. Some forms of diarrhœa and dysentery have been ascribed, with a less degree of probability, to the same cause. In this case, as in that of emanations from other organic sources, the impurities received by the air are both gaseous and particulate.

(b) The Air of Graveyards contains an excess of carbonic acid. The older intramural graveyards appear to have been a cause of illness; but modern graveyards, kept under good regulations have never been shown to cause illness.

(c) The Effluvia from Decomposing Carcases, especially of horses on the battle-field, have led to outbreaks of diarrhœa and dysentery among the soldiers.

(d) The Effluvia from Manure and Similar Manufactories do not seem to injure the workmen as a rule, but attacks of diarrhœa have been produced in the neighbourhood when the wind has wafted the effluvia towards any particular part. Sore throat, and occasionally diphtheria, have been ascribed to the inhalation of London manure taken into Essex.

(6) The Effluvia from Certain Manufacturing Processes seem to be rather nuisances than actually productive of ill health. The vapours given off by tallow-making and bone-burning processes are most disagreeable, but there is little or no positive evidence of their direct insalubrity.

The air of brickfields and cement works is peculiarly disagreeable.

The Degree of Moisture and the Temperature of air are of great importance in relation to health. Air which is unduly moist or dry, hot or cold, may be injurious apart from any foreign matters it contains.

The relative amount of moisture is of greater importance than its actual amount. An atmosphere which contains aqueous vapour up to the point of saturation is very oppressive; the normal evaporation of insensible perspiration (and with it of the organic impurities removed from the skin) is interfered with; and consequently the "oppressiveness of the day" is complained of.

An unduly hot air is generally productive of pallor and ill health, though it is difficult to know how much to ascribe to the high temperature, and how much to the commonly coexistent vitiated atmosphere. The temperature of living-rooms ought not to be over 60° to 65° Fahr., and of bedrooms not over 60° Fahr.

The devitalising influence of extreme cold is well known. Its effects are more particularly seen in young children and the very old, who require to be carefully tended during severe and long-continued cold weather. Dry, cold weather, with the temperature near the freezing point of water, and a cutting east wind prevailing, is not uncommonly described as "bracing." This is so far from being the case, that it requires all the vital powers of the strong and healthy to resist its depressing influence, and the feeble of both extremes of age succumb.

CHAPTER XVII

TRADE NUISANCES

Many occupations are the source of considerable danger to the workers engaged in them. They are chiefly injurious by the inhalation into the lungs of some foreign agent, which produces serious local inconveniences and irritation, and may be also absorbed into the circulation and produce more remote effects.

The injurious agents may be classified under four heads:—
(1) Insoluble particles or dust.
(2) Soluble or partially soluble substances.
(3) Injurious gases or vapours.
(4) Effluvia from offensive trades.

It is evident that, as regards the effluvia named under (4), they might generally be included under the three previous heads, though it is convenient for our present purpose to keep them separate.

The occupations in which dust and soluble substances are productive of injurious effect have already been described, pages 107 to 109.

Injurious gases and vapours have received consideration on pages 111 and 112. The special offensive trades still require attention.

Offensive Trades.—The legal enactments relating to offensive trades are contained in sect. 112 of the Public Health Act, 1875, which states, any person who, after the passing of this Act, establishes within the district of an urban sanitary authority, without their consent in writing, any offensive trade, that is to say, the trade of—

> *Blood boiler, or*
> *Bone boiler, or*
> *Fellmonger, or*
> *Soap boiler, or*
> *Tallow melter, or*
> *Tripe boiler, or*

any other noxious or offensive trade, business, or manufacture,shall be liable to a penalty not exceeding fifty pounds in respect of the establishment thereof, and a penalty not exceeding forty shillings for every day on which the offence is continued.

These provisions can only be enforced in rural districts with the sanction of the Local Government Board.

The "other noxious or offensive trades," in order to be brought within the operation of the section, must be analogous to those which are specially enumerated.

The most exhaustive and authoritative report on this subject is by the late Dr. Ballard, whose report is largely quoted in the following remarks.

We may consider (1) the extent to which the public is inconvenienced by various effluvium nuisances. The majority of the nuisances arise from trade processes in which animal matters are chiefly used. Among the most disgusting are the effluvia from gut-scraping, and the preparation of sausage skins and catgut, the preparation of artificial manures from "skutch" (the refuse matter of the manufacture of glue), the manufacture of some kinds of artificial manures, and the melting of some kinds of fat. Manufacturing businesses dealing with vegetable substances are often offensive, but rarely give out disgusting effluvia. The most offensive vegetable effluvia are probably those thrown off during the heating of vegetable oils, as in the boiling of linseed oil, the manufacture of palmitic acid from cotton oil or palm oil, the manufacture of some kinds of varnish, the drying of fabrics coated with such varnishes, and the burning of painted articles, such as disused meat-tins.

Occasionally offensive effluvia arise in connection with industries in which neither vegetable nor animal matters are used; as in the manufacture of sulphate or chloride of ammonia, and some other processes in which sulphuretted hydrogen is copiously evolved; and in the making of gas and the distillation of tar. The fumes from the manufacture of alkali and bleaching powder are acid and irritating, and produce very injurious effects on vegetation in the neighbourhood.

The distances to which nuisances extend vary greatly according to circumstances—as, for instance, the elevation at which the effluvia are discharged into the air. Discharge from a high chimney may relieve the immediate vicinity of the works at the partial expense of those living at a greater distance. With a damp and comparatively stagnant atmosphere, effluvia have a much greater tendency to cling about a neighbourhood.

(2) The industrial processes in which offensive effluvia are produced are classified by Dr. Ballard as follows:—

1. The keeping of animals.
2. The slaughtering of animals.
3. Other branches of industry in which animal matters or substances of animal origin are chiefly dealt with.
4. Branches of industry in which vegetable matters are chiefly dealt with.
5. Branches of industry in which mineral matters are chiefly dealt with.
6. Branches of industry in which matters of mixed origin (animal, vegetable, and mineral) are dealt with.

(3) It is important to inquire to what extent offensive trade effluvia

111

are injurious to the public health. It is impossible to bring statistics to bear on the inquiry, as other influences, apart from occupation, can scarcely be eliminated. The term "injurious to health" is capable of a double interpretation. It might mean either serious damage to health, or the mere production of bodily discomfort or other functional disturbance by the offensive effluvia, leading by its continuance to an appreciable impairment of vigour, though not to any actual disease.

In the latter sense offensive effluvia have a deleterious effect on health. Such symptoms as loss of appetite, nausea, headache, occasionally diarrhœa, and general malaise are produced by effluvia of various kinds, but agreeing in being all offensive. "A condition of dis-ease or mal-aise is produced."

There is little difficulty in proving bad effects on the workmen, though the invariable defence of manufacturers is an appeal to the condition of health of their workmen. The workmen only remain such so long as they are healthy, and as they become disabled they necessarily cease to rank among workmen. The decomposition of putrefying organic matters is unquestionably dangerous. The general doctrine of sanitation that filth is one of the chief factors in producing disease is certainly applicable to trade effluvia as well as to general sanitation. It has been alleged on behalf of such effluvia as chlorine sulphurous acid and tar vapours that they are useful disinfectants; but modern research has shown that disinfectants, in order to be of practical use, must be in such a concentrated condition that the air containing them is irrespirable. Probably such septic diseases as erysipelas are favoured by organic trade effluvia.

(4) The means available to prevent or minimise the nuisances arising from trade effluvia vary with the character of the processes. The general principles on which treatment must be founded depend, as Dr. Ballard points out, on a recognition of the following kinds of effluvia:—

Effluvia dependent—

1. On the accumulation of filth on or about business premises, or on its removal in an offensive condition.

2. On a generally filthy condition of the interior of buildings and premises and utensils generally.

3. On an improper mode of disposal of offensive refuse, liquid or otherwise.

4. On insufficient or careless arrangements in reception of offensive materials of the trade, or in removal of offensive products.

5. On an improper mode of storing offensive materials or products.

6. On the escape of offensive gases or vapours given off during some part of the trade processes.

It is evident that under the first two headings the proper remedy is cleanliness. Filth should be removed in impervious covered vessels, at regular intervals. Structural arrangements should be made, which will facilitate cleansing operations. Solid refuse should, as far as possible, be separated from liquid refuse, as thus putrefaction is retarded.

Under the last head important remedies are applicable. In many cases a careful selection of the materials of manufacture will form an effective remedy. Thus much of the nuisance connected with soap or candle works arises from the putrid condition of the fat collected from butchers and marine store dealers, and might be obviated by more regular and more frequent collection of the materials of manufacture. The offensive vapours arising during processes of manufacture may be intercepted before reaching the external air, and so treated that they lose their obnoxious character. Various methods of interception are adopted, according to the processes involved. Occasionally it is necessary to have the air of the entire workshop drawn by means of artificial ventilation in a special direction; usually the interception of air from special chambers suffices. When thus collected, the offensive air may be dealt with by (1) passing it through water or some other liquid capable of absorbing the offensive materials; or (2) passing it through some powder with which it has chemical affinity; or (3) if its offensive materials are capable of condensation by cold, passing them through an appropriate condensing apparatus; or (4) if the evolved matters are organic in nature, conducting them through a fire. (5) Occasionally it is sufficient to discharge the offensive gases into the air from a high chimney; and this always produces a mitigation of nuisance, as compared with discharge at a low level.

It is usually found that the adoption of one or other of these methods is directly or indirectly profitable to the offender.

Nuisances from the Keeping of Animals.—The 47th section of the Public Heath Act prohibits the keeping of pigs in towns so as to be a nuisance, and, as a general rule, it is possible to obtain a magistrate's order, entirely prohibiting the keeping of pigs in towns. The excreta of the pig have a very offensive and penetrating odour, and however carefully kept, pigs in towns form an intolerable nuisance.

Not only is there nuisance from the accumulation of manure and dirtiness of the piggeries, but also from the storage and subsequent preparation of food. The boiling of hog-wash is often an even greater nuisance than the filth of the styes.

Cow-keeping and horse-keeping in towns are still allowed and, as compared with pig-keeping, form a small nuisance. Mews, if kept clean and well drained, need not be offensive, though it is objectionable for persons to sleep over stables. The removal of manure also constitutes a difficulty. The manure should not be allowed to accumulate in deep wet pits, but in an iron cage-work over a cement paving at or above the ground-level, thus allowing free drainage, and keeping the manure dry, and reducing ammoniacal decomposition to a minimum.

Cowsheds are generally very badly ventilated, as the cowkeeper finds that more milk is produced by the cows when the temperature of the shed is maintained at 65° or higher; and he does not see the necessity for providing artificial means of warmth. The grains which are used so largely for food are stored in a wet condition, and speedily give rise to nuisance. Cowsheds and stables should be well paved and well drained. At least 800 cubic feet should be allowed for each cow in the shed.

Cowsheds are regulated under the Dairies', Cowsheds', and

Milkshops' Order of the Local Government Board. This order provides for and insists on the registration of cowkeepers, dairymen, and purveyors of milk, by the local authority. It also provides that no cowshed or dairy shall be occupied as such, unless provision is made to the satisfaction of the local authority, for the lighting and ventilation, including air-space, and the cleansing, drainage, and water-supply of the same; and for the protection of the milk against infection or contamination. With the view of preventing contamination of milk, no person suffering from an infectious disorder, or having recently been in contact with a person so suffering, is allowed to milk cows or take any part in any stage of the business of a milk-seller. The milk of a cow suffering from cattle plague, pleuro-pneumonia, or foot and mouth disease must not be mixed with other milk, must not be sold or used for human food, nor for food for swine or other animals, unless it has been boiled. By the order of 1899 this regulation is made to extend to tubercular disease of the udder.

Slaughtering of Animals.—Nuisance may arise in slaughter-houses from various causes:—(1) the uncleanly way in which animals are kept in the pound or lair before being killed; (2) the insanitary condition, bad paving, lack of lime-whiting of walls, etc., of the slaughter-house; (3) the accumulation of hides, blood, fat, offal, dung, or garbage on the premises; (4) the uncleanly condition of the blood-pits, or the receptacles for garbage; (5) the flowing of blood or offal into the drains and thence into the public sewer.

Private slaughter-houses ought to be abolished, and all animals intended for human food slaughtered in public abattoirs under efficient supervision. When a large number of private slaughter-houses exist in different parts of a large town, it is impossible for the sanitary officials to properly supervise the slaughtering, or to ensure that diseased meat shall not enter the market. The inspector may only have the opportunity of examining the flesh, the internal organs which more particularly show the presence of a diseased condition having been concealed. Such concealment and the consequent foisting of diseased meat upon the public, can only be efficiently prevented by forbidding the slaughtering of any animal intended for food in a private slaughter-house.

Most local authorities have bye-laws regulating the slaughtering of animals. These provide for a cleanly condition of the lairs, and prevent keeping the animals longer in the lairs than is necessary for the purpose of preparation for slaughtering. They also insist on the provision of proper covered receptacles of iron or other non-absorbent material for the reception of garbage, and similar receptacles for blood; for cleansing of the floor, etc. after slaughtering; for lime-whiting of the walls four times a year; and for other matters of detail.

For knackers' yards similar regulations are applicable. The flesh should not be kept until it becomes putrid before being boiled, and the boiling of the flesh and fat should be so arranged as to avoid the escape of offensive vapours into the external air.

In smoking bacon, the singeing has formed a serious nuisance. Fish-frying in small shops is often a most troublesome nuisance. A hopper over

114

the pan in which the frying is conducted has not been always successful in carrying the fumes up the chimney. The frying should preferably be done in a closed outhouse, close to a chimney with a good up-draught.

The fellmonger prepares skins for the leather-dresser, the chief operations being taking off the wool, liming the skins, etc. The skins deprived of wool are called "pelts." The pelts are thrown into a pit containing milk of lime, and thence sent direct to the leather-dresser. Nuisance may arise from (1) the odour of the raw skins; (2) the ammoniacal odour from the lime-painted skins hanging in the yard; (3) the emptying and cleansing of the "poke" or tank in which the hides are washed; (4) the foul condition of the waste lime taken from the exhausted lime pits; (5) the odour from the dirty unpaved yards.

The leather-dresser only deals with "pelts," derived from sheep-skins; the tanner with bullocks'-hides. The skins brought from the fellmonger to the leather-dresser are first deprived of lime, and then soaked in a solution of dog's dung, called "pure," until they become soft. In winter this "pure" solution is warmed for use. The odour is very abominable, both from the "pure" tub, and from the discharge of the exhausted "pure" liquid into the drain.

At each stage of tanning nuisance may arise unless great precautions are taken, as when the hides are soaked in lime and water, when the hair is being removed, when the loose inner skin of the hide is being removed, and especially when the hides are soaked in pits containing pigeons' or other dung. Nuisance may arise again during the passage of offensive hides through the street. Cleanliness is the great rule. If every process is carried on with due precaution, including frequent washing out of receptacles and the free use of disinfectants, little complaint need arise.

The manufacturers of glue and size boil out the gelatine from bits of hides and "fleshings" from leather dressers and tanners, from damaged "pelts," ox or calves' feet, horns, and other similar substances. The raw material is apt to be offensive in collection or while accumulating on the premises. The process of boiling causes offence by the effluvia from the steam. The residue remaining after the process is known as "scutch," and this, unless frequently removed, is a most serious source of nuisance.

Prussiate of Potass is manufactured by heating carbonate of potass with refuse animal matters. In order to avoid nuisance the pot in which the boiling is done should have a pipe to conduct away the steam, first running horizontally and then vertically down to the back part of the fire.

Fat-melting and Dip-candle-making, as usually carried on, give rise to nuisance. The fat which is melted down usually comes from butchers and marine-store dealers in a rancid or even putrid condition, and it may be stored on the premises for some time before it is boiled. The vapours from the melting-vat are very offensive. They should be carried by means of a pipe down until they discharge just under the boiler-fire. The residue from the fat-melting process (known as "greaves") requires frequent removal to avoid nuisance.

Bone-boiling, in order to extract the fat and gelatine, is most offensive, and most difficult to deal with. After boiling, the bones are apt to

115

give off offensive smells. The vapours from the closed boiler should be condensed as far as possible in a worm condenser, and the remainder passed through a furnace fire.

In the manufacture of artificial manures nuisance is apt to arise (1) from the reception and accumulation of the raw materials, as putrid fish, putrid blood, scutch (the residue from the manufacture of glue), recently boiled bones, etc.; (2) from the preparation of the raw material for use. Thus the drying of condemned fish or meat on open kilns is very offensive; similarly the drying of sewage sludge. (3) From the process of mixing the materials of manufacture, irritant and offensive vapours being evolved, as for instance in the manufacture of manure by crushing bones, and converting into super-phosphate by the addition of sulphuric acid. (4) From the removal of the manure from the hot den, after it has been dried. When sulphuric acid is mixed with coprolites or other mineral phosphates, most irritant and offensive vapours are produced, which may be perceived in some cases at the distance of a mile.

Blood-boiling is now almost obsolete, having been replaced by albumen-making and clot-drying. Nuisance may arise from the blood collected from slaughter-houses being in a putrid state; and from the effluvia evolved during the drying process.

Gutscraping, gut-spinning, and the preparation of sausage-skins are very closely akin. In gut-scraping the putrid intestines are deprived of their interior soft parts by scraping with pieces of wood, and are then, after being cleansed, ready for sausage-skins. In gut-spinning the prepared gut is twisted into a cord. The small intestines of hogs and sheep are used for this purpose. The stench from these establishments is indescribably horrible. Extreme cleanliness is desirable. Immersion of the guts in common salt is useful; so also the use of impervious vessels, early removal of all refuse material, etc.

Brick and ballast burning are a frequent source of complaint in the neighbourhood of towns. Brick burning is conducted either in kilns or clamps. When bricks are burnt in closed kilns comparatively little nuisance arises; but when they are burnt in open clamps the effluvia are very irritating, partly owing to the fact that very commonly house refuse, containing vegetable and animal matters, is burnt with the bricks. Clamp burning should be absolutely prohibited in the neighbourhood of large towns.

In Ballast burning stiff clay is converted by the agency of heat into a brick-like material, which is of use in road-making. The clay is usually burnt in heaps, mixed with ashes and breeze from dust-bins. The process is offensive unless carried on with precautions similar to those for brick-burning.

CHAPTER XVIII

THE EXAMINATION OF AIR

There are various methods of ascertaining the quality of the air in enclosed spaces, of which not the least useful is the information furnished by the sense of smell, on entering a room from the external air. Besides the evidence given by the senses, chemical and microscopical examination of the air gives important information, while the thermometer and hydrometer ascertain the temperature and degree of moisture.

Examination by the Senses.—The dull grey haze hanging over a town, when it is viewed from a distance, indicates comparative impurity of its atmosphere, and the presence of a considerable amount of suspended matter, including smoke.

The smell of a stagnant atmosphere is a good preliminary guide to its condition. The fact that a room has been occupied for some time without efficient ventilation can be at once detected on entering a room from the external air. The sense of smell is extremely delicate; it has been estimated that the 3/100,000,000 part of a grain of musk can be apprehended by it. But nothing is so soon dulled as the sense of smell. An atmosphere which did not appear to be unpleasant while remaining in a room, is intolerable when one returns to it after a few minutes in the open air. It is important not to confound the "closeness" perceived by the sense of smell, with the oppression due to the high temperature of a room. The two are easily distinguished (unless the two co-exist) by a reference to the thermometer, which ought always to be placed in rooms inhabited during the evening. The remedy for a close room is to allow free entry of fresh air, and not allow the fire to go down, as is so commonly done, under the impression that the closeness is due to heat.

De Chaumont has made many experiments, shewing how accurate is the information given by an acute sense of smell. Carbonic acid is destitute of odour, but as its amount is usually proportionate to that of the organic matter producing closeness, it may be taken as an index of the amount of impurity present in living rooms. De Chaumont found that the limit of smell is reached when carbonic acid amounts to 6 parts in 10,000 of air, or half as much again as in the external air. In the following extracts from his experiments, there was a close accordance between the evidence of his sense of smell and the amount of carbonic acid:—

At 14·80 per 10,000	Extremely close and unpleasant.
„ 10·90 „	Extremely close.
„ 9·62 „	Very close.
„ 9·21 „	Close.
„ 8·43 „	Not very foul.
„ 8·04 „	Close.
„ 6·58 „	Not very close.
„ 5·68 „	Not close.

He also found that humidity of the air had marked influence in rendering the smell of organic matter perceptible, even more than a rise of temperature. The sense of smell is doubtless aided in detecting impurities in the air, by the besoin de respirer, a feeling of oppression caused by the deficiency of interchange between the blood and air. The state of cleanliness of the room as well as of the persons in it influences smell; hence there may not be in particular instances exact correspondence between excess of carbonic acid and of organic matter.

Chemical Examination.—The estimation of nitrogen and oxygen in air is usually unnecessary, as these vary but little. The oxygen is, however, reduced in frequently re-breathed air. The ill effects of an often-breathed atmosphere are due not only to deficiency of oxygen, but also to the addition of carbonic acid and organic matters, rendering difficult the interchange between oxygen and the blood.

The Estimation of Carbonic Acid is of great importance, as under ordinary circumstances, its amount is a fairly exact indication of the amount of contamination in the air.

Pettenkofer's Method.—A carefully dried glass vessel containing a gallon of water is filled with the air to be examined, by emptying the water in the room, the air of which is to be examined. Fifty cubic centimetres of clear freshly prepared baryta water are then added, and the stopper of the bottle then replaced. It is then well shaken, and afterwards allowed to stand for an hour. The carbonic acid combines with part of the baryta to form barium carbonate; and the baryta water remaining is consequently diminished in alkalinity. Given the alkalinity of the baryta water before and after the experiment, and the difference will give the amount of baryta which has combined with carbonic acid.

The alkalinity of the baryta is estimated by a standard solution of oxalic acid, of such a strength that 1 c.c. is the equivalent of 0·5 c.c. of CO_2. The indicator used in making this test is phenolphthalein, which colours baryta water red, but its colour disappears when neutralization is reached.

The following example is taken from "Pakes' Laboratory Text Book of Hygiene," p. 292:—

The jar is found to contain 3,950 c.c.

As 50 c.c. baryta water were run into the jar, the air experimented on = 3,950-50 = 3,900 c.c.

On titrating 25 c.c. of the original baryta water, 22·50 c.c. standard acid solution were required to neutralise it.

The baryta water in the jar required 19·35 c.c.

22·50-19·35 = 3·15 c.c. = difference of acid used.

But 1 c.c. acid = 0·5 c.c. CO_2 at 0° C. and 760 mm. of mercury.

Therefore CO_2 taken up by 25 c.c. of baryta = 3·15/2 = 1·575 c.c.

As 50 c.c. were used the CO_2 absorbed by the baryta = 3·15 c.c. This was present in 3,900 c.c. of air. Therefore the CO_2 = 0·80 per cent.

Correction may be required for variations from the normal pressure of 760 mm. and normal temperature of 0° C., in accordance with ordinary rules.

In Lunge and Zeckendorf's Method, the air to be examined is pumped through a glass bottle in which is 10 c.c. of a N/500 solution of Na_2CO_3 containing phenolphthalein as an indicator. The air is pumped by a hand pump through this solution until the phenolphthalein is decolourized. The number of times the ball of the pump has been squeezed indicates the amount of CO_2 present in accordance with a table prepared from separate experiments by Pettenkofer's method.

Dr. Angus Smith's plan for the estimation of carbonic acid in air is similar in principle to the last calculations. It is based on the fact that the amount of carbonic acid in a given volume of air will not render turbid a given amount of lime water, unless the carbonic acid is in excess.

TABLE.—To be used when the point of observation is "No precipitate." Half an ounce of lime water containing ·0195 gramme lime.

Air at 0° C. and 760 M. M. Barometric pressure.

118

CARBONIC ACID IN THE AIR PER CENT	VOLUME OF AIR IN CUBIC CENTIMETRES	SIZE OF BOTTLE IN CUBIC CENTIMETRES	SIZE OF BOTTLE IN OUNCES AVOIRDUPOIS
·03	571	584	20·63
·04	428	443	15·60
·05	342	356	12·58
·06	285	299	10·57
·07	245	259	9·13
·08	214	228	8·05
·09	190	204	7·21
·10	171	185	6·54
·11	156	170	6·00
·12	153	157	5·53
·13	132	146	5·15
·14	123	137	4·82
·15	114	128	4·53
·20	86	100	3·52
·25	69	83	2·92
·30	57	71	2·51

The foregoing table shows how to apply this method. The first and second columns state the ratio of carbonic acid in a quantity of air which will give no turbidity or precipitate in half an ounce of lime water; the third column gives the corresponding size of the bottle in cubic centimetres; and the fourth column gives the same in ounces. Thus different sized bottles, each containing half an ounce of lime water, will indicate with a fair degree of accuracy the ratio of carbonic acid in the air containing them, by giving no precipitate when the bottle is well shaken. For instance, if a pint bottle is used and there is no precipitate with half an ounce of lime water, it indicates that the ratio of carbonic acid does not amount to ·03 per cent.; if an eight-ounce bottle be used, and there is no precipitate, it indicates that the ratio does not amount to ·08 per cent., and so on. The air of a room ought never to contain more than six parts of carbonic acid in 10,000 of air, or ·06 per cent., i.e. a 10½ ounce bottle full of the air shaken up with half an ounce of clear lime water ought to give no precipitate.

Dr. Haldane has recently described (Journal of Hygiene, No. 1, 1901) a method of estimating CO2, which, although it appears complicated, is really both simple and convenient. For particulars, see the above Journal.

The Estimation of Organic Impurities may be accomplished approximately by drawing a definite amount of air by means of an aspirator, through a dilute solution of permanganate of potassium of known strength. The result is stated by giving the number of cubic feet of air required to decolourise .001 gramme of the permanganate in solution. Sulphuretted hydrogen, sulphurous acid, and other substances in air likewise decolourise the permanganate; these ought to be separately tested for, and allowance made.

The Estimation of Ammonia, whether free or derived from albuminoid impurities, is a matter requiring very delicate processes. It is accomplished in the same way as the estimation of ammonia in water, the air being drawn through perfectly pure distilled water, and then the analysis proceeded with as a water analysis. The mere presence of free ammonia may be determined by exposing to the air strips of filtering paper dipped in Nessler's solution, which become brown if there is any ammonia in the air.

Microscopical Examination is required for the detection of suspended matters. These are the most potent for harm, containing sometimes the germs of infectious diseases. The suspended matters scattered throughout the air may be collected by Pouchet's aeroscope. This consists of a small funnel drawn out to a fine point, under which a slip of glass is placed moistened with glycerine. Both funnel and glass are enclosed in an air-tight chamber, connected by tubing with an aspirator, by means of which when water is allowed to escape from it, air is drawn through the funnel and its particles impinging on the glycerine are there arrested. Glycerine may be objectionable from the foreign particles previously contained in it. Various other plans have been devised, one of which is to draw the air through a small quantity of pure distilled water and then examine a drop of it. By microscopic examination large particles can be detected. For the detection of bacteria and their spores more delicate methods are required.

The Bacteriological Examination of air is usually conducted as follows. Air is drawn through a wide glass tube (Hesse's tube), which has been previously sterilised, and on the inner side of which liquid gelatine has been allowed to solidify. The air as it passes over the gelatine deposits any germs present in it. The entrance of any further germs is prevented by closing the tube, and it is then left to stand for two or three days. Moulds and colonies of bacteria will develop in the gelatine, and these can be counted and differentiated by their appearance and by further tests. In closed rooms the number of microbes (i.e., bacteria and moulds) ought not to be more than 20 per litre of air in excess of those in the outside air; and the ratio of bacteria to moulds ought not to exceed 30 to 1.

Examination of Temperature and Moisture.—The temperature should be observed at the point most remote from an open fire-place, and compared with the external temperature.

It may be useful to recapitulate at this point the desiderata in an inhabited room. The temperature should be 60-62° Fahr., the amount of carbonic acid should not exceed ·06 per cent. and the humidity should range between 73 and 75 per cent. of the amount required to produce saturation. The dry bulb thermometer should read 63-65° Fahr., the wet bulb 58°-61° Fahr., and the difference between the two should not be less than 4° or more than 8°.

CHAPTER XIX

THE PURIFICATION OF AIR

In addition to the artificial measures which will be discussed in the next chapter, various natural agencies are constantly at work for the removal of the impurities discussed in preceding chapters. Of these, the most important are the action of plants, the fall of rain, natural methods of ventilation, and certain natural constituents of the atmosphere.

1. Plants, by virtue of the chlorophyll contained in their green parts, absorb carbonic acid from the atmosphere, liberating oxygen in an active

condition. In addition, ammonia and nitrous and nitric acids are dissolved from the air by rain-water, and assimilated by plants. During the night plants only give off carbonic acid.

2. The Fall of Rain clears the atmosphere of any solid particles contained in it, the impurities being transferred to rain-water which generally contains an appreciable amount of ammonia as well as other impurities. Rain not only washes and purifies the air, but by washing the ground, diminishes dust, and prevents its escape into the air. It is the great natural scavenger.

3. Ventilation—that is, the interchange of pure and impure air, is constantly being effected. Before entering on the details of ventilation, we must consider the physical causes at work which tend to purify the air, apart from all artificial contrivances. These are three in number—namely, diffusion, winds, and differences of temperature of masses of air.

(1) Diffusion causes the rapid mixture of gases placed together. Every gas diffuses at a certain rate—namely, inversely as the square root of its density. In any room which is not air-tight, diffusion is constantly occurring, air passing in and out at every possible point. Through chinks and openings in the carpentry-work of a room, the air diffuses rapidly. Bricks and stone commonly allow air to pass through them; diffusion occurs to a slight extent even if the wall is plastered, but very little through paper. Diffusion alone is quite insufficient to purify a room under ordinary circumstances; and solid particles including the organic matter evolved from the skin and lungs, not being gaseous, are unaffected by it. To remove these, the room must be periodically flushed with air, and washing of all dirty surfaces must be carried out.

Diffusion sometimes produces evil results, when the sanitary arrangements of a house are bad. If there is a leakage of sewage under the kitchen floor, the foul gases from it diffuse upwards; occasionally foul air diffuses from the dust-bin through the wall into the rooms of a house. These results are helped by the fact that the internal temperature of a house is commonly higher than the external.

(2) Differences of Temperature cause active movements of air. In fact winds are caused by movements between large masses of air of unequal temperature and consequently of unequal density. Light gases ascend, as familiarly illustrated by the smell of dinner perceived in bedrooms, or the smell of a cigar lit in the hall perceived in the attic. In rooms differences of temperature of the air are caused by the heat of fire, gas, and our own bodies. Currents of air result; the warmer and lighter air ascends up the chimney or towards the ceiling, while colder and denser air rushes in under the door or through the floor, etc. The lighter gases carry with them solid particles in suspension and thus tend to remove the most important impurities. Assuming that the external air is colder, if admitted into the lower part of a room, it produces a draught; if admitted at the top of a room, being heavier, it falls by its own weight on the heads of those in the room. The problem of ventilation is to secure a sufficient interchange of air without the production of perceptible currents.

Movements of air are constantly occurring, so long as the

121

temperature of the air is subject to changes. This cause alone will suffice to ventilate all rooms in which the air is hotter than the external air. It may thus happen that a room with windows and doors closed in winter, may possess purer air than the same room in summer with these thrown widely open. The value of diffusion of air through the walls, and the influence of temperature on this diffusion are well illustrated by some experiments of Pettenkofer.

When the difference between the outside and inside temperatures was 34° Fahr. (66° inside and 32° outside), and the doors and windows were shut, an ordinary room in his house, of the capacity of 2,650 cubic feet, which was built of brick, and furnished with a German stove instead of an open fire-place, had its entire atmosphere changed once in an hour. With the same difference of temperature, but with the addition of a good fire in the stove, the change of air rose to 3,320 cubic feet per hour. On lessening the difference between the external and internal temperature to 7° Fahr. (64° and 71°), the change of air was reduced to only 780 cubic feet per hour. In these experiments, all crevices and openings in doors and windows were pasted up.

It is instructive to note the greater amount of ventilation effected through the walls, etc., than by the draught of the stove.

The amount of ventilation through walls varies with the material of which they are built. Mortar is exceedingly porous when dry; sandstones and bricks are easily permeated by both water and air. Limestone is almost impervious to air, but requires much mortar in building, which effects a partial compensation (see page 206).

The rise of temperature caused by the bodily heat and by the combustion of illuminating agents, is well shown by some figures of Dr. Angus Smith. He found that the rise of temperature of 170 cubic feet of air in one hour, produced by the bodily heat of one man was 5°·6 Fahr.; by the combustion of a candle 3°·8 Fahr. Thus, in a room 8 feet high, 4 feet broad, and 6 feet long, a man burning a candle would in an hour raise the temperature from 60° to 70° Fahr. This rise in temperature would not only cause currents of hot air towards the upper part of the room, but would probably make the room uncomfortable, and so lead to the opening of a door, etc.

(3) Winds are of great value in flushing rooms with fresh air. They ought to be utilised as often as possible, by throwing windows widely open; without, however, taking the place of constant ventilation in the intervals. They are especially valuable in getting rid of organic matters which are unaffected by diffusion.

The wind will pass through wood, and even brick and stone walls. When it is allowed to pass directly through a room, as from window to door, it produces a more powerful effect than can be produced in any other way. The average rate of movement of winds in this country is 10 feet per second, or about 7 miles an hour. If the surface which a man exposes to this average wind = 6' × 1½' = 9 square feet, then 90 cubic feet of air flows over him in one second, and 324,000 in an hour. If 3,000 cubic feet were the allowance for each person indoors—a much greater allowance than is usually given—he only receives 1/108 of the air with which he is supplied in the open.

Winds act as a ventilating agent in two ways—directly by perflation, driving impure air before them, or freely mixing with it; and indirectly by aspiration, drawing the impure air along with them. In the last case, the wind causes a partial vacuum on each side of its path, towards which all the air in its vicinity flows. Thus, the wind blowing over the top of a chimney causes a current at right angles to itself up the chimney. In a spray-producing apparatus we have a familiar instance of the same principle, the current of air or steam along the horizontal tube causing the fluid to rise in the vertical tube till it is scattered in spray. In Sylvester's plan of ventilation, both these forces are used.

4. Certain Constituents of the Atmosphere have an important purifying effect. Of these oxygen is by far the most important. By its means organic impurities become oxidised, and thus rendered harmless. It is probable that much of this oxidation is effected by means of ozone—a peculiarly active and concentrated form of oxygen. A large part of this ozone is probably produced during thunderstorms and similar electrical disturbances of the atmosphere. The ammonia and organic impurities in air become changed into nitrites and nitrates—chiefly of ammonium—and being washed down by rain, form an important part of the food of plants.

5. For Chemical Measures of purification of the atmosphere see page 297.

CHAPTER XX

GENERAL PRINCIPLES OF VENTILATION

The Amount of Air required.—Ventilation is chiefly concerned with the removal of the products of respiration, just as sewage is chiefly concerned with the removal of the solid and liquid excreta.

In a less degree it is required for removing the impurities produced by the burning of gas, candles, and lamps. The main problem, however, is the removal of the respiratory products.

The amount of carbonic acid in air is usually fairly proportional to that of the other respiratory products. It may therefore be taken as a measure of the impurity of the air. There are, however, certain fallacies in this test. In soda water manufactory, for instance, there would be a comparatively harmless excess of carbonic acid. In dirty rooms, and in hospitals and other institutions where rooms are not vacated for a considerable period, the amount of organic matter present is often in excess of what would have been anticipated, judging by an estimation of the carbonic acid. This is strikingly shown by some valuable researches at

Dundee, which are summarised in the following table. If we take the average amount (in excess of outside air) of carbonic acid, organic matter, and micro-organisms respectively in houses of four or more rooms as unity, then in one or two-roomed houses or tenements we have as follows:—

	HOUSES OF FOUR ROOMS AND UPWARDS	TWO-ROOMED HOUSES	ONE-ROOMED HOUSES
Carbonic acid	1	1·5	2·0
Organic matter	1	1·6	4·4
Micro-organisms	1	5·1	6·7

It is evident that in these cases the carbonic acid did not increase in the same proportion as the organic matter and micro-organisms, and that it alone does not form a sufficient test of the impurity of any given atmosphere. The amount of carbonic acid, however, is a valuable and convenient test of the condition of the air of a room, and the problems of ventilation, of which examples are given on page 123, are based on its amount.

The Standard of purity is somewhat difficult to fix. The external air ought only to contain 4 parts of carbonic acid to 10,000 parts; but it is almost impossible to maintain this degree of purity in inhabited rooms. The experiments made by Drs. Parkes and De Chaumont showed that when the carbonic acid is 06 per cent., or in the proportion of 6 parts in 10,000 of air, the air begins to be perceptibly stuffy; this may therefore be taken as the limit of impurity. Pettenkofer has adopted the limit of 07 per cent.[7]

The problem then is to discover the amount of pure external air (containing 04 per cent. of carbonic acid) that will be required to pass hourly through a room, for every person in that room, in order to keep the carbonic acid at the ratio of 06 per cent.

This may be ascertained by actual observation of the air of rooms in which a given number of persons are placed; or by calculations from physiological data.

As the result of numerous experiments on the atmosphere of prisons, barracks, etc., where the amount of fresh air supplied per hour is exactly known, it is found that in order to keep the carbonic acid at ·06 per cent., 3,000 cubic feet of pure air are required per head per hour; 2,000 cubic feet keep the carbonic acid at ·07 per cent.; 1,500 cubic feet at ·08 per cent.; and 1,200 cubic feet at ·09 per cent.

For the removal of the products of combustion of gas, an additional supply of air is required, for the amount of which, see page 106.

---

[7] In practice one has frequently to be contented if the CO_2 does not exceed 1 part per 1000 of air; and if the room is clean and free from dust, this higher limit may be accepted.

Where a number of sick persons are collected, as in hospitals and workhouses, a much freer supply of air is required. Much depends, however, on the cleanliness of the wards, and on whether the ventilation is constant in character. In St. Thomas's Hospital, the space allotted to each ordinary patient is 1,800 cubic feet, and to each patient in the fever wards 2,500 cubic feet. Thus, by changing the air of the wards twice in the hour, an abundant supply of fresh air is ensured. The mortality after operations, and in all fevers, is much diminished by a free supply of air.

Soldiers are allowed 600 cubic feet of space per head in their sleeping rooms, which involves a change of the air five times per hour, in order that the carbonic acid may be maintained at ·06 per cent. The limit of overcrowding for lodging-houses is usually fixed at 300 to 500 cubic feet, but this is too little.

The amount of pure air required in order to keep the carbonic acid in a room at ·06 per cent., may also be ascertained from physiological data.

An average adult expires 3/5 (·6) cubic foot of carbonic acid per hour. Now as the carbonic acid in air to be breathed must not contain more than two parts in 10,000 (·02 per cent.) in excess of what is present in external air (·04 per cent.), it follows that if x = the amount of fresh air required by an adult per hour in order to keep the carbonic acid in the room down to .06 per cent., then:—

$$·02 : ·6 :: 100 : x.$$
$$x = 3,000 \ cubic \ feet.$$

Relation of Air Required to Cubic Space of Room.—If we accept 3,000 cubic feet of air as the amount required per head per hour, this may clearly be furnished by having a large room with comparatively little circulation of air, or by having a small room with frequent interchanges. Thus, supposing the cubic space allowed to each individual is 1,000 cubic feet—that is, 10 feet in every direction—the atmosphere will require changing three times per hour.

Now, it is found that when a current of air, at the temperature of 55°-60° Fahr., is moving at the rate of less than one mile per hour, it is not perceptible—that is, produces no draught. The rate of a breeze, which is just perceptible, is 18 inches per second, or one mile per hour. As draughts are objectionable, ventilation, in the best sense of the word, means the supplying of abundant fresh air at a rate of less than one mile per hour, or warmed air at a higher rate. Air moving at the rate of 2½ miles per hour, or 3½ feet per second, is perceived as a slight draught by all, at the average temperature of our climate (about 50° Fahr.)

Where natural ventilation is employed, the difficulties of thoroughly ventilating a small space, without draught, are very great.

A change of air three or four times in an hour is all that can be borne under ordinary conditions in this country, and this necessitates a supply of 1,000 or 750 cubic feet of space respectively for each individual. And a change of this frequency is commonly not effected; the ventilating apparatus may fail temporarily, or may be wilfully stopped up, or there may be no means of ventilation; it is essential therefore to have as large a

125

cubic space as possible. A large cubic space, does not obviate the necessity for efficient circulation of air. It is, however, advantageous, not only on account of the initial longer time before the air reaches the limit of impurity, but also because there are less draughts, and there is a larger wall surface and larger windows for unperceived ventilation.

Common Errors as to Ventilation.—(1) In relation to the cubic space of a room, it is most important to note that a lofty ceiling does not compensate for deficiencies in floor-space. One hears, "lofty" and "airy" rooms spoken of as though the two terms were necessarily synonymous. This is by no means the case. The impurities produced by respiration tend to accumulate about the persons who have evolved them, although it is true that in rooms heated by gaslight, a large amount of hot and impure air collects near the ceiling. The necessity of an abundant floor-space is shown by the fact that a space enclosed by four high walls and without a roof, will, if crowded, speedily become offensive. Twelve feet is quite high enough for large rooms in schools, hospital wards, etc., and nine feet suffices for the rooms of a private dwelling-house. There is no objection to a greater height, if it is remembered that in reckoning the practical cubic dimensions of a room, the height should only be reckoned as twelve feet. Supposing 500 cubic feet is the amount allowed per individual, then the floor-space should be forty-two square feet, which would be furnished by a room about 8½ feet long and 5½ feet wide. In barracks, soldiers are allowed fifty square feet of floor-space. In school-rooms the Education Code requires that at least ten square feet of floor-space, and at least 120 cubic feet shall be allowed for each child in average attendance.

(2) It is commonly supposed that a large room compensates for a deficient circulation of air. The cubic space of a room is really of less importance than the capacity for frequent interchanges of air. Even the largest enclosed space can only supply air for a limited period, after which the same amount of fresh air must be supplied, whether the space be small or large. Thus, supposing that as large a space as 10,000 cubic feet per head were allowed, the limit of purity would in the absence of ventilation be reached in three hours, and after that time an hourly supply of 3,000 cubic feet of air would be just as necessary as if the space were only 200 cubic feet.

(3) It must not be overlooked that the furniture in a room must be deducted from the breathing space, as the amount of air is diminished by the space occupied by the furniture. About 10 cubic feet ought to be allowed for each bed, and 3 to 5 cubic feet for each individual in a room; projecting surfaces must be allowed for by subtraction, and recesses by addition. The deductions to be made for furniture are not of any great consequence, if there is a free interchange of air; as the cubic space is of less importance than free ventilation.

General Rules respecting Ventilation.—The two great objects in ventilating being to remove all impurities from the air, and to avoid draughts, it is important that—

1. The entering air should be, if possible, of a temperature of 55° to 60° Fahr. Whenever the temperature of a room differs from the external

126

temperature by 10° Fahr., a draught is certain to ensue. It is impossible at all times to ensure the incoming air being of the temperature of 60°, without some artificial means of warming it. In this country it is seldom necessary to cool the incoming air, but this may be managed in artificial systems of ventilation by passing the incoming air over ice, or by using compressed air which becomes cooled on expansion, or by passing the incoming air through subterranean tunnels.

2. The entering air should be pure. When a room is hotter than the passages and kitchens, air from the latter, whatever may be its character, is drawn into the room. Similarly the ground-air under the kitchen-floor or the air from ash-pits may be drawn into the house, when no other means of ventilation are provided; and this is often followed by evil results.

3. No draught or current should be perceptible from the incoming air, except when it is wished to flush the room with air, by opening the windows wide. It is a common complaint that a room is draughty, and, to remedy this, keyholes are stopped up, and mats are placed at the bottom of the door, etc. The draught can often be remedied by increasing the size and number of the openings through which air is admitted, so that the current of air is not concentrated and rapid. When this does not remedy it, the incoming air should be warmed. A feeling of draught is very often due to the radiation to and from a window, and disappears when a curtain or screen is placed between the radiating surface and the occupant of the room.

4. The entry of air should be constant, not intermittent. The occasional opening of a window or door will not compensate for the lack of a constant interchange of air, although it forms a very valuable adjunct, especially in the removal of organic particles which do not follow the law of diffusion.

5. An exit should be provided for impure air, as well as an entrance for pure air. The chimney furnishes this in most living-rooms, and diminishes the necessity for other means of exit.

If the openings in a room for entrance and exit are properly regulated, a rate of 5 feet per second (about 3½ miles per hour) will provide sufficient air without any unpleasant draught in a room. For instance, if the opening measure 1 square foot, then a rate of 5 feet per second will give five cubic feet of air per second, that is, 18,000 cubic feet per hour. But as only 3,000 cubic feet are required, it follows that an opening one-sixth this size, i.e. 24 square inches, is sufficient for each individual. Reckoning the same amount for means of exit, 48 square inches is the size of the ventilating orifices required by each individual.

6. A number of small divided openings are not collectively equal in ventilating power to one large one having the same area. Thus, when a ventilating orifice is divided into four parts, which have the same collective area as the original orifice, it is found that only half as much air passes through these as through the original orifice. In order to obtain as much air, therefore, each opening must be equal in size to half the original opening. This is in accordance with the rule that the friction for air passing through openings is inversely to the diameter of these openings, i.e. inversely to the square-root of the area of the openings.

7. The most important requirements of perfect ventilation may be recapitulated as follows:—

1st. The maximum impurity of air vitiated by respiration should not exceed 6 parts carbonic acid per 10,000 volumes.

2nd. To ensure the maintenance of this standard, 3,000 cubic feet of pure air must be supplied per head per hour.

3rd. In order to supply this amount of pure air, with ordinary means of ventilation, 1,000 cubic feet at least must be allowed per head in buildings always occupied.

CHAPTER XXI

PROBLEMS AS TO VENTILATION

The following formula enables many problems relating to ventilation to be solved. Let p = the amount of poison (carbonic acid) in every cubic foot of fresh air, viz. ·0004 cubic foot. Let A = the number of cubic feet of fresh air delivered or available, P = the amount of carbonic acid exhaled, and x = the amount of carbonic acid per cubic foot in the room at the end of a given time. Then—

$$x = p + P/A, \text{ whence } A = P/(x - p).$$

If the carbonic acid in the air of a room is ·75 per 1,000 volumes (that in the outer air being ·4 per 1,000 volumes), and there are five persons in the room, how much air is entering the room per hour?

Here x = ·00075.

p = ·0004.

P = ·6 (*i.e. number of cubic feet of carbonic acid expired by each person per hour*).

Now x = p + P/A.

·00075 = ·0004 + ·6/A.

Therefore A = about 1,700.

Thus 1,700 cubic feet are required for each individual to keep the air within the given limit, and five times this amount will be required for five persons = 8,500 cubic feet.

A room has been occupied for one hour, at the end of which the total carbonic acid present was found to be 1·1 per 1,000 parts. The carbonic acid in the open air amounting to ·0004 per cubic foot, find the quantity of air supplied per hour.

Here x = ·0011.

p = ·0004 and P = ·6.

Hence ·0011 = ·0004 + ·6/A.

Therefore A = 857 cubic feet.

If six persons are in a room containing 3,000 cubic feet, and there is a supply of 2,000 cubic feet of air per head per hour; how much carbonic acid is there in the air of the room at the end of 4 hours?

Here $p = \cdot0004$.
$P = \cdot6 \times 6 \times 4 = 14\cdot4$.
$A = 2,000 \times 6 \times 4 + 3,000 = 51,000$.
$x = \cdot004 + 14\cdot4 / 51,000 = \cdot000682 = 6\cdot82$ parts CO_2 in 10,000 of air.

The air of a room occupied by 6 persons and containing 5,000 cubic feet of space, yields 7·5 parts of CO_2 per 10,000 parts of air. How much air is being supplied per hour?

$A = P/(x - p) = \cdot6 \times 6/(\cdot00075 - \cdot0004) = 10,280$ cubic feet.

In the same room what would be the condition of the air at the end of 4 hours?

$x = \cdot0001 + \cdot6 \times 6 \times 4/(10280 \times 4 + 5,000)$
$= \cdot0004 + 14\cdot4 / 46,120 = \cdot000712 = 7\cdot12$ of CO_2 in 10,000 of air.

Given two sleeping rooms, Y 10 ft. by 15 ft. and 10 ft. high, Z 15 ft. by 20 ft. and 12 ft. high, with three adults in each; how much fresh air would you supply in each? What would be the condition of the air of each of the rooms after, ¼;, ½, 1, and 2 hours respectively?
Amount of fresh air to be supplied in Y—

$A = P/(x - p) = \cdot6 \times 3/(\cdot0005 - \cdot0004) = 9,000$ cubic feet per hour.
Condition of air in Y after ¼ hour—

Here $p = \cdot0004$.
$P = \cdot6 \times 3 / 4 = \cdot45$.
$A = 9,000 / 4 + 1,500 = 3,750$.
$x = \cdot0004 + \cdot45 / 3,750 = \cdot00052$.
At the end of 2 hours—
$x = \cdot0004 + 3\cdot6(18,000 + 1,500) = \cdot000584$.
And similarly for Z.

Suppose two rooms, one 10 feet cube, the other 50 feet by 20 feet and 15 feet high, have continuously admitted into each of them a volume of fresh air containing ·04 parts carbonic acid per 100 parts, amounting to 2,000 cubic feet per hour, so as to replace to that extent the air of the room; suppose also that an average adult be placed in each room: show by detailed calculation what would be the condition of impurity of air in each room, as measured by carbonic acid, at the end of 4 hours and 12 hours respectively.
In the case of the first room—

$P = \cdot6 \times 4 = 2\cdot4$.
$A = 2,000 \times 4 + 1,000 = 9,000$.
$p = \cdot0004$.
$x = \cdot0004 + 2\cdot4 / 9,000 = \cdot000667$.

The amount of impurity at the end of 12 hours, and in the second room may be similarly ascertained.

Ventilation in relation to Temperature.—The temperature of a given atmosphere is a most important factor in determining the ease with which it is replenished from the external air. Speaking generally, the greater the difference between the temperature of two masses of air the more rapidly an interchange occurs.

129

Air has weight. A column of it one inch square and extending to the uppermost limit of the atmosphere weighs about 14·6 lbs., and exerts this pressure on all substances at the surface of the earth. This pressure is exerted uniformly in all directions; but for this fact our chests would be crushed in by the external pressure on them, which amounts to over four tons. If the atmospheric pressure is diminished at any point, it is evident that the surrounding air will tend to press in this direction. Now, when air is heated it expands, and consequently the heavier fresh air flows in from all sides and pushes the lighter air upwards.

The expansion of air for every increase of 1° Cent. is ·003665 (1/273), for every increase of 1° Fahr. is ·00203 (1/492). Thus if the air in a room is 20° F. warmer than that outside, it will be expanded to 1/25 additional bulk.

Thus if M = volume of a given air at 32°, with the barometer at 30 inches, and

M1 = volume at temperature t° above 32°, while a = co-efficient of expansion for each degree of elevation of temperature, then the dilatation effected by heat will be expressed by the formula—

$$M1 = M (1 + at).$$

When the temperature is decreasing

$$M1 = M (1-at).$$

If the air in a chimney flue is cooler than the air of the room with which it communicates, it will flow down into the room. It is the object of an economical fire-place to cause the chimney to act as an outlet for the products of combustion and for the impurities of the air of the room with the smallest possible waste of heat. Short of producing a down draught of cold air and smoke, the smaller the difference between the temperature of the air of a room and of the air escaping near the top of the chimney, the greater the economy of fuel.

The movement of air in flues and other outlets is governed by general laws, like those governing the general movements of fluids, but allowances require to be made for friction in the channels of entrance and outlet.

The theoretical velocity, when friction is not taken into account, may be calculated by a formula based on what is known as the law of Montgolfier, or the law of spouting fluids. According to this law, fluids pass through an opening in a partition with the same velocity as a body would attain in falling through a height equal to the difference in depth of the fluid on the two sides of the partition, i.e. to the difference of pressure on the two sides. Thus, if AB equals the height of a column of air at, say, 50° F., and AC is the height of the same quantity of air heated to 60°, then the velocity with which the warmer air ascends will be that which a body would acquire in falling from C to B.

Now the velocity in feet per second of falling bodies is about eight times the square root of the height from which they have fallen; and the formula for determining this is—

C

$$v = c \sqrt{(2gh)} = 8·2c \sqrt{h}.$$

$g = 32·17$ feet per second;

h = distance fallen through by the body;

B

c = a constant determined by experiment, and expressing the proportion of the actual to the theoretical velocity.

Adapting this formula to the special circumstances under which Montgolfier's formula holds, we find that the force which drives the warm air up the flue is the force of gravity, i.e. of the excess of the weight of a column of cold air over the weight of a column of warm air of exactly the same size (represented by BC in the preceding diagram). The difference of the two weights or pressures is found by multiplying the distance from the point of escape of heated air out of the room (fire-place or elsewhere) to the point of escape into the outer air (top of chimney or other point of exit), by the difference in temperature inside and outside, and again multiplying this product by 1/492 for degrees of Fahrenheit temperature, or 1/273 for degrees Centigrade.

Thus omitting c for the present, we have—

$$v = \sqrt{(2gh(t - t_1)/492)} = 8{\cdot}2\sqrt{(h(t - t_1)/492)}$$
Where t = temperature in the chimney,
t_1 = temperature of the external air, and
h = height of chimney.

Example.—The chief means of ventilating a given room is by its open fire-place. The temperature in the chimney is 100° F., that of the external air 40°, and the height of the chimney 50 feet; what is the velocity with which air is leaving the room?

$$v = 8{\cdot}2 \sqrt{((100 - 40) \times 50/492)}$$
$$= 20{\cdot}$$

This gives the theoretical velocity, but the real velocity will differ from the theoretical by an amount varying from 20 to 50 per cent.

It will be evident, from what has been said, that the movements of the air in a confined space are dependent upon (1) the difference between the internal and external temperatures; (2) the area and friction at the apertures through which air enters and leaves the room; and (3) the height of the column of ascending warm air. The higher the chimney (assuming it to contain warm air), the greater the draught and the more efficient the ventilation of the room communicating with it. Hence ventilation is more difficult in upper rooms of large houses and in single-storeyed houses than in the lower storeys of large houses.

Allowance for Friction.—Practically the friction varies greatly according to the size, form, and material of outlet for air. A rough or sooty or angular chimney greatly impedes the outgoing current of air.

It is usual to reduce the theoretical velocity by 20 to 50 per cent. Apart from the friction which is governed by roughness and length of channels, that due to bends in the channel may be calculated by the formula $1/(1-\sin^2 \theta)$, θ being the angle at any bend in this channel.

(It may be convenient to note that—

$$\sin^2 90° = 1,$$
$$\sin^2 60° = \tfrac{3}{4}$$
$$\sin^2 45° = \tfrac{1}{2},$$
$$\sin^2 30° = \tfrac{1}{4}.)$$

Thus every right angle in a bent shaft reduces the velocity in it by one-half.

The loss by friction in two similar tubes of equal sectional area varies (1) directly with the square of the velocity of the air currents; and (2) directly with the length of the outlet channel. In two similar tubes of unequal size the loss by friction is (3) inversely as the diameter of the cross-section in each.

When two tubes are of different shapes, the loss by friction is inversely as the square roots of the sectional areas.

Owing to the variable value of the co-efficient of friction (called c in the first formula given), it is usually preferable to measure the actual rate of progress of air through a given flue by means of an anemometer (wind measure). Then the velocity of the current of air and the area of the cross section of the flue being

131

given, the volume of air discharged in a given time is represented by the product of these two and the time which has elapsed.

$$\text{Thus, } q = a \times v.$$

Where q = quantity of air discharged in a given time, a = area of cross section of flue, v = velocity of current.

By means of this formula, the area of chimney required to discharge a given volume of air at a given average velocity can be ascertained. Thus—

$$a = q/v.$$

The application of the preceding principles and formulæ will be rendered clearer by the following examples.

How much inlet and outlet area per head will be required to give 10 persons in a room of 5,000 cubic feet capacity, 2,000 cubic feet of air per head per hour, supposing that the outside temperature is 40°, while the internal temperature is 60°, and the height of the heated column of air 20 feet?

First ascertain the velocity of entrance and exit of air.

$$v = 8\cdot2\sqrt{(h(t - t_1)/492)}$$
$$= 8\cdot2\sqrt{(20(60 - 40)/492)} = 8\cdot2 \times \cdot902.$$
$$= 7\cdot3964 = velocity\ in\ feet\ per\ second.$$

If we allow one-fourth for friction, then there remains a velocity of 5·5473 feet per second.

$$5\cdot5473\ feet\ per\ second = 19700\cdot8\ feet\ per\ hour.$$
$$Now,\ a = q / v$$
$$= 2{,}000 / 19700\cdot8 = \cdot1015\ square\ feet.$$
$$= 14\cdot6\ square\ inches.$$

Thus the size of the outlet required per head is 14·6 square inches. The size of the room and the number occupying it do not enter into the question, except for a short time at the beginning. (See page 135.)

The amount of inlet required will also be 14·6 square inches per head. Theoretically it ought to be slightly less than that required for outlet, as the outgoing air is more expanded than that entering the room; but practically no allowance need be made for this fact.

The total amount of inlet and outlet required per head = 29·2 square inches.

If the mean temperature of a room is 61°, the external temperature 45°, while the heated column of air is 50 feet, and the required delivery of air 2,000 cubic feet per hour, find the size of inlet and outlet.

$$v = 8\cdot2\sqrt{(h(t - t_1) / 492)}$$
$$= 8\cdot2\sqrt{(50(61 - 45) / 492)}$$
$$= 10\cdot55\ feet\ per\ second.$$
$$= 37{,}980\ feet\ per\ hour.$$

If we make no allowance for friction, then

$$a = q / v$$
$$= 2{,}000 / 37{,}980\ square\ feet.$$
$$= 2{,}000 \times 144 / 37{,}980 = 7\cdot58\ square\ inches.$$

This gives the required size of outlet. The size of inlet and outlet together = 15·16 square inches.

If 3,000 cubic feet of air are supplied in one hour through an aperture of 12 square inches to a room containing 1,000 cubic feet of space, at what rate does the air enter the room?

132

12 square inches = 1/12 square foot.
a = q / v
1/12 = 3,000 / v
Therefore
v = 36,000 feet per hour.
= 10 feet per second.

If a room is supplied with 3,000 cubic feet of air per hour, through a single opening, what must be its area, if the rate of movement of the air is 5 feet per second?

5 feet per second = 18,000 feet per hour.
a = 3000 / 18000 = 1/6 square foot.
= 24 square inches.

As already stated, the difficulties connected with the estimation of amount of friction greatly detract from the practical value of the formulæ just given. Even the results given by anemometers are not always trustworthy, but by comparing the results given by them with those obtained by the use of Montgolfier's formula an approximation to the truth can be obtained.

The ordinary anemometer consists of four tiny vanes fixed to a spindle, so that revolutions are caused by the current of air the velocity of which is to be measured. The revolutions are counted by a mechanical arrangement. The value of the revolutions of the vanes has to be first determined by direct experiment; a known bulk of air being forced through a channel of known size at a uniform rate, and the instrument graduated accordingly. In Fletcher's anemometer a modification of the manometer or pressure-gauge has been used for the same purpose.

Inlets and Outlets.—Having given the average velocity of the wind, the size of a room, and the number of persons occupying it, the size of inlet opening required can easily be calculated.

Find the size of inlet for air in a room occupied by one person, the air moving at the average velocity of 5 feet per second, assuming that 3,000 cubic feet of air are to be supplied per hour.

Let x = size of inlet.
Then x × 60 × 60 × 5 = 3,000.
Therefore x = 3000 / 18000 = 1/6 square foot.
= 24 square inches.

Given that the air moves at a velocity of 10 feet per second, and that the area of the inlet aperture into a room is 12 square inches, find how much air enters the room in an hour.

Let y = amount of air.
Then 10 × 60 × 60 × 12 / 144 = y.
Therefore y = 3,000 cubic feet of air.

Calculations as to supply of air in a room founded on the average velocity of air-currents are, however, much less trustworthy than when the velocity is determined, as previously explained, by means of Montgolfier's formula, or, better still, by an anemometer.

The Commissioners on Improving the Sanitary Condition of Barracks and Hospitals, in their report (1861) recommended for inlets, one square inch for every 60 cubic feet in the contents of the room; or one square inch for every 120 cubic feet in the contents, if warm air is admitted round the fire-grate. For outlet

133

shafts on lower floors, one square inch to every 60 cubic feet, slightly increasing for the higher storeys.

Amount of Air-space required.—We may take 3,000 cubic feet of air as the average amount of air required hourly by each individual, and inasmuch as the air of a room cannot be changed oftener than three times an hour without producing an unpleasant draught, it follows that at least 1,000 cubic feet of space must be allowed per person.

This may be compared with the amount actually supplied under various circumstances.

In the British Army for each soldier—

In permanent barracks	600	cubic ft.
In wooden huts	400	„
In hospital wards at home	1,200	„
In hospital wards in the tropics	1,500	„
In general hospitals	1,000-1,500	„
In fever hospitals	2,000-3,000	„
In workhouse hospitals	850-1,200	„
In common lodging houses	300 or 350	„
Do., if occupied night and day	350 or 400	„
In workhouses	300	„
In schools—		
London School Board requires per scholar	130	„
English Educational Code per scholar (minimum), in old schools	80	„
Do., in new schools	120	„

Floor-space has an important bearing on ventilation. In calculating the available cubic space of a room, the height over 12 feet should be disregarded. Thus, if 500 cubic feet is allowed for each individual, the floor-space should be 42 square feet. In barracks, soldiers are allowed 50 square feet of floor-space.

In the Government regulations for workhouses it is stated that there must not be more than two rows of beds, and that the height of rooms above 12 feet must not be reckoned. This gives a minimum floor-space of 25 square feet per occupant, or with dormitories 17 feet wide, a bed-space of about 3 feet.

In hospitals, the question of floor-space is extremely important, as it regulates the distance between the sick inmates and the convenience of nursing. Assuming each bed to be 3 feet wide and 6½ feet long, the distance between any two beds should be at least 5 feet. This makes the wall-space for each bed 8 feet long, and allows from 80 to 96 square feet of floor-space per bed. At St. Thomas's Hospital, London, the floor-space is 112 square feet, and in fever hospitals it is from 150 to 300 square feet per bed. In regard to the ventilation of hospitals, it has been well said that nothing less than too much is enough.

Means of ascertaining Cubic Space.—Circumference of a circle = Diameter (D) × 3.1416.

Area of circle = D2 × .7854.
Area of square = square of one of its sides.

134

Area of rectangle = product of two adjacent sides.
Area of triangle = base × ½ height, or height × ½ base.
Area of ellipse = product of the two diameters × ·7854.
Circumference of ellipse = half the sum of the two diameters × 3·1416.
Area of any polygon found by dividing into triangles, and taking the sum of their areas.
Cubic capacity of a cube found by multiplying the three dimensions together.
Cubic capacity of a cylinder = area of base × height.
Cubic capacity of a cone or pyramid = area of base × 1/3 height.
Cubic capacity of a dome = area of base (circle) x 2/3 height.
Cubic capacity of a sphere = D3 x ·5236.
Area of segment of a circle found by adding to ⅔ of product of chord and height, the cube of the height divided by twice the chord.
(Ch x H x ⅔) + H3 / (2 Ch)

Give the dimensions of a circular ward for 12 patients, each to have 1,750 cubic feet of available air-space.
Capacity of ward = 1,750 X 12 = 21,000 cubic feet.
If we allow 120 square feet floor-space for each patient, then the total floor-space will be 1,440 square feet. Consequently the height of the ward = 21000 / 1440 = 14·75 feet.

> *Area of circle = D2 x ·7854.*
> *1,440 / ·7854 = D2.*
> *Therefore D = 43·2 feet.*
> *Circumference of circle = D x 3·1416.*
> *= 43·2 x 3·1416.*
> *= 135·7 feet.*

The dimensions of the circular ward required are therefore a height of 14·75 feet, diameter of 43·2 feet, and circumference of 135·7 feet.
Find the cubic capacity of a circular hospital ward 28 feet in diameter, 10 feet high, and with a dome-shaped roof 5 feet high.

> *Area of floor-space = D2 x ·7854.*
> *= 614·8 square feet.*
> *Cubic capacity of the cylinder below the dome is 614·8 x 10 = 6,148 cubic feet.*
> *Cubic capacity of dome = 614·8 x ⅔ x 5 = 2049·3 cubic feet.*
> *Total cubic capacity of the ward = 8197·3 cubic feet.*

In practical measurements of rooms, deductions must be made from the cubic space for the furniture contained in it and for its inmates. About 10 cubic feet ought to be allowed for each bed and bedding, and 2½ to 4 cubic feet for each individual. Projecting surfaces must be allowed for by subtraction, and recesses by addition.
A circular ward with a diameter of 36 feet has a dome-shaped roof, the height of whose centre is 18 feet. The height to the dome is 12 feet. Find the floor-space and total cubic contents. How many patients ought the ward to accommodate?

> *Area of floor-space = (36)2 x ·7854.*
> *= 1017·8784 square feet.*
> *Cubic capacity of cylinder below dome = 1017·87 x 12 = 12214·5 cubic feet.*

Cubic capacity of dome = $1017 \cdot 87 \times \frac{2}{3} \times 6 = 4071 \cdot 48$ cubic feet.
Total cubic capacity of the ward = $16285 \cdot 98$ cubic feet.

Assuming that 1,500 cubic feet are required for each patient, then the ward is large enough for 10 patients. It is well to test this conclusion by calculating whether sufficient floor-space has been allowed for each patient. The floor-space has been found to be about 1,018 square feet, which would give 100 feet for each of 10 patients and more than the minimum standard previously stated.

What number of people should be allowed to sleep in a dormitory 40 feet long, of which the accompanying sketch is a section?

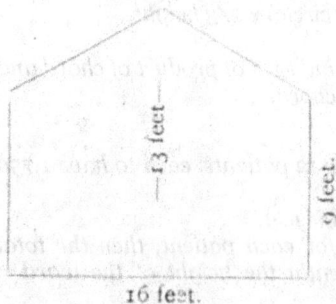

The cubic capacity of the quadrilateral space below the roof = $16 \times 9 \times 40 = 5,760$ cubic feet.

Area of floor = area of base of roof = $40 \times 10 = 640$ square feet.

Cubic capacity of roof = $640 \times \frac{1}{3}(13 - 9)$.

= $853 \cdot 3$ cubic feet.

Total cubic capacity of dormitory = $6613 \cdot 3$ cubic feet.

If we take the low standard of common lodging houses and allow 350 cubic feet of space for each inmate, then 18 persons may be allowed to sleep in the dormitory.

How much space would a man occupy supposing him to weigh 175 lbs.? How much is usually allowed for a man with his clothes, bed and bedding?

The space occupied by a man is stated by Parkes to be from 2½ to 4 cubic feet (say 3 for the average). He gives the following rule: The weight of a man in stones divided by 4 gives the cubic feet he occupies. Thus, a man weighing 175 lbs. would occupy 3⅛ cubic feet of space.

About 10 additional cubic feet must be allowed for clothing, bedding, and bed for each person.

What size of inlet and outlet aperture should be allowed per head? How large should each individual inlet be made? If an inlet aperture 100 square inches in area is divided into four, with apertures of 25 square inches each, what is the loss by friction?

A size of 24 square inches per head for inlet and the same for outlet meets common conditions.

It is desirable to make each individual inlet not larger than 48 to 60 square inches in area, i.e. large enough for two or three men; and each outlet not larger than one square foot, or enough for six men (Parkes). This ensures more uniform diffusion of the air throughout a room. On the other hand, the loss by friction is greatly increased by having a number of small openings instead of one large opening. This loss is inversely to the square roots of the respective areas. Thus the square root of 100 is 10; the sum of the square roots of the four apertures of 25 square inches each is 20. The loss by friction is double in the second case what it was in the undivided opening. It is evident, therefore, that in order to get as much air through the four openings as through the original large opening, each must be equal in size to half the original opening.

Why is ventilation more difficult in upper rooms of large houses and in single-storied houses than in the lower storeys of large houses?

Cold external air being heavier than the internal warm air presses downwards to the lowest point, and pushes up the warmer air. If there were a

136

vacuum in the room, air would rush into it with a velocity which, as seen before, is represented by the formula—

$$v = \sqrt{(gs)}$$

Where g = 32, s = height of column of air, which we may take as roughly 5 miles.

From this formula we obtain v = 1,306 feet per second.

It is evident that in such a case the velocity of entry of air into a vacuum on the ground floor would be greater than into a vacuum on any of the higher storeys, owing to the greater velocity acquired through the increased action of gravity.

And the same increased facility of entry of air into lower rooms must hold good under ordinary circumstances, inasmuch as by Montgolfier's formula (which is founded on the fundamental formula v = √2(gs))

$$v = \sqrt{2(gh(t-t_1)/492)}$$

h = distance between top of chimney and floor of room in question, and thus the velocity with which air enters is governed by the difference between the internal and external temperature, and the height from which the cold air descends in order to take the place of the air which has escaped.

CHAPTER XXII

METHODS OF VENTILATION

In most houses no special means of ventilation are provided, windows, doors and fire-places being trusted for ensuring a sufficient supply of fresh air. These do not suffice in well-built houses, unless the inhabitants train themselves into enduring the currents of air necessarily associated with open windows and doors. They are, however, aided in the majority of houses by the porosity of walls, by currents of air through crevices of wood-work, and so on. It is desirable that adequate special provision for ventilation should be made for every house when it is built, and that as much care and forethought should be exercised in this respect as in the laying on of a water-supply or sanitary appliances connected with drainage.

Whatever the system of ventilation adopted, it is wise to flush rooms frequently with fresh air. This is best effected by throwing the windows wide open whenever a room is left unoccupied. In this way a much more thorough and complete purification is effected than by any other means. This is especially important in the case of bedrooms, in which organic impurities are most prone to accumulate.

Not only should rooms be ventilated, but likewise the furniture they contain. This again is most important for bedrooms. Beds should not be "made" till sometime after using; and in the interval, should be freely exposed to the air. The same applies to night apparel.

It is well to allow rooms to lie fallow at intervals. Organic matter accumulates about a room, and devitalises any air which enters. If the room is vacated, and flushed with air for a continuous period, it becomes sweeter and purer. The importance of this is now well recognised in the case of hospital wards. Such temporary disuse of rooms must not, however, be regarded as sufficient without thorough cleansing of every surface in them, in order effectively to remove all organic and other dust.

An Inlet and Outlet for air should both be provided. According to some an inlet only is required, while others would only provide an outlet; but a perfect system of ventilation requires both. As heated air expands, the outlets should theoretically be larger than the inlets; but as the average difference of temperature is only 10°-15° Fahr., the expansion is only slight, and may be practically neglected.

The necessity for both inlets and outlets may be illustrated by a single apparatus like that shown in Fig. 11. A taper is burning at the bottom of the jar, in the stopper of which two tubes, A and B, are placed. So long as both tubes are kept open the candle will keep alight, but if A be blocked, the candle goes out.

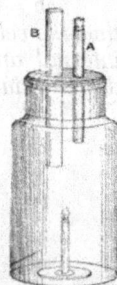

Fig. 11.
Illustrating Necessity of Inlet and Outlet.

Inlets should bring air from a pure source, and should be arranged at intervals in large rooms. Externally, inlets should be protected from the wind; and the shorter the inlet tubes the better, as thus a current is ensured, and they can be easily cleaned. The position of inlets should not be too near the outlets, otherwise the fresh air may escape immediately. The best position for inlets is at the floor, but this necessitates warming the entering air, as otherwise it would be intolerable, except in summer time. If the air cannot be warmed, it should he admitted about seven feet above the floor, and directed upwards. For size of inlets, see page 133.

Outlets, under ordinary circumstances, are best placed near the ceiling. They should be enclosed as far as possible within walls, so as to prevent the outgoing air being cooled; and should have smooth walls, reducing friction to a minimum. Where artificial warmth increases the temperature of the air, the discharge of outlets is much more certain and constant. The chimney with an open fire forms one of the best outlets. Gas, again, may be made to heat an outlet tube, which carries off the products of combustion.

Two forms of ventilation are usually described—natural and artificial. The former term is used to describe any plan not requiring heating apparatus or the motive power of steam, or gas, or electricity, while the latter implies the use of some such motive power or source of heat. Obviously, however, there is no sharp line of demarcation between the two. A lighted fire is strictly an artificial plan of ventilation, but inasmuch as no apparatus intended for ventilating purposes is required, it is hardly a means of artificial ventilation.

Natural Ventilation.—The most important means of natural ventilation are the window and the chimney; but openings in outer walls and over the door may form valuable adjuncts.

The Window is perhaps the most important agent in purifying a room—both the light and air it admits being essential for health. The window is invaluable (1) for flushing the room with fresh air at intervals. Where possible, opposite windows should be opened, or window and door. Cross-ventilation by opposite windows open at the top forms one of the best means of natural ventilation, in large rooms, such as school-rooms. This can, as a rule, be borne without discomfort, while the room is occupied, unless the wind is very high.

(2) The Upper Segment of a window may be made to workinwards on a hinge, and turned so that the current of air may be upwards. Where this plan is adopted, triangular pieces of glass should be placed at the two sides to prevent cold air from falling directly down at the sides of the opening.

(3) A Block of Wood, two or three inches wide, may be inserted at the bottom of the window sash at A (Fig. 12), and then the window pulled down on this. The consequence is that air is admitted between the two sashes at B, its current being necessarily directed upwards (Fig. 12). This plan answers admirably in admitting pure air; but it possesses a disadvantage common to all the plans in which external air much colder than the internal is admitted into a room. The current of cold air passes upwards for some distance, but may then fall down on the heads of those occupying the room.

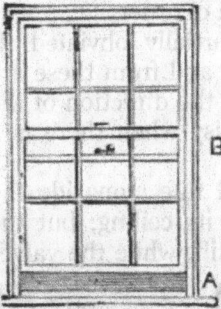

Fig. 12.
Window Ventilation

(4) The top sash of the window may be opened, and some zinc gauze fastened across the open part. This is practically the same as the last arrangement, except that the air is admitted through the apertures of the zinc, and the amount admitted is greatly diminished.

(5) In Louvre Ventilators, a number of parallel pieces of glass, each directed upwards, are substituted for a pane of glass. They may be fixed or made movable, as in Moore's ventilator. The incoming current of air may be similarly directed upwards, in an open window, by arranging Venetian blinds with the laths inclined upwards.

(6) In windows that will not open, Cooper's Ventilators are often used. Each of these consists of a circular disc of glass, having five oval apertures in it, which works on a pivot through its centre, close in front of one of the panes of a window, which has five similar holes pierced in it. Consequently, when the disc is turned, so that its holes are opposite those of the window, fresh air is admitted. The amount thus admitted is necessarily small.

139

The Chimney forms the best means of escape of foul air. No room ought to be built without a fire-place, which should never subsequently be boarded up. In bedrooms the chimney forms a most important means of ventilation. If there is no fire, the chimney occasionally furnishes an undesirable source of air; but as a rule the current is upwards, owing to the aspirating action of winds at the top of the chimney. The downfall of air from a chimney chiefly occurs when there is an insufficient inlet for pure air. This is the explanation of smoky chimneys in nine cases out of ten; then the cure is easy by laying on a pipe from the outside of the house to the hearth. When the smoky chimney is due to the contiguity of higher buildings, the chimney must be raised, or a cowl placed over it.

(1) The action of the chimney in carrying impure air away from the room may be considerably increased by narrowing the two ends, so as to produce a more rapid current at the entrance and exit of air.

(2) The heat of the chimney may be utilised by having a separate smaller flue alongside it, with openings from the rooms on each floor. The air in this being heated aspirates the air from each room in succession.

Openings may be made into the chimney-flue at a higher point than the fire-place. These are very valuable for carrying off the heated and impure air resulting from the combustion of gas, as well as for carrying off the respiratory products, which, in their warmed condition, tend to rise towards the ceiling.

(3) Dr. Neil Arnott first devised a valve for this purpose. An opening being made through the upper part of the wall into the chimney, an iron box was inserted, in which was placed a light metal valve capable of swinging towards the chimney flue, but not towards the room. The objections to this apparatus are that it is apt to make irregular clicking noises, and to admit blacks from the chimney when out of order.

(3) In Boyle's Valve these objections are partially obviated. It consists of an iron frame, across which lie iron rods; and from these are suspended thin talc plates, only capable of moving in the direction of the chimney (Fig. 13). Even this apparatus is rather noisy when there is a strong wind.

Neither of these plans answers so well as a second flue alongside the chimney flue, communicating with each room near its ceiling; but the latter can only be arranged for when the house is built, while the valves may be inserted at any time.

View from room. View from chimney.
Fig. 13.
Boyle's Mica Flap Ventilator.

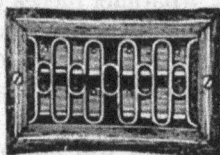

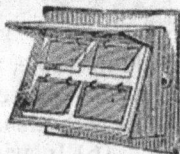

The Ceiling may be utilised for removing foul air; and thus serve to diminish the draught which is often produced by the currents of air towards the chimney, when this forms the only means of outlet.

In large rooms (1) a sunlight gas-burner forms an important means of ventilation. It causes a strong up-current from every part of the room. If there is a fire in the room, the burner is apt to become an inlet for air, or the chimney to smoke, according to the relative strength of the two currents.

(2) Benham's and other forms of Ventilating Gas Burners serve the same purpose. In each of them the products of combustion are conveyed by special ducts above the ceiling to the outer air.

(3) McKinnell's Ventilator is useful in single-storied buildings, like certain barracks. It consists of two tubes encircling one another, the inner forming an outlet tube, because the casing of the outer tube maintains the temperature of the air in it. It is made higher than the outer tube, and is protected by a hood. The outer tube forms the inlet for fresh air. The entering air is thrown up towards the ceiling and then to the walls by a flange placed at the bottom of the inner tube. The air after traversing the room, and becoming heated, passes upwards to the inner tube. When doors and windows are open, both tubes become outlets; if there is a fire in the room, they may both become inlets; but this may be prevented by closing the outlet tube.

(4) Various other means have been devised for carrying foul air from the ceiling through channels between the ceiling and the floor of the room above. All share the disadvantage that the channels become dirty and are difficult or impossible of access for cleaning.

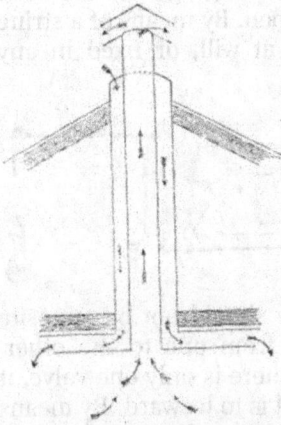

Fig. 14.
McKinnell's Roof Ventilator.

(5) Various cowls connected by metal tubes with the ceilings of rooms have been placed on roofs, and their aspirating effect used in ventilating these rooms. When a room is furnished with a chimney such cowls are most undesirable. In large rooms without a fireplace they are helpful, but much more confidence can be placed in cross-ventilation by hinged windows. It is doubtful if any of the advertised fixed cowls produce materially greater aspiration of air from rooms than a simple open tube of the same size. It is desirable that the tube should be protected at its upper end against the entry of rain, and that a grating should be provided to prevent birds building their nests in the tube.

In the preceding plans of ventilation, the ceiling serves almost entirely as an outlet for impure air. In the following plan, it is used as an inlet for pure air.

(6) In Sylvester's Method of Ventilation, the perflating force of the wind is employed to produce an abundant entry of fresh air. A cowl is placed, always turning towards the wind; the air received is conducted to the basement, where it is warmed by a stove or hot-water pipes, and then passed through tubes into the upper rooms. From these it is carried by tubes above the roof, these tubes being covered with cowls turning from

141

the wind, so that in this way the aspirating power of the wind is likewise used.

Ships are often ventilated in a somewhat similar manner. The tube to which a windward cowl is attached above, ought to be bent at right angles, so as to lessen the velocity of the entering air. By covering other air-shafts with movable cowls, turning from the wind, the aspirating action of the wind is brought into action to aid the escape of foul air.

The Walls of a room, unless covered with an impervious material, are constantly traversed by gentle currents of air, which play an important part in the ventilation of rooms. Special apertures may be made to furnish a freer supply, and these may be in various forms.

(1) A Simple Grating, may be inserted; but this is apt to become blocked with dirt, and does not allow a large amount of air to enter. Louvred openings in the walls are objectionable, except for very large rooms.

(2) Sheringham's Valve is the most convenient means of ventilating through the wall. An opening in the external wall is made by a ventilating brick or grating; into the wall is fixed an iron box, which has in front of it an iron valve hinged along its lower edge, so that it can open towards the room. On the sides of the valve cheeks are attached, which fit into the box when the valve is shut. A heavy piece of iron pressing against the valve from within the box, tends to keep it constantly open. By means of a string and pulley, the valve can be opened or closed at will, or fixed in any intermediate position.

Fig 15.
Sheringham's Ventilator

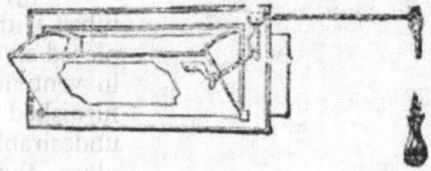

In a very large room, it is better to have several medium-sized valves, than a few larger ones, the air being thus more completely diffused. If there are two valves, they should not be opposite one another, as the air may then simply pass from one to the other, without becoming diffused through the room. If there is only one valve, it may occasionally serve as an outlet when the wind is to leeward. By means of this form of valve, the air is projected upwards in a diverging current towards the ceiling. The valve should be placed above the level of one's head, but not too near the ceiling; as in the latter case, the current of air is driven hard against the ceiling, and falls thence with considerable force towards the floor. A combination of Sheringham's inlet and Boyle's mica outlet into the chimney at the opposite side of the room ensures efficient ventilation in a dining-room. Better than the outlet into the chimney is an opening into a special flue alongside the chimney-flue, if this be available.

(4) Ellison's Inlet consists of a brick pierced with conical holes, the apex of the cone being towards the external air. By this means any great draught is avoided, and the air is distributed over a considerable area. In order that this may prove an efficient means of ventilation, a considerable number of bricks are required.

142

The Floor of a room is always the source of considerable currents of air, even when well carpeted. Air mounts up through the crevices of the wood-work, being aspirated into the room when its temperature is higher than that of the rooms below. In the case of rooms on the ground floor, air is often drawn from the subjacent soil, or through dust-bins, etc.

Theoretically, in all measures of ventilation, the floor would be the best point for the entry of cold air. This, however, is intolerable when the incoming air is cold, and the floor must therefore be abandoned as a means of ventilation, apart from heating apparatus.

The floor may be used as a means of entry of fresh air in a modified manner, by directing the air entering at the floor-level for some distance up a tube at the side of the wall. This apparatus is known as Tobin's tube. It consists of a rectangular or cylindrical tube from 4 to 6 feet high, which communicates at the lowest point with the external air by means of a perforated brick or grating. The air enters the room in an upward direction, and is consequently sent towards the ceiling, where it becomes mixed with warmer air, before diffusing itself throughout the room. But when the incoming air is very cold, it may fall more rapidly, causing cold draughts on the heads of those in the room.

As the air enters directly from outside the house, it often carries with it particles of dirt, soot, etc. This may be remedied by placing a pan containing a shallow layer of water at the lowest part of the tube, or by placing cotton wool at the point of entry of the tube into the room. The tray of water soon dries up and is rarely replaced, while the cotton wool diminishes the amount of entering air. It is very useful however in cold weather, or when fogs occur. A gauze funnel is sometimes inserted in the tube, or a sheet of gauze arranged diagonally across the tube from its highest to its lowest point. The gauze does not keep out minuter particles of dust, and requires occasional cleaning. All Tobin's tubes, like other ventilating openings, should be made to open, so that their interior can be frequently cleaned.

Summary as to Domestic Ventilation.—Open windows, doors, and fire-places may be in most instances trusted. If gas is used as an illuminant, they should be combined with special arrangements for carrying off the products of combustion from the room. For delicate people, and especially in small rooms, outlet ventilation into the chimney breast combined with a Sheringham's valve on the opposite wall is desirable.

Artificial Ventilation.—Artificial ventilation may include two important and very different measures. In one of them currents of air and an exchange of pure for impure air are effected by means of various forms of heating apparatus. In the other mechanical measures are used for the same purpose,—the air being either driven out of the room or drawn out of it. In this chapter we shall consider only the mechanical means of artificial ventilation. There are two kinds, the first being known as ventilation by aspiration, or the vacuum system; and the second as ventilation by propulsion, or the plenum system.

In Ventilation by Aspiration the foul air is drawn out of the room by

143

machinery, its place being supplied by fresh air, which may be warmed before entry or not. This plan and the next have been employed chiefly in connection with large buildings, such as hospitals, etc., and in mines.

The extraction of foul air may be effected by—(1) a steam-jet, which is allowed to pass into a chimney, and sets in motion a body of air more than 200 times its own bulk. Tubes from each room of the building are connected with this chimney, and the strong upward current extracts the air from them. This plan is useful in factories, where there is a superfluous supply of steam.

(2) A fan or screw may also be used. The vanes of the fan, when set in motion by electrical or some other motive power, produce a powerful current of air, which can be regulated according to requirements. As in the last plan, the aspirating influence of the fan may be exerted over a system of rooms, by means of connecting tubes.

In Ventilation by Propulsion a fan is used as in the last plan, the air being propelled along conduits leading from it into the room to be ventilated. The size of the conduits being known, the amount of air to be discharged can be regulated by timing the rapidity of the revolutions of the fan.

This plan is suitable for crowded places, where a large amount of air is required in a short time. It is excellent for large schools, churches, and theatres. Its superiority for large elementary schools has been proved at Dundee by the experiments of Drs. Carnelley, Haldane, and Anderson, the results of which are summarised in the following table:—

	NO. OF SCHOOLS	NO. OF ROOMS	CUBIC FT. ALLOWED PER PERSON	CARBONIC ACID IN 10,000 OF AIR	MICRO-ORGANISMS PER LITRE	
					BACTERIA	MOULDS
Mechanical ventilation by warmed air	6	32	160	12·3	17·5	1·0
Natural ventilation and hot pipes	17	43	176	16·3	96·5	1·1
Natural ventilation and open fires	33	84	145	19·2	153·2	4·8

The air to be admitted may be warmed by passing it over hot-water or steam-pipes. In large establishments, as in hospitals, theatres, etc., it has been arranged so that the incoming air is passed through a screen of coarse cloth, which is kept wet by water trickling down each cord. The air is thus kept moist and freed from dust.

The great advantage of the plan of propulsion, is its certainty. By it the temperature, moisture, and freedom from suspended matters of the

144

incoming air can be exactly regulated and controlled. Its chief disadvantages are that (1) it is somewhat costly, and (2) the apparatus requires skilled supervision. On the other hand it maintains the air in crowded rooms in a condition which cannot be secured by any other method. When combined, as is done in the Houses of Parliament, with the use of a flue for the extraction of foul air, this plan answers admirably.

The Relative Value of Artificial and Natural Ventilation scarcely needs to be discussed. They are both valuable, but under different circumstances. In dwelling-rooms natural ventilation by doors, windows and chimney usually suffices, especially if the products of combustion of gas are removed through a special flue. Natural ventilation is always occurring, and only needs a little aid in domestic life. For large rooms occupied by many persons artificial ventilation is necessary to maintain pure air.

Whatever method of ventilation is adopted, the atmosphere will remain to some extent polluted, if the room and its occupants are dirty. In certain experiments made by Carnelley in schools, it was found that dirty children increased the number of micro-organisms per litre of air more rapidly than dirty rooms. Thus:—

DEGREE OF CLEANLINESS OF CLEAN. MEDIUM. DIRTY.

	CLEAN.	MEDIUM.	DIRTY.
Children	63	99	159
Rooms	85	94	139

Number of micro-organisms per litre of air.

Hence cleanliness of rooms and of their occupants is quite as important as a good system of ventilation.

CHAPTER XXIII

VENTILATION BY THE INTRODUCTION OF WARMED AIR

Ventilation by the Burning of Coal. In winter and at any time of the year when the out-door temperature is below 50° Fahr., the warming and ventilation of a room are necessarily combined. If air is admitted unwarmed it will produce draughts, unless directed upwards by Tobin's tubes or otherwise. In dwelling-rooms such contrivances may suffice; but in any larger building, in order to ensure sufficient ventilation, it is necessary to warm the incoming air.

The Open Fire-place forms the most common means of ventilation by heat. The ascent of warm air up the chimney, causes cold air to rush along the floor to the fire-place from all parts of the room, especially the door. Part of the air thus approaching the fire is carried up the chimney with the smoke, while the remainder, after having been warmed, flows upwards towards the ceiling near the chimney-breast. It passes along the ceiling, and cooling in its progress towards the opposite wall, descends, and is again drawn towards the fire-place. Thus there is a continuous circulation of the air in a room.

In the experiments of the Barrack Commissioners (1861), it was found that the amount of air passing up the chimney while a fire was lit, ranged from 5,300 to 16,000 cubic feet per hour, the mean of 25 experiments being 9,904 cubic feet. We may conclude, then, that with an ordinary grate, a chimney provides outlet for impure air sufficient for four or five persons. Its lack of economy as a heat-producer will be considered later. Its efficiency as a ventilator within the above limits is evident.

When a fire is burning in the grate, all other openings in the room, except openings into the chimney, serve as inlets. If the room is insufficiently supplied with openings, a double current may be established in the chimney, with the result that occasional down-puffs of smoke occur.

As a rule the chimney serves only as an outlet for impure air. It may by appropriate means be made to serve as an inlet for pure and warmed air, the heat which would otherwise escape up the chimney being utilised for this purpose. Galton's stove is one of the best for this purpose. At the back of this stove is an air-chamber, communicating with the external air, and in which the fresh air is heated before it enters the room. On the back of the stove broad iron flanges are cast, in order to present as large a heating surface as possible. They project backwards into the air chamber; and their heating surface is aided by the iron smoke-flue, which passes through the air-chamber. The warmed fresh air enters the room by a louvred opening above the mantel-piece, or by an opening in each side of the chimney breast. By this stove one-third of the total heat of the fire is utilised, as against one-eighth in an ordinary fire-place.

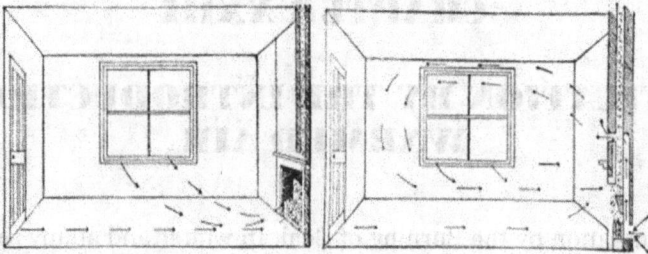

Fig. 16.
Vertical Section through Two Rooms, showing—A. Currents of cold air with an ordinary fire; B. Direction of currents of warmed fresh air with a Galton's Ventilating Stove.

Shorland's Manchester and other stoves are constructed on the same principle as Galton's.

146

The Ventilation of Mines is effected by lighting a fire at the bottom of a shaft. The air for the combustion comes down another shaft (the intake shaft), or down another half of the same shaft separated by a partition. The consequence is that constant up and down currents of air are produced. The air from the intake shaft is made to traverse the galleries of the mines, its course being directed by partitions, before it is allowed to reach the fire and s be carried up out of the mine.

In addition to, or instead of, an ordinary coal-fire, the power for extracting impure air may be obtained from Hot Water or Steam Pipes. There are various plans founded on this principle.

When hot-water pipes are used for baths, etc., they may also be utilised for ventilation, in two ways:—1st. The hot-water pipe may be made to coil round the tube by which fresh air is admitted into a room, thus warming the air as it enters. 2nd. The hot-water pipe in its course upwards may be enclosed in a shaft, which opens into the external air above. The air in this shaft being heated, the impure air may be collected and removed from the different rooms by tubes connected with it. Thus, a hot-water apparatus, when well arranged and complete, may furnish pure warm air, and carry away impure air. The ventilation by this plan is found in practice to be somewhat irregular.

The plan proposed by Drs. Drysdale and Hayward of Liverpool is similar in principle:—Fresh air is warmed by a coil of hot-water pipes in the basement, and is admitted into the staircase and landings, when it is supplied to the different rooms by openings provided with valves. From the rooms, special outlets converge to a foul-air chamber under the roof. This is connected with a shaft leading from the kitchen-fire, the latter, therefore, acting as an extraction furnace.

Lighted Gas may be employed to produce a current for ventilating purposes, as well as fire or hot-water.

Sunlight and Benham's Ventilating Gas-burners, have already been mentioned in this connection. They are extremely valuable means of ventilation, producing powerful currents of air from all quarters of the room unless they are specially enclosed.

In theatres and similar buildings the Chandeliers may be made to extract vitiated air. Where a number of chandeliers exist, they may be connected by tubes with a main shaft, and all made to contribute to the same object. According to the experiments of General Morin, the discharge of 1,000 cubic feet of air is produced by the combustion of one cubic foot of gas.

Various forms of gas-stoves are now sold, which act as ventilators as well as sources of heat. Among these is George's Calorigen Stove (Fig. 17). It can be obtained in various forms suitable for burning coal-gas, or coal, or oil. Within its outer case is contained a special iron tube, which communicates at its lower end with the outer air, and opens at its upper end into the room. The heat generated in the stove warms the air in the spiral tube, which accordingly ascends into the room. The ascent of warm air causes a draught from below, and the consequence is, that so long as the combustion is going on, a current of warm air continues to ascend into the room. The products of combustion are carried out of the room by the pipe F. This stove is free from most of the objections appertaining to gas-stoves; it can be fixed into an ordinary fire-place, and made to keep the temperature of a room uniform.

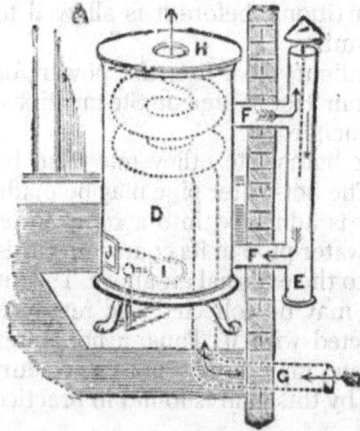

Fig 17.
George's Calorigen Stove.
A—The interior of the room.
B—Exterior of building.
C—Wall.
D—The Calorigen.
E—A cylinder.
FF—Pipes communicating with stove and cylinder to supply air for combustion, and to carry off the products of combustion.
G—Pipe for passage of fresh cold air to Calorigen. Can be carried above the floor between the joists, as may be more convenient.
H—Outlet for air into the apartment after being made warm.

Bond's Euthermic Stove is similarly constructed to the above, but is open below so that the air needed for the gas combustion is drawn from the interior of the room, and the continuous change of air is thus favoured.

Objections to Ventilation by Heating Apparatus.—When warmed air is admitted into a room, it is very apt to be dry and irritating. This can be usually avoided by having water standing in the room, so as to allow evaporation. A more difficult problem is to ensure the complete absence of all products of combustion, particularly of the products of incomplete combustion.

CHAPTER XXIV

THE WARMING OF HOUSES

Physiological and Physical Considerations.—The warmth of our bodies is naturally kept up by the oxidation changes constantly going on in the system. In Chapter XL., p. 265, are discussed the modes in which heat is lost by the system, and the influence of clothing in controlling the amount of this loss. Artificial warming of houses has a similar action to clothing. It diminishes the demand on the system, and so economises the amount of food required.

148

The degree to which this diminution of loss of heat by clothing and artificial warming of houses may be carried varies with circumstances. There can be no doubt that if food be abundant, exposure to external cold, if not too extreme, is on the whole beneficial, for vigorous people. But for old people and young children, means of artificial warmth require to be more carefully provided. Severe cold is for them often the harbinger of death.

The Degree of Temperature at which living-rooms should be kept will vary with circumstances.

For healthy adults, any temperature between 50° and 60° Fahr., will be moderately comfortable; for delicate children and old people it may be 65° with advantage.

For sick rooms and hospitals the temperature of 60° is usually adopted, but this is by no means always necessary. A temperature of the room as low as 50°, except for such diseases as whooping cough and bronchitis, suffices if the patient is well covered with warm personal and bed coverings.

Convalescents from any acute illness bear low temperatures badly.

The Different Kinds of Heat.—Heat may be communicated by radiation, conduction, and convection. By radiation of heat is meant the process by which heat passes from a fire or other source of heat, through a vacuum, dry air or any other medium, without heating any of the media through which it passes, but only the bodies against which it finally impinges. The solid bodies (including ourselves) which are warmed by radiant heat, by a process of conduction then warm the surrounding air. This method is the nearest imitation of the natural warmth of the sun.

Conduction of Heat is the passage of heat from one particle to another, whether it be of a gas or solid. It is an extremely slow process when air is concerned, and may be practically ignored.

Convection of Heat is the process by which a gas or liquid actually carries the heat in itself from one part to another. The heated particles are relatively lighter, and ascend to the higher parts of a room, while colder and heavier particles descend, and are subjected to the same process. Heat can be carried by convection only by gases and liquids. It is quite possible, therefore, for a person to be cold in a room filled with warm air, if the walls, etc., are cold; and on the other hand, to feel comparatively warm in a room filled with cold air, if more heat is radiated from an open fire-place or the warm walls to his body than he radiates to his surroundings. The feeling of "draught" when sitting near a wall is sometimes caused by radiation of heat from the body to the colder wall. The ideal arrangement, were it practicable, would be to have cool air to breathe, but to be surrounded by warm walls, floors, and furniture. A room warmed by an open fire is more comfortable than a room warmed by hot air from a furnace, assuming the temperature of the air is the same in both instances, because the walls of the room are several degrees lower in temperature in the latter than in the former. For warming walls as well as the air high pressure steam pipes are more efficient than hot-water pipes. The great advantages of radiant heat are that—(1) it heats the body without

149

appreciably heating the air; while at the same time (2) there is no possibility of impure gases being added to the air.

It has, however, considerable disadvantages. (1) It is costly, though its expense may be greatly diminished by a well-constructed fire-place. (2) It only acts on bodies near it to any useful extent. Its effect lessens as the square of the distance; thus, its warming effect at five feet distance, is twenty-five times less than at a distance of one foot. It is evident, therefore, that for long rooms, and for large assembly-rooms, a single source of radiant heat is quite inadequate. The immense loss of heat in our ordinary fire-places is slowly leading to their modification; and although it is probable that radiant heat will always be the favourite source of warmth in dwelling-houses, it will be used for larger buildings chiefly as an adjunct to convection of heat.

The different sources of heat are employed, either singly or combined, in the following methods of warming our dwellings and other buildings:—

1. *Warming by the open grate.*
2. *Warming by closed stoves.*
3. *Warming by hot-water pipes.*
4. *Warming by steam in pipes.*
5. *Warming by hot air.*
6. *Warming by electricity.*

Warming by the open Grate.—In the open fire-place radiation is the source of heat chiefly employed.

The position of the fire-place is important. It should not be on the external wall of the house, as thus a large proportion of heat is lost; but should be placed where the heat from the flue may be utilised in keeping up the temperature of the house.

The construction of a fire-place is commonly faulty in several respects. (1) The fire-place may be too far included in the wall, so that the heat at once passes up the chimney. (2) It may be composed chiefly of iron, which rapidly conducts away the heat, and does not furnish a surface for radiation. (3) The bars and bottom of the grate may be so arranged, that coal and cinders fall out in an incompletely burnt condition.

It has been estimated that with an ordinary fire-place, seven-eighths of the possible heat is lost, one-half being carried up the chimney with the smoke, one-quarter carried off in the ascending current of warm air, and one-eighth of the combustible matter remaining unconsumed, forming the solid matter of the smoke.

The defects which have been indicated may be remedied by bringing the fire-place rather further out into the room; by substituting fire-brick for iron behind and at the sides of the fire, and by having a layer of fire-brick at the bottom of the grate, or the grate lowered, so that as in Teale's stove, it lies on a bed of fire-brick at or below the floor level.

The shape of the grate is important. The width of the back of the grate should be about one-third that of the front, the sides sloping out towards the front of the recess. The depth of the grate from before

150

backwards should be equal to the width of the back. The sides and back of the fire-place must be made of fire-brick, thus ensuring the heat being retained in the grate. And finally, the chimney throat must be contracted so as to ensure more complete combustion. The chief objections to an open fire-place are (1) the great waste of fuel involved, even after the improvements indicated have been carried out. (2) The unequal heating at different distances from the fire. (3) The smoke and dust always produced to some extent, from accidental smoking of the fire, or from the escape of ashes. (4) The trouble involved in frequently replenishing the fire. (5) The cold draughts produced by the currents of air towards the chimney. These travel chiefly along the floor, when, as is commonly the case, the space between the bottom of the door and the floor forms the chief place for the entry of fresh air.

Many patents have been brought out for the introduction of the fuel at the lowest part of the fire. The uppermost part of the fuel being first burnt, and the remainder attacked from above, the smoke is consumed in passing through the red part of the fire. Thus a comparatively smokeless fire is produced, and the amount of heat evolved is greatly increased. So far none of these have been altogether satisfactory. The production of a comparatively smokeless fire is a great boon. Smoke means so much unburnt fuel, and not only so but the sooty particles float about in the atmosphere, rendering it impure, and changing comparatively harmless mists into town fogs, which are loaded with soot and the products of combustion, and do incalculable mischief to health and property. The prevention of this smoke nuisance demands more consideration than it has yet received. The Public Health Acts constitute the emission of black smoke from the chimneys of manufacturing premises a nuisance; and manufacturers can if they use proper boilers, especially those in which mechanical stokers are employed, almost completely obviate this nuisance. The great principle is to prevent the escape of smoke before it is completely burnt. This may be accomplished by careful stoking, by keeping the unburnt coal at the front of the fire, and by ridges exposing the smoke to red-hot fire-clay before it escapes. In domestic fires, gas is gradually replacing coal for cooking, with a corresponding reduction of the smoke-nuisance.

The Utilization of the Heat Produced in the fire-place to warm the air on its way into the room, as in Galton's and other similar stoves has been already described.

A larger amount of heat can be obtained out of a given quantity of fuel by cutting off some of the cold air, which rushes through the fire, and carries the half-burnt gases and much of the heat up the chimney. This is effected by having a solid fire-brick bottom to the grate, or by closing up the front of the open chamber under the grate, by means of a close-fitting shield or door. These "Economisers," as Mr. Teale calls them, appear to answer better than solid fire-brick bottoms, as they do not prevent the ashes falling under the grate.

151

The Fuel burnt in an open fire-place may be either coal or coal-gas. Occasionally coke is also employed. Coke and coal-gas have the advantage over coal, that (1) no smoke is produced. Coal-gas presents the additional advantages, that (2) it can be turned on at any moment, without having to go through a tedious process of lighting the fire; and that (3) the amount of heat can be exactly graduated by regulating the supply of gas. A gas fire is however, as a rule, more expensive than a coal fire.

Open Gas-stoves are made in various forms. In the common one, small jets of gas are lit under the grate, which is filled with pieces of asbestos. These become red hot, and radiant heat is emitted. To obtain the greatest value from the heat generated by the combustion of gas, a stove should be chosen in which the heat generated is brought into contact with a large surface of the grate before the products of combustion are allowed to escape to the flue.

Gas stoves which are advertised as not needing a flue, should be avoided. A large amount of carbonic acid is discharged by them into the room, and the sulphurous acid also produced by the combustion of gas is not completely absorbed in the water of condensation which collects in a tray under such stoves.

Closed Stoves form the most economical and efficient warmers for rooms of moderate size, and coal, coke, coal-gas or paraffin may be burnt in them.

The advantages rightly claimed for coal stoves of this type are that (1) the amount of fuel consumed is small; (2) by adjusting the damper, combustion may be rendered as slow as desired, so that but little heat is lost by the flue or chimney; and (3) heat radiates from all parts of the stove into the room, and not simply from a small area of fire-front.

The chief objections to closed stoves are, that (1) they dry the air excessively, rendering it somewhat unpleasant. (2) They produce a peculiar close smell, apparently caused by the charring of minute particles of organic matter in the air, coming in contact with the stove. If the air of the room is not heated above 75° Fahr., no smell is produced, and the relative humidity is not lessened to any appreciable extent (Parkes). But when the heat produced by the stove is excessive, these results do follow. The unpleasantness may be modified though not entirely removed, by placing shallow pans of water near the stove.

(3) Portions of the products of combustion may pass through cracks or fissures in the stove, or even through the joints of the stove. Independently of such accidental cracks, cast-iron stoves, when red hot, appear to allow gases to pass through them with comparative ease. Thus carbonic oxide and other gases may find their way into the room, and it is probable that this rather than the dryness of the air, is the cause of the unpleasant symptoms sometimes complained of in rooms where closed stoves are in use. This escape of carbonic oxide does not occur with earthenware stoves properly encased with fire-clay.

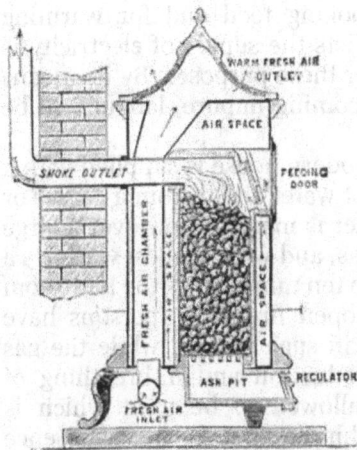

Fig. 18.
Slow Combustion Stove.

Many modifications of the older closed stoves are now in common use. In the stove shown in Fig. 18, excessive heating of the air is prevented by the presence of two air chambers, only the outer one, which brings external air to be warmed, having its air emptied into the room.

Warming by open grates or closed stoves is specially applicable to the rooms of private houses; warming by hot air or steam, or hot water, is chiefly used for large buildings. It is quite possible that these methods will be applied at some future time on a large scale to the warming of private houses. In some large towns of the United States this has been already done, blocks of a hundred or more houses being warmed from the same centre, by the same system.

But apart from such a central system, hot air and hot water lend themselves to the heating of houses on what may be called the Whole House System (page 146). We have mentioned in the last chapter some methods of doing this, and shall now describe others.

Hot-water Pipes are probably the best means of carrying heat to various parts of a large house, and hot water is more thoroughly under control and less dangerous than either hot air or steam. There are two systems of heating by hot water.

In the first, which we may call the low pressure system, there is a boiler from which water circulates through pipes to every part of the building, and as it cools down returns again to the boiler. At the highest points of the pipes, outlets are provided for air. In this system the water is not heated above 200° Fahr., and there is consequently no great pressure on the pipes.

In the high pressure system (Perkin's patent), the pipes have an internal diameter of about ½ an inch, and have thick walls made of two pieces of welded iron. There is no boiler, but one portion of the tube passes through the fire and the water is heated to 300-350° Fahr., thus subjecting the pipes to great pressure. In dwelling-houses with the low pressure system, for every 1,000 cubic feet of space to be warmed to 50°, 12 feet of 4-inch pipe should be given; with Perkin's pipes, probably about two-thirds of this will suffice.

Steam Distributed by Pipes may be employed instead of hot water. This method has been used in factories in which there is a surplus supply of steam.

Warming by Hot Air is only applicable on a large scale, and should only be used in association with a system of ventilation by propulsion, in which the temperature, humidity, and freedom from dust of the entering air are carefully regulated.

153

Warming by Electricity both for cooking food and for warming rooms has a large future, but in most districts the supply of electricity is not hitherto sufficiently cheap to be used for these purposes. By its means the atmosphere will be prevented from becoming impure, labour will be reduced, and life rendered more pleasant.

Hot Water Supplies.—Nearly every modern house is supplied with a bathroom, and this may be supplied with hot water either from a geyser or from the kitchen boiler. In a geyser the water is made to flow over a large heating surface furnished by burning coal-gas, and with the best varieties a bath of 98° F. can be supplied in from five to ten minutes. As the bathroom is usually small and unprovided with an open fire-place, persons have occasionally been suffocated by remaining in such a room while the gas continues burning. This is due to the production and in-breathing of carbonic oxide. No geyser ought to be allowed to be used which is unprovided with a flue passing into the chimney flue or in its absence through an external wall of the house. Short of fatal poisoning, violent headaches often occur when a warm bath obtained by means of a geyser is taken, unless such a flue is provided. In Ewart's lightning geyser, additional protection is furnished by the fact that a dual valve is so arranged, that immediately the water is turned off or the supply fails from any cause, the supply of gas is also cut off.

Hot water supplies from kitchen boilers, unless carefully arranged, may be responsible for serious explosions during severe frosts.

Four plans are in common use. (1) The worm-boiler system. This system is unsafe unless the supply of water to the boiler is attended to; and as the hot water supply to the kitchen is drawn from the boiler itself and not from the worm, the hot water supply for the rest of the house may be deficient. Usually the small feed cistern for the boiler in this system is too near the boiler to freeze.

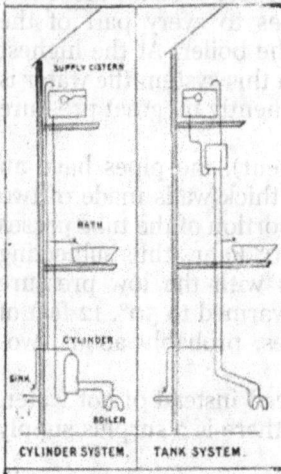

CYLINDER SYSTEM.   TANK SYSTEM.

(2) The cylinder system is very effective. In this system a metallic cylinder, capable of withstanding a pressure of 20 lbs. to the square inch, is placed in the kitchen or bathroom between the cold and hot supplies, its contained water being heated by circulation from the boiler, hot water ascending and cold descending. On the top floor of a house is a cistern from which cold water is supplied. Both the supply pipe and escape pipe for hot water may become frozen during frost. Then the supply of water is stopped, and the boiler and reservoir may boil dry. This would not occur without some indication in unusually vigorous boiling. Boilers sometimes explode, and cylinders sometimes explode. This can be effectually prevented by (3) A Double-cylinder apparatus one within another. In this the water in the outer cylinder supplied from the main cistern can only be heated to 212° F., and the water in the boiler and inner cylinder supplied from a lower feed cistern can only be heated to 214° F., on account of the small head of water. Two escape pipes give free communication with the atmosphere. (4) In the tank system, which being cheap, is usually

154

adopted in poor houses, the tank is placed high up in the system. The hot water branch pipes are usually taken from the flow-pipe between the boiler and tank. Hence when the supply fails, as during frost, the tank is drained empty, the circulation of water ceases, and the system is changed from a circulation system to a high-pressure one.

Safety valves cannot always be relied on to prevent explosions. If they lead to the lighting of fires in frosty weather, when pipes are frozen, they may cause explosions. Explosions from frost only occur when both pipes are blocked. Incrustation of the boiler and pipes increases the danger of explosions; hence the necessity for their periodical cleaning.

CHAPTER XXV

HOUSE DRAINAGE

The Removal of Impurities.—In order that health may be maintained in any inhabited house, it is essential that the impurities produced by animal life should be removed. These impurities may be divided into two classes—the first including the gaseous and volatile products evolved from the lungs and skin; and the second, the liquid excretion from the kidneys, and the solid from the bowels. The former are got rid of by efficient ventilation and by cleanliness; the latter, ought to be as quickly removed, but require more elaborate arrangements to ensure this.

The average daily amount of solid excreta is about 4 ounces, and of fluid excreta about 50 ounces for each adult male. Taking all ages and both sexes into consideration, the amount per head is about 2¾ ounces of fæces and 32 ounces of urine. When dried, the daily fæces amount to 1·04 oz., the daily urine to 1·74 oz., so that the manurial value as well as the possible polluting power of urine is much greater than that of the fæces.

After a variable interval urine and fæces begin to decompose, ammonia and foetid gases being disengaged in large quantities. Urea the chief constituent of urine is decomposed into carbonic acid and carbonate of ammonia. Thus

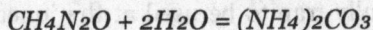

$$CH_4N_2O + 2H_2O = (NH_4)_2CO_3$$

In addition to the excreta, house-slops have to be got rid of, and "dust." House-slops vary greatly in quantity, but probably amount to as much as sixteen gallons per head daily. They consist chiefly of the water used in cooking and washing and for baths. It would be a mistake to suppose that only urine and fæces need careful disposal. There are masses of decaying epithelium from lavatories and baths, organic matters from soiled apparel, and various organic matters from culinary operations, all of which may cause serious nuisance unless promptly disposed of.

155

The Dust consists chiefly of the ashes from fires; but the dust-bin also forms a favourite refuge for kitchen refuse, composed of various animal and vegetable matters, as well as for broken pots and tins. It is dealt with apart from the house-slops and excreta, except in certain dry methods of disposal of sewage.

Two chief plans of getting rid of the sewage have been proposed, though there are many varieties of these. They are—

    1. The Water Method, and

    2. The Dry Methods.

For towns the water carriage of sewage is indispensable, and in this chapter we shall confine ourselves to the part of this system which relates to the Drainage of the House.

The chief sanitary appliances of a house, which empty their contents into the drain and thence into the street sewer, are—(1) Rain-water Pipes; (2) Bath-room and Sink-pipes; (3) Water-closets; (4) Soil-pipes; and (5) The House Drain. We will consider these in detail.

Rain-water Pipes collect the water from the roof by means of gutters, and carry it down to the house drain, except in the few cases in which the rain-water is collected for use. The rain-water or stack pipe was formerly joined directly at its base with the underground drain. This was evidently bad, because the upper end of the pipe was frequently near windows, and foul gases from the drain might be conducted by it into the house. It is equally objectionable to connect the rain-water pipe with the soil pipe and for the same reasons as above.

The general rule with regard to all pipes carrying away water from the house, with the sole exception of the soil-pipe, is that they must be disconnected from the underground drain and discharge into the open air over a gulley-trap. This rule applies to

    rain-water pipes, and to

    waste pipes from baths,

    lavatories,

    sinks.

It does not apply to the soil-pipes leading from

    water-closets and

    slop-sinks,

Overflow or waste-pipes from cisterns for drinking water or from cisterns for flushing w.c.'s or to safe trays under the seat of water-closets should all be made to discharge into the open air, where the leakage can at once be discovered.

The form of gully-trap to be used at the junction with the drain is described on page.

Other Waste-pipes as from bath, lavatories, and sinks, must be similarly disconnected from the drain, and made to discharge over gully-traps. When the pipe leading from the bath, lavatory basin, or sink, is long, it is apt to become foul from the accumulation on its inner surface of slimy matter, consisting of soap, dirt, and other offensive matter. For this reason it is wise to have a syphon bend in the waste-pipe near its junction with the sink or basin. Such a trap is shown in Fig. 19.

The syphon bend alone in the waste-pipe without disconnection from the drain at its lower end would not suffice to ensure complete absence of nuisance, especially for sinks and lavatories which may be disused for a considerable period. Under these circumstances the water in the syphon trap may become evaporated, and then foul drain gases be wafted into the house. Furthermore, even if the water in the syphon trap remained, foul gases may be absorbed from the drain and given out at the end nearest the house (a, Fig 19). Hence it is always best to disconnect all waste-pipes from the drain, except the soil-pipe which cannot be treated in this way. The waste-pipe from the upstairs lavatory or bath may be made to discharge over a hopper-head and thence into the rain-water pipe, which is disconnected below from the drain. This plan should only be adopted when the hopper-head is not close to a bedroom window.

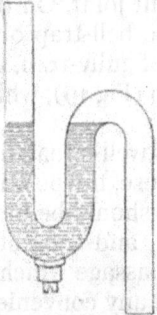

Fig. 19.

Syphon Trap under Sink, with Screw-opening for Cleansing.

Syphon Trap under Sink, with Screw-opening for Cleansing.

Under the bath is usually placed a leaden tray, called a safe, to catch any accidental spillings of water. The overflow pipe from this safe should discharge direct into the open air. Formerly much evil was caused by allowing waste-pipes from baths, sinks, and lavatory-pipes, or overflow pipes from drinking-water cisterns or from the bath-safe, to be connected directly either with the trap of the w.c., or with the soil-pipe beyond it.

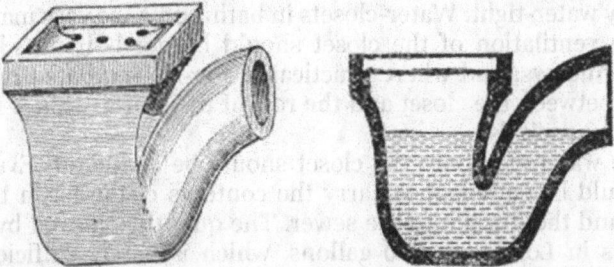

Fig. 20.

A Stoneware Gully-trap.   B Section of the same, showing a Water-seal 3 inches in Depth.

Sinks are not uncommonly the source of offensive smells, when made of wood or stone. A hard glazed sink should be provided; as this is non-porous and can be kept clean. The sink should be placed against an external wall, so that the waste pipe can be carried through the wall to a gully-trap outside the house. Formerly the sink-pipe was joined below

157

directly into the drain, the only obstacle to the entry of sewer or drain gases into the kitchen being a bell-trap at the sink. This is quite insufficient for the purpose. The waste-pipe from the sink should have a syphon trap under it, with an inspection opening at its lowest point (Fig. 19), and should discharge in the open air over a gully-trap (Fig. 20), as in the case of rain-water and bath-waste pipes. It is usually stated that the waste-pipes from sinks, etc., should discharge at least 18 inches distant from the grating of the gully. This is too far, because some of the foul water may become dried up in the channel, and its solid particles be blown about. They may be allowed to discharge directly over the grating of the gully (Fig. 20) or even into the side of the gully below the grating, but above and on the house side of the water-seal shown at B. Fig. 20.

The gully-trap is connected with the socket of the first drain-pipe, and the junction is made water-tight by means of a cement joint. On this account, and because it gives a better water-seal than the bell-trap or D trap, the gully-trap should be always used. The best form of gully-trap, the P trap, is shown in Fig. 20 B. This is better than the S trap (Fig 19), which involves a bend in the drain at its junction with the trap.

Water-closets require to be skilfully constructed and well-situated, if they are not to become a serious nuisance. In building a house, the position of the closet should be carefully considered. In all cases it should be in an out-standing part of the house, against an external wall, and separated from other parts of the house by a passage, preferably a passage which is cross-ventilated. Instead of this, one commonly finds it in any convenient recess, abutting on a bedroom, or where it cannot be properly ventilated. Usually the closet is placed at the back of the house; and as the main-sewer is generally situated in the front street, it follows that the drain must in terrace houses pass under the house. Hence the importance of having it completely water-tight. Water-closets in bathrooms are very inadvisable.

The ventilation of the closet should be good—if possible, by two opposite windows; and where practicable a cross-ventilated lobby should intervene between the closet and the rest of the house. This is now always provided in hospitals.

The water-supply to the closet should be abundant. Every flush of water should be sufficient to carry the contents of the basin through the soil-pipe and the drain into the sewer. The quantity allowed by the Water Companies in London is two gallons, which is barely sufficient for this purpose, unless the form of closet pan is good, and the down-pipe to it of sufficient diameter. Each closet should have a separate cistern, the best being the so-called "water-waste preventer," by means of which a certain quantity of water, and no more, can be discharged each time the handle is pulled. One of the best of these is shown in Fig 21. When the handle of this is pulled, the whole of the water in the cistern is syphoned out by the syphon and carried down to the water-closet, whether the handle be held down or not.

The amount of fall from the cistern to the closet should not be less than four feet, and the pipe should be free from bends in order to ensure a thorough scouring of the trap and soil-pipe; and the flushing-pipe should have an internal diameter of not less than 1½ inches. It is commonly supposed that a small flow of water, trickling continuously down a closet, tends to keep it clean, and prevent smells; but the water thus used is simply wasted. Others fasten up the handle of valve-closets so as to allow a large flow of water. This does not answer the desired end, and renders the offending person liable to a penalty for wasting water.

Many different forms of water-closet are in use. In all of them the main requisites are that there should be (1) a good flush of water, (2) a rapid removal of the excreta, and (3) no possibility of reflux of gases. The chief varieties of closets are the pan, valve, wash-out, and wash-down closets.

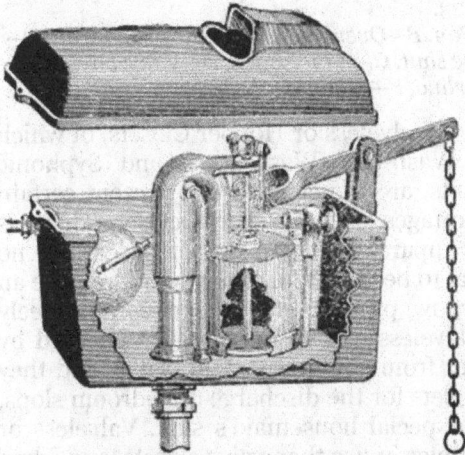

Fig. 21.
Syphon Flushing Cistern

In Fig. 21 a portion of the bell of the syphon is shown cut out, so as to display the movable plug at the bottom of the cistern. An objectionable feature in most cisterns is their noisiness in use. In the above cistern, the pipe admitting water is carried down to within an inch of the bottom of the cistern, thus ensuring noiseless entry of water.]

Pan-closets (sometimes called double-pan closets) are essentially bad, though largely employed in the past. The construction is shown in Fig 22. Below the conical basin there is a metal pan capable of holding a certain amount of water, the lower end of the basin dipping into this water. By means of a pull-up apparatus the contents of the pan can be tilted into a second larger pan or container, and the bottom of the container is connected by means of a short pipe with a leaden [bowl-shaped symbol] shaped trap, from the side of which the soil-pipe passes out to be carried down to the drain. The arrangement insures the production of nuisance. The container and [bowl-shaped symbol] trap always arrest a certain amount of foul matter; and each time the handle of the closet is pulled up a puff of foul air comes into the operator's face. Occasionally the [bowl-shaped symbol] trap becomes corroded by the filth it contains, and foul gases from the drain escape into the house.

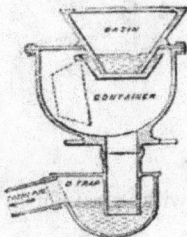

Fig. 22.
Insanitary Pan Closet, showing D Trap below.

Valve Closets differ from the last in having no container, but only a small box containing a movable water-tight valve, exactly fitting the lower edge of the basin (Fig. 23). They are much superior to the pan-

159

closet, but require an overflow pipe in order to avoid accidental flooding of the closet. The overflow pipe should be made with a syphon bend in it, and the flushing of the closet should be so arranged that each time it is performed water enters the overflow pipe. (See Fig. 23.) The trap below the valve should be in the form of a syphon (see under traps, page 179), as this is not easily fouled. It is preferably made of lead, securely jointed to the soil-pipe and to the valve box of the closet. A lead tray or "safe" is required on the floor beneath a valve closet, in view of accidental spillings or overflow; and this should be provided with an overflow pipe discharging into the open air.

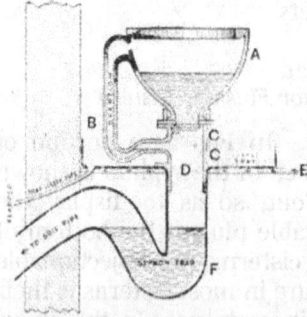

Fig. 23.
A—Pan. B—Overflow pipe with syphon trap. C—Valve shut. C₁—Valve open. D—Valve box. E—Floorline. F—Water-seal of trap.

Valveless or Hopper Closets, of which the Wash-out, Wash-down and Syphonic Closets, are the chief forms, present certain advantages over the valve closet. There is less apparatus to get out of order and no metal to become foul. They do not require an overflow pipe, as water can escape freely through the trap of the closet. Valveless closets need not be encased by wood-work, thus ensuring freedom from spillings of foul water, and they are more easily used than valve closets for the discharge of bedroom slops, thus obviating the necessity for a special housemaid's sink. Valveless or hopper closets are cheaper and simpler in use than valve closets, and when in use are equally sanitary. If a house is left empty for a considerable time, the water in the trap may, however, become evaporated, an event much less likely to occur with a valve-closet. The latter are furthermore less noisy when flushed. With a valve to hold up the water in the pan, as in the valve-closet, a much larger quantity of water can be retained than with a hopper closet. Hence the importance of the latter having such a shape as shall prevent fouling of the basin by fæces.

One of the older hopper closets was the long hopper shewn in Fig. 25. In this form the pan is conical in shape, its sides necessarily becoming fouled by its use, and the spiral flush, the point of entry of which is shewn in the figure is quite insufficient for cleansing the pan.

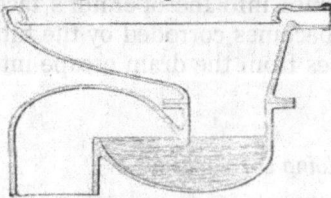

Fig. 24.
Rim Flushing Wash-down Basin.

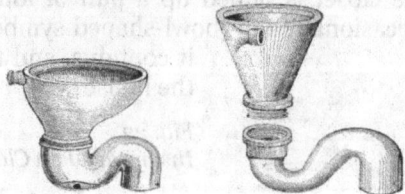

Fig.25.
Short Hopper Closet.
Long Hopper Closet with Spiral Flush.

Of Short hoppers the best has a nearly vertical back as shewn in Fig. 24, a rim-flush, by means of which at least two gallons of water are discharged with the fæces, and the pan is thoroughly cleansed.

The wash-out closet is shewn in Fig. 26. In it a certain amount of water is kept in the upper part of the pan by a ridge over which the fæces have to be driven before entering the trap. The force of the flush is thus broken. In this closet a large area is liable to be fouled, and it is now almost entirely disused.

Syphonic water-closets are wash-down closets, in which the flushing out is aided by syphonic action. They need to be fitted with a flushing cistern, giving an after-flush as well as a flush; otherwise the basin is left untrapped. One of the most elaborate closets of this type is Jennings' Closet of the Century. Fig. 27 shows that the flushing cistern has two connections with the closet, one in the usual manner with the flushing rim of the pan, the other connected to the long arm of the syphon (A Fig. 27). B is a puff pipe allowing the escape of air from this syphon when started. Thus while one part of the flush scours the basin, the other expels the air from A through the puff-pipe B, fills both arms of the syphon with water, and thus starts the syphonic action by which all the contents of the basin are sucked out of it. In this form of w.c., syphonage is intended to be produced, and the after-flush prevents the w.c. from being left untrapped.

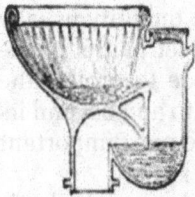

Fig. 26.
Wash-out Closet.

Syphonic water-closets appear to me to be unnecessarily elaborate and complicated, and the only advantage over the wash-down closet is the deeper layer of water in the basin. With a well-shaped wash-down closet this is of little importance.

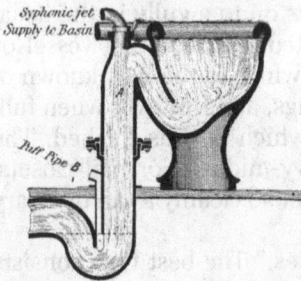

Fig. 27.
Syphonic Closet.

In other forms of wash-down w.c., unsyphoning may also occur, for instance, by pouring the contents of a slop-pail into the pan. This is particularly apt to occur, when two or three water-closets are on different floors of a house, one over another. This unsyphoning is prevented in the case of the highest w.c. by the soil-pipe ventilator, but not always for the lower w.c.'s. For these it may be necessary to carry a pipe from the highest point of the trap of the closet, where it joins the soil-pipe, through the wall into the external air. Such a pipe is called an anti-syphonage pipe (Fig. 28). It effectually prevents the water being sucked out of the trap of a lower w.c. when the w.c. on a higher floor is being flushed.

161

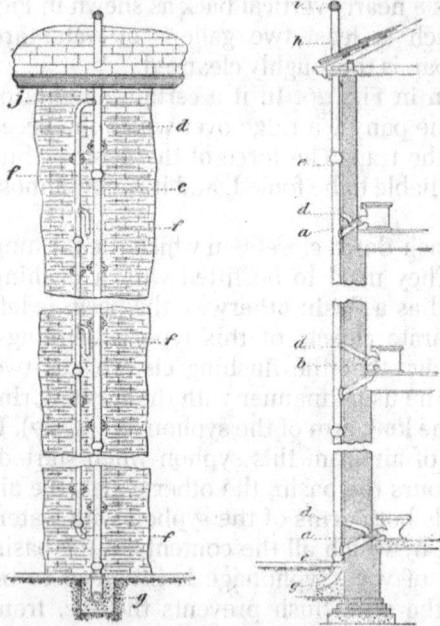

Fig. 28.
A
B
A—Elevation. B—Section through wall of house, showing connection of w.c.'s on three floors, with soil-pipe and anti-syphonage pipe. b—Junction of closet trap with soil-pipe, a being a P and b an S trap. c—Junction of soil-pipe with earthenware drain. d—Anti-syphonage pipe, seen best in elevation A. e—Soil-pipe. f—Anti-syphonage pipe. g—Underground drain. h—Soil-pipe ventilator. i—Cage-work protecting top of h. j—Point at which anti-syphonage pipe is connected with soil-pipe ventilator, above the highest w.c.

In the forms of w.c. already described, clean water is used for flushing, and we have seen that two gallons, the quantity usually allowed, does not suffice for this purpose, unless the closet pan is of the best possible shape, and the service pipe sufficiently wide to project the water by means of a rim-flush forcibly over the pan and into and beyond its trap. Other forms of w.c. have been employed of which the most important are slop-water closets, and trough-closets.

In Slop-Water Closets the waste water from sinks and baths is utilised for flushing, and thus a saving of water is effected. This form of closet is used considerably in manufacturing districts, and is less liable to freeze than an ordinary w.c. The sink discharges on to a gully in the usual manner, but the outlet of this gully is connected with a tilting vessel or tipper, holding 3½ gallons in Duckett's closet, which is the best known of this type. The tipper is balanced on brass bearings, and tips over when full, discharging its contents into the closet trap, which is thus flushed. The slop-closet is a great improvement on the privy-middens or pail-closets, which in some towns it has superseded, but is not so cleanly as an ordinary w.c.

Trough Closets are also known as "latrines." The best type consists of a glazed earthenware trough under a series of w.c. seats. The trough is slightly inclined towards the outlet, at which is a weir, beyond which is a trap. An automatic flushing tank connected with the upper end of the trough and five to six feet above it, discharges water at intervals and drives the fæcal matter over the weir and through the trap. This form of closet is only suitable for factories. It is to be deprecated for schools, and even for factories, unless there are exceptional reasons for its continuance, as fæcal matter possibly of an infectious character may be retained a considerable time in the trough.

The domestic Slop Closet or "housemaid's sink" must not be confused with slop-water closets mentioned above. The slop-closet or sink is used for emptying the contents of bedroom pails. These being necessarily foul and liable to early putrefaction must be treated exactly like other sewage matters. An ordinary pedestal w.c. with a lift-up seat answers excellently as a slop-closet; but in large houses and public establishments a separate slop-sink is desirable with a larger surface than most water-closets. The slop-closet must be connected with the soil-pipe, just in the same way as a w.c.

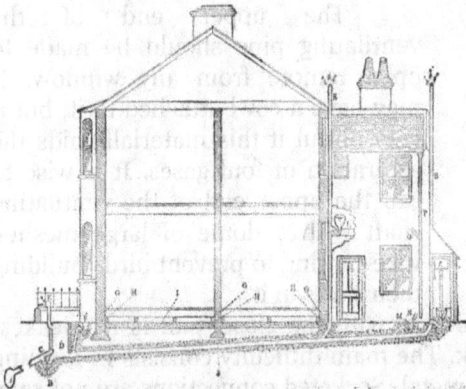

Fig. 29—Section through a House from Front to Back shewing Drainage Arrangements.

A.—Sewer;   B.—Intercepting trap; C.—Cleaning eye for pipes between chamber and sewer; D.—Inspection chamber; E.— Inlet ventilator; F.—Gully-trap for forecourt; G.—Air-bricks for ventilation under floors; H.— Damp-proof course; I.—Concrete 6" thick over site of house; J.— Drain, fall 1 in 24, imbedded in concrete; K.—Soil-pipe carried up full size above eaves; L.—Upstairs w.c.; M.—Gully-trap receiving water from N scullery-sink, O bath and P rain-water stack-pipe; S.—Ventilating pipe at upper end of drain; T.—Pipes leading to same.

The soil pipe is the vertical pipe carrying the contents of the water-closets in the drain. It must be distinguished from the drain, which is chiefly, if not entirely, underground. The exact position of the soil-pipe and its relation to the drain can be seen in Fig. 28 and 29, which should be carefully studied. The soil-pipe should be made of drawn lead without seam, of uniform thickness throughout, and of at least 7 lbs. or better 8 lbs. weight per superficial foot. Any joints in the lead pipe should be of the kind known as "wiped," not a "slip" joint. The outside of a wiped joint is shewn in Fig. 30B. Iron pipes if used must be 3/16 inch thick, and have sockets sufficiently wide and strong to permit of the joints being caulked with molten i.e. "blue" lead, in the same way as water-mains are laid.

The soil-pipe should be throughout its course under observation. It should not be built into a wall, where it might be accidentally pierced by nails, nor within the house, allowing foul gases to escape from weak points in the joints. It should be carried through the wall of the house immediately beyond the closet trap.

The soil-pipe should not be more than four inches in diameter. It should be continued from its highest point at the junction with the closet-trap above the roof by a pipe of the same diameter, with its end wide open

(Fig. 29 K). This ventilation of the soil-pipe is essential (a) to prevent the entry of foul effluvia into the house, especially when the water in the closet-trap is dried up; (b) to prevent unsyphoning of the upper by the lower water-closets in a house. (On this point see p. 172).

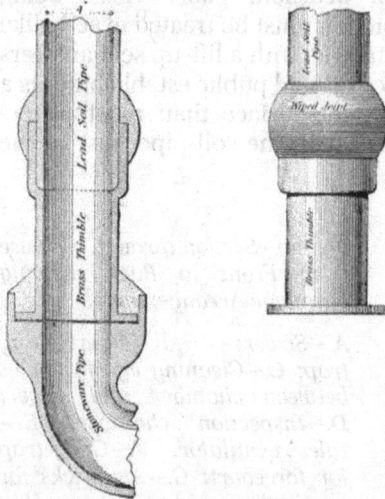

Fig. 30. A. B.
A.—Section showing a Good Method of connecting Soil-pipe to Drain by Brass Thimble.
B.—Outer View, showing Brass Thimble wiped on to Soil Pipe.

The upper end of the ventilating pipe should be made to open remote from any window. It may have a cowl attached to it, but it is doubtful if this materially aids the aspiration of foul gases. It is wise to cap the upper end of the ventilating shaft with a dome of large meshed wire-netting to prevent birds building their nests in it.

The connection of the soil-pipe with the closet-pan is its weakest point, and the most liable to leak. The main difficulty consists in forming joints between earthenware and metal. Socketed connections are not safe. The use of an india-rubber ring inserted between the lead and earthenware flanges and bolted together by means of a brass collar and hooked bolts makes a fairly good connection. Various screwed connections are made. In another form the earthenware collar is covered outside with lead, so that a soldered joint can be made between the earthenware trap and the soil-pipe. In the "metallo-keramic joint" the earthenware joint is painted over with a metallic solution and fired. To the metal film thus formed, lead or other metal can be firmly soldered.

The connection of the soil-pipe into the socket of the first pipe of the earthenware drain requires also to be carefully made. This pipe is curved, and at its upper end has a socket, into which the soil-pipe enters. A length of brass or copper tubing known as a "thimble" (about a foot long) should be soldered to the bottom of the soil-pipe; the rim of this thimble rests in the socket of the drain-pipe and the space between the two is filled with Portland cement (Fig. 30A). With the ordinary connection between lead soil-pipe and drain, the former is apt to become dented by blows, and the latter is very liable to be partially blocked by the dropping of cement inside the pipe when making the joint.

The House Drain under ordinary circumstances receives waste water from sinks and baths, rain-water, and the discharge from the closets.

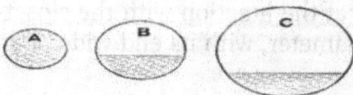

164

Fig.31.

Showing Depth of Fluid and consequent Flushing Force of Three Drains containing an Equal Quantity of Sewage.

We may consider drains under the following heads: material, form, joints, gradient, ventilation, trapping. The first essential is that they should be water-tight, so that their contents do not percolate into the surrounding soil. Socketed glazed stoneware pipes and iron pipes best fulfil this condition. The best material for making stoneware pipes is Devon or Dorset, or similar fine clay, which makes a very strong pipe. Tested pipes free from cracks and flaws must alone be used. The pipes should be laid in straight lines, each pipe being arranged with the spigot and not the socket end directed towards the flow of sewage. The fall should not be less than 1 foot in from 40 to 60. If the fall is less than this amount, artificial flushing from the upper end of the drain is necessary. Usually branch drains are made 4 inches in diameter, the main house-drain having a diameter of 6 inches. A larger size than this is seldom necessary. Thus if A, B, and C be three drains with an equal fall and conveying an equal amount of sewage, the rate of travel and therefore the flushing force will be greater, because the depth of the fluid is greater, in A than in B, and in B than in C. Small drains are more completely self-cleansing than large drains. The water-tightness depends on the character of the joints. In this respect iron drains present the great advantage over earthenware that there are fewer joints and that these can be rendered permanently water-tight without difficulty by being run with blue lead and well caulked. To render an earthenware drain water-tight, (a) it must be laid on a solid bed of cement concrete at least 6 inches thick, so as to prevent sinking, and under the house it should be covered with an equal thickness of cement concrete (I, Fig. 29). (b) The joints must be made with extreme care, the best Portland cement being used for the purpose. Clay is inadmissible, as the fibrils of tree-roots easily find their way through it. The inside of the joint must be raked by the workmen, before the next pipe is laid, to make sure that no fragments of hard cement are left projecting in its interior. Such projections are not uncommon causes of subsequent blockage. Various patent joints have been used, but they are no better than the above when properly laid. Just before the drain leaves the curtilage of the house and near its junction with the sewer, it is trapped, and on the house-side of the trap (E, Fig. 29) an inlet ventilator is provided. The general arrangement should be studied in Fig. 29.

Ventilation of the house drain from end to end is important, a free escape of foul gases out-of-doors being induced. The exit is provided by carrying the soil-pipe up full bore above the eaves, and remote from windows. One opening alone would not induce a current of air, and the other end of the drain being trapped from the sewer (B, Fig. 29) it is necessary to provide an inlet for fresh air at E. This may be placed a few feet above the ground or at the ground-level. Usually a mica-flap valve is provided at its upper end, which closes whenever a puff of foul air attempts to escape from the drain. The necessity for this is doubtful. Ordinarily air enters at the inlet and circulates through the drain, escaping at the upper end of the soil-pipe ventilator.

It has been advocated that the soil-pipe ventilator should form a means of ventilating the sewer as well as the house-drain, the intercepting trap in the latter (B, Fig. 29) being removed. This is inexpedient, an element of risk being introduced, in view of the possibility of the drain or some of the connections of internal sanitary fittings being defective.

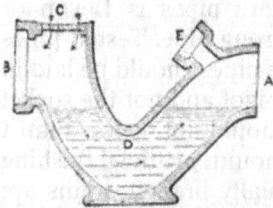

Fig. 32.
Weaver's Intercepting Trap.

The drain as ordinarily arranged is trapped from the sewer by an intercepting trap. This is not merely a trap, but a trap provided with ventilation at its end nearest the house. A form commonly employed is shown in Fig. 32. B is the junction with the house-drain, at D is the water-seal, while at C fresh air enters the house-drain. E is a cleaning eye, through which any chokage can be cleared towards A, leading to the public sewer. It is important that the intercepting trap should be accessible in the event of accidental stopping. This is provided by an inspection chamber or man-hole. This if close to the house is provided with an air-tight cover, the inlet ventilator being conveyed above ground to a convenient point. The man-hole itself is built with brick set in cement and lined with cement. Note that in the man-hole itself half-channel pipes convey the sewage instead of complete pipes.

Sometimes more than one drain-pipe converges to the same man-hole, and then a more elaborate arrangement than that shown in Fig. 29 is required, the branch-pipes converging into half-channel pipes in the man-hole.

Varieties of Traps.—Traps are placed at various points of the house-drainage system to prevent the admission of currents of foul air into the house. They are all constructed so as to intercept a water-seal between the drain and the house or yard at the upper end of the trap. Traps are placed in four positions in connection with the drainage of a house: (1) near the junction of the house-drain with the sewer; (2) under the pan of each w.c.; (3) in the open air at the ground level to receive waste water from bath, sink, and lavatory basin; and (4) in the waste-pipe close under the bath, sink, or lavatory, when the waste-pipe is long and apt to become foul; (5) inside sinks at the upper end of their waste-pipes.

Intercepting traps between the drain and sewer have already been described. They must always be ventilated (C, Fig. 32 and Fig. 29). A syphon shape with a water-seal of 3 inches is required, and the trap should be self-cleansing, that is, whenever the w.c. is used, the fæces ought to be carried beyond the intercepting trap into the sewer. Other forms of intercepting trap were formerly used, one of the worst of which is shown in Fig. 33. With such a trap as this, an accumulation of filth is inevitable.

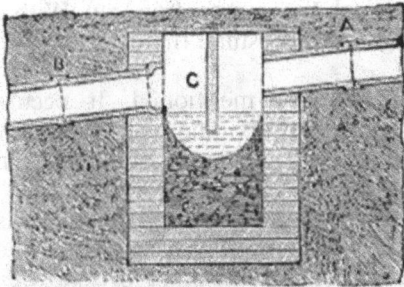

Fig.33.
Deep Dipstone Trap, with Accumulation of Filth in it.
A—*Drain entering trap.* **B**—*Drain leaving trap.* **C**—*Dipstone.*

Water-Closet and Slop-Closet Traps are of the syphon or anti-D type. The water-seal in these must be at least 3 inches deep, and the trap must be ventilated by an upright extension of the soil-pipe, otherwise the water in the trap may be syphoned out when the w.c. is used. Hellyer's "anti-D" trap is a lead syphon trap, the calibre of which is diminished at its bent portion, while the portion of the trap nearest the soil-pipe or drain is square instead of circular. The constriction increases the force of the flush of water and thus cleanses the whole trap, while the square shape impedes the free flow of water, and thus diminishes the risk of syphonage. Various forms of trap are shown in Fig. 19 to 34. The most objectionable of these is the old-fashioned D trap (Fig. 22), the corners and angles of which become fouled, and consequently the lead becomes corroded.

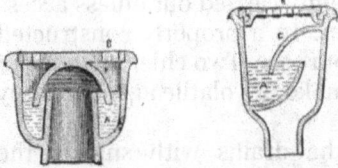

Fig.34.
Bad Form of Trap: Bell Trap. Bad Form of Trap: Antill Trap.

Gully-traps are placed in the yard, for the discharge over them of waste-pipes (Fig. 20). A complete disconnection from the drains is thus effected. Formerly bell-traps were used for this purpose. In the Bell-trap not much water can get through, the space A becomes blocked with dirt, the cover B is often taken off and lost, and then the drain is untrapped; and even without this, the water-seal is very slight, and the water quickly evaporates.

Traps under sinks, etc., have been already described.

Traps were formerly placed at the upper end of the waste-pipe of the sinks when this was directly connected with the drain. Of these the Bell-trap and Antill's trap were most common. The Bell-trap has been described above. In the Antill-trap the trap is not removable, and the water-seal is deeper than with a bell-trap. This trap is sometimes used instead of a gully-trap, but is not so good.

Efficiency of Traps.—Eassie has said "honestly speaking, traps are dangerous articles to deal with; they should be treated merely as auxiliaries to a good drainage system."

(1) The trap may have been imperfectly laid to begin with.

(2) It may be emptied by evaporation.

(3) Unless the precautions already mentioned are adopted, the flushing of one trap may empty another.

(4) The water of the trap may become impregnated with foul gases, and these then escape on the house-side of the trap. When a sewer becomes suddenly charged with a large amount of water, as during heavy

rain, sewer-gases may force their way through the intercepting trap. With a ventilated drain and soil-pipe these dangers are so small that they may be ignored.

Unsyphoning of traps has been already mentioned. It occurs particularly when there are several water-closets one over another, connected with the same soil-pipe. The method of preventing it is shown in Fig. 28.

The Examination of Drains and Sanitary Appliances.—This examination will involve the detection of (a) any deviations from the details of construction and ventilation of drain and soil-pipe, form of w.c., disconnection of waste-pipes, already insisted on; and (b) any defect or leakage in any part of these.

1. Testing of Water-closet.—The interior of the basin or pan may be painted with a mixture of lamp-black, size and water. If the usual flush applied immediately afterwards clears this off, the form of pan and the flushing power are satisfactory. By removing the wood-work around the w.c., leakage or spillings of slop-water around the w.c. can be detected.

2. Testing of the soil-pipe may be effected by one of the volatile tests named under the next heading. To give the test a fair trial, the upper end of the ventilating pipe should be temporarily sealed over.

3. Testing of the drain cannot be efficiently carried out unless access can be obtained to the drain near the sewer. In a properly constructed house-drain a man-hole is provided for this purpose. Two chief methods of testing drains and soil-pipes are in use, by smoke or volatile agents and by water.

The smoke-test consists in filling the drains with smoke, the assumption being that this will find its way through any faulty joint or trap, thus indicating the site of the defect. Various arrangements are employed for pumping the smoke into the drain from the combustion chamber of a pumping apparatus; or smoke is produced by means of specially prepared rockets. All outlets or ventilating pipes must be carefully stopped during the operation, and the place where the smoke is smelt will then indicate any leaky point.

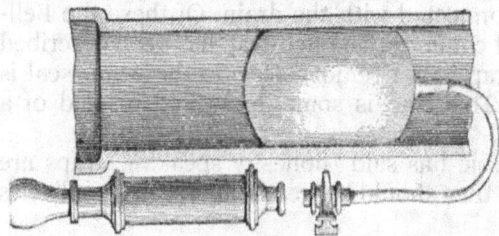

Fig. 35.
Showing Stopper for Water-testing of Drains.

Drain grenades are largely employed for the volatile testing of drains, the essential constituent being phosphide of calcium. The grenade, which is attached to a piece of string, is passed beyond the trap of the w.c., and as the string unwinds the grenade opens and discharges its contents into the soil-pipe. Or a tablespoonful of strong oil of peppermint, mixed with hot water, is poured down the highest water-closet in the house. If this is smelt by another person in the lower closets, it indicates defective traps or soil-pipe.

All volatile and smoke tests have but a limited utility. They are

168

useful in detecting defective joints in traps and in the soil-pipe. They may detect defects in an underground drain; but if no smell or smoke is perceptible when a drain is tested by this means, the drain may still be seriously defective. The only absolutely trustworthy test for drains is the hydraulic or water test. The lower end of the drain is stopped up by a suitable water-tight stopper. Then the drain is filled with water by means of a tap in the yard, the amount of water used being approximately estimated by the rate of flow from this tap. The drain is filled up to the level of the gully-traps in the yard. If it remains at this level for half an hour, the drain is sound. More often it leaks so rapidly that it will not fill, or the level of the water falls quickly after filling, and it is necessary to strip and repair, or more generally to relay the drain so as to make it water-tight.

Rats are an important indication of defective drains. The presence of rats in a house should always lead to a thorough investigation of its drains.

CHAPTER XXVI

CESSPOOLS AND MAIN SEWERS

The terms Sewer and Drain are used somewhat confusedly. The term drain should be used to designate the pipes bringing the sewage from the house into the street-sewer, or any pipes by which the subsoil is drained; the term sewer being confined to the trunk canals into which the house drains empty their contents.

Where the water-carriage system of sewerage is adopted, involving the use of water-closets as described in the last chapter, the sewage may be carried from the house either into cesspools or into the main sewer.

Cesspools are only permissible in isolated country-houses supplied with water-closets. They should always be situated a considerable distance from the house, and should be emptied at regular intervals, the sewage being placed in shallow trenches on the land.

The construction of the cesspool requires careful attention. Its walls should be of brickwork set in cement, lined inside with cement, and surrounded by clay puddle. The bottom should have a fall towards one side, where a pump can be fixed, to remove the more liquid contents. The depth of the cesspool should never exceed 7 feet. The drain emptying into the cesspool should be trapped and ventilated, near its junction with the cesspool; and the cesspool itself should be ventilated.

In connection with many old houses in towns, cesspools still exist, sometimes under the basement or near the house, and so built as to allow soakage in every direction. The surrounding soil becomes contaminated

169

for a considerable distance, the water in any neighbouring well is tainted, or leaky water-pipes receive the soakage. The cleansing of cesspools is always a disgusting process, and even dangerous to the workmen employed. They incur the risk of suffocation, and are very subject to ophthalmia. To avoid these dangers a pump and hose connected with a partially exhausted barrel is employed, but even with this provision some nuisance arises. In the Bexley cart, which is used for this purpose, a hose is used to connect the cesspool with an air-tight cylinder in the cart, into which the contents of the cesspool are pumped.

A modification of the cesspool system, called the Pneumatic System has been proposed by Captain Liernur. In it the cesspool is not placed under the house or the courtyard of the house, but under the street at the angle of junction of several streets. It is made of cast-iron and air-tight, and is connected with all the houses of several streets by iron pipes. By means of a powerful air-pump worked by steam, the cesspool is emptied into barrels in which it is sent directly to farms; and the barrels being placed on ploughs of peculiar construction, the manure is discharged from the bung-hole of each barrel and covered over with earth in the progress of the plough. The pipes tend in this and similar systems to get clogged with fæcal matter, and large quantities of water are required to keep them clean, so that the system merges into that of the use of water-closets, but without the thoroughness of the latter.

Cesspools have been almost improved out of existence in some continental towns, by the introduction of movable cesspools,—fosses mobiles,—to which would correspond strictly the tubs and pails used in some of our large towns. Such movable receptacles have been still further "improved" by the adoption of separators, by which the liquid parts are allowed to escape into the sewer, while the solid parts remain comparatively inoffensive. But when this is done, the cesspool may be as well abolished, as the foulness of the sewage is not greatly increased by allowing solid as well as liquid excreta to enter it.

Sewers are built of glazed stoneware or of impervious brick laid on a bed of concrete to prevent sinking of any part, the parts being most solidly put together with cement. Iron and steel pipes are also used especially when extra strength is required, as when there is some danger of the pipes sinking. For most small streets circular stoneware sewers suffice. Oval brick sewers are more suitable for main streets in which the amount of flow varies greatly. The cross-section of these should be an egg-shaped oval with the small end downwards, as this ensures the most rapid current. Sewers should be laid in as straight a line as possible, and with a fall which will ensure a flow of at least 2½ feet per second. The following rule gives approximately the fall required for smaller sewers and drains:

A 4-inch pipe requires a fall of 1 in 40.
A 6-inch pipe requires a fall of 1 in 60.
A 9-inch pipe requires a fall of 1 in 80.

For further particulars as to the velocity of flow see page 173.

Where a town is very flat, and a proper fall of sewer impossible, Shone's ejectors are sometimes used to raise the sewage. The sewers are laid in sections, each section falling to a certain point, from which the sewage is raised by the ejector to a higher level and so carried to the next section of sewers. Each section has a separate system of ventilation. The provision of manholes for inspection of an intercepting trap and of ventilation of the house drain near its junction with the sewer has already been considered.

As sewers have commonly to carry away the rain-water in addition to the waste matter from houses, their size must be regulated accordingly. The rainfall being very various, the sewers may occasionally become overcharged and flood the basements of houses. During heavy rainfall large quantities of road grit are washed into the sewers, the intercepting gully tanks at the road sides being insufficient to prevent this.

In addition to the above disadvantages associated with discharging storm water into sewers, the sewage owing to its increased bulk is more difficult of disposal, whatever method of disposal be adopted. The size of the sewers and of storm-outfalls into the nearest river or the sea must be regulated so that they are equal to these sudden strains on them; or the Separate system, by which the rain is carried in special conducts to the nearest river, must, in the alternative be adopted. The objections to this plan are that it necessitates a double system of sewerage, and does not allow of the useful scouring effect of rain on sewers. Where it is feasible, and particularly in small country towns, its adoption is advisable. In such cases the old brick drains are used for carrying off rain-water, while new pipe-sewers are employed for carrying the sewage. Such pipe sewers are not liable to become fouled, and on account of the decreased dilution of the sewage can be made smaller than brick-sewers.

Sewers being closed conduits containing sewage, it is highly desirable that the gases resulting from decomposition should be freely diluted. Such gases in unventilated sewers may find their way through intercepting traps into the house drain. The danger from this source has been considerably exaggerated. Ventilation of the sewer is, however, desirable. This has been commonly accomplished by gratings opening at intervals directly into the middle of streets. In narrow streets, the stench from street-grids is occasionally a source of complaint, and may cause malaise and ill-health. Charcoal traps placed below sewer grids to intercept offensive gases have been found to be of little use. The best plan is to do away entirely with surface ventilators, and carry up iron shafts or brick shafts lined with stoneware pipes above the level of all neighbouring houses. The only difficulty in adopting this plan is the difficulty in securing premises to erect such shafts up houses, although no danger attaches to the practice.

Ventilating shafts should be erected at intervals and particularly at the highest points of the sewage system of a town, the upper end of these shafts being remote from the windows of any dwelling-house. When sewers are laid with too steep a gradient, they act as chimneys, the gases mounting to the higher part of the town, and frustrating attempts at ventilation on lower levels. Various attempts have been made to ventilate sewers by artificial means, as by the aspirating effect of street lamps, etc., but these efforts have not been successful, as the effect of the up-current only influences a short length of sewer. The usual method of combined up-shafts and street grids answers fairly well, but when any complaint of smell from street-grids occurs they should be replaced by up-shafts. In Bristol and a few other towns no provision is made for sewer-ventilation, and no ill effects have apparently resulted. There can be no question that the importance of sewer-ventilation has been exaggerated. If the sewer has a sufficient gradient, and is properly laid, and efficiently flushed, so that no offensive deposits occur, the provision of up-shafts at favourable points is all that is necessary. Sewer effluvia have been credited with causing enteric fever, diphtheria, and other diseases. These diseases rarely if ever owe their origin to this cause. The microbes discovered in sewer-air have always been those of the outside atmosphere, and not derived from the sewage. Sewer effluvia might, however, predispose to such diseases, if exposure to them were frequent or protracted, by lowering the powers of resistance of the constitution.

Flushing of Sewers is required at intervals, in order to remove any deposits of grit or other solid matter. Flushing is effected by filling special flushing shafts placed at intervals in the sewers with clean water and then suddenly releasing this.

Whenever there is stagnation, a foul odour is certain to be emitted. The cardinal rule with regard to sewage is to keep it in rapid onward motion, until it has passed the outlet of the sewer. The introduction into a sewer of hot water or waste steam is an occasional cause of nuisance.

The Outfall of a sewer requires to be large and perfectly free in order that the progress of the sewage may not be impeded. When the sewage is discharged into the sea above the low water level, it becomes backed up in the main sewers when the tide is high. The same condition of things has occurred when the outfall is into a river below the water line, or into a tank out of which the sewage has to be pumped. In all these cases the ventilation of the sewers requires to be perfect, and great precautions taken to prevent obstruction of the outflow.

In low-lying sewers where the outfall is impeded, mechanical aids are required to prevent blocking of the sewers. This may be obtained by pumping at the outfall, to enable sewage to escape at all conditions of the tide, or to raise the sewage on to land for irrigation. In the Shone system the sewage is raised to the required height by means of compressed air. In this system the sewage is received into "ejectors." These are cylindrical reservoirs, in which is a float on a counterpoised lever. When a certain quantity of sewage has entered, a valve opens admitting the compressed air, which forcibly raises the sewage into a higher length of sewer or to the outfall.

CHAPTER XXVII

PROBLEMS AS TO FLOW IN SEWERS

In order to prevent deposit of solid matter, sewers should be constructed with a sufficient gradient, and of a shape which presents the least surface for friction in proportion to the amount of liquid to be conveyed.

All brick sewers should be egg-shaped, with the narrow end downwards. The egg is formed by two circles touching one another, the diameter of the upper circle being twice that of the lower.

This shape possesses the great advantage that when the depth of the stream is diminished the amount of wetted surface of sewer (wetted perimeter) is diminished in equal proportion, whereas in every other form of sewer it is relatively increased. Thus the friction, which depends on the extent of the wetted perimeter, is kept down to a minimum. Where, as in outfall sewers, the volume of sewage is large, and does not vary greatly in amount, the circular form may be preferable, as it is cheaper and stronger than the egg-shaped sewer. Below 18 inches internal diameter, sewers should be circular in section, and made of stoneware, not brick.

The velocity of flow depends upon (1) the hydraulic mean depth of the stream, and (2) its inclination or fall.

The hydraulic mean depth means the depth of a rectangular channel whose sectional area (and therefore the volume of whose current) equals that of the curved sewer or pipe, concerning which the calculation is made, and whose width equals the entire wetted perimeter of the sewer or pipe. It is thus equal to sectional area/wetted perimeter.

In the case of circular pipes, if we take the diameter to be 1, and assume the pipe to be running full, the sectional area = $\pi r2$, where $\pi = 3\cdot1416$ and r = half diameter.

The wetted perimeter = $2\pi r$, that is, the circumference of the circle formed by the pipe.

Therefore hydraulic mean depth = h = $\pi r2/2\pi r$ = ¼;

Similarly when the pipe runs half full—

$$h = \frac{\pi r^2/2}{2\pi r/2} = ¼$$

The solution of problems where a smaller arc of a circle is occupied by fluid requires trigonometrical methods, and is not usually needed in practice.

The quantity of fluid discharged in a given time is represented by the product of the sectional area of the stream into its velocity. The greater the hydraulic mean depth the greater is the velocity, if the inclination remains the same.

The velocity of flow is determined by Eytelwein's formula, which states that the mean velocity per second of a stream of water similar in form to those now under consideration is nine-tenths of a mean proportional between the hydraulic mean depth and the fall in two English miles, if the channel were prolonged so far.

Thus if f = the fall (in feet) in two miles,
h = hydraulic mean depth in feet,
V = mean velocity per second,
Then V = ·9√(hf),
or if v = velocity per minute, then
v = 55√(hf).

It is more convenient to let f = fall in one mile.

Then the formula becomes v = 55√(h × 2f).

How much sewage will a circular drain 3 feet in diameter running half full convey, the fall being 1 in 400?

Here h = (πr2/2)/(2πr/2) = r/2 = ¾.

1 in 400 = x in 5,280 feet (i.e. a mile).
f = 13·2 in a mile.
v = 55 × 4·4 = 242 feet per minute.
= 55√h × 2f.
S = πr2/2 = 3·1416 × 9/(4 × 2) = 3·5343.
v × S = 242 × 3·5343 = 855·8 cubic feet, discharged per minute.

In what way does the size and shape of a sewer affect the velocity of the sewage flowing through it? If a 12-inch pipe sewer, laid at a gradient of 1 in 175, gives a velocity of 3½ feet per second, what would be the velocity if the sewer had a gradient of 1 in 700 (the pipe running half full in each case); and would this latter velocity suffice to keep the sewer clear of deposit?

An elliptical sewer gives greater velocity to flow of small quantities of sewage than a circular one because it exposes a smaller surface for friction.

By formula = v = 55√h × 2f.

h = ¼ ∴ √h = ½.
f = 1 in 175 = 30 feet in one mile.
v = (55/2)√60 = 212·85 ft. per min., i.e. slightly over 3½
ft. per sec.

In the second case f = 1 in 700 = 7·56 feet in one mile.

v = (55/2)√15·12 = 106·97 feet per minute.

Thus in the first case there is a velocity of 3·55 feet per second, and in the second case of 1·78 feet per second. The latter velocity is quite insufficient to keep the sewer free from deposit, 3 feet per second being the minimum velocity required for that purpose.

Given a sewer 3 feet in diameter, with a fall of 1 in 1,760, what would be the relative discharge if the fall were 1 in 5,280?

In the first case, 1 in 1,760 = 3 in mile.

1 in 5,280 = 1 in mile.

h = r/2 = ¾.

v = 55√(h × 2f)
= 55√(¾ × 6) = 165/√ = 118.
In second case v = 55√(¾ × 2) = 55√(3/2) = 67·9.
Thus the velocity of the two streams would be as 118: 67·9.

Supposing a sewer to have a gradient of 1 in 300, how much would the velocity and discharge be increased by altering the gradient to 1 in 100?

1 in 300 = 17·6 in mile.
1 in 100 = 52·8 in mile.

As h is not given, we must assume it = ¼;, as it does in circular sewers running full or half full.

v = 55 √(h x 2f)
= 55 √(35·2 / 4) = 163 feet per minute.
v1 = 55 √(104 / 4) = 281 feet per minute.

The increase in discharge may be similarly calculated.

Describe the relation existing in a sewer between gradient, volume, velocity, and size.

By the formula v = 55 √(h. f.)

Where v = velocity in feet per minute.

h = hydraulic mean depth = (area of cross section of stream)/(wetted perimeter).

f = fall in feet in two miles.

In circular sewers h = diameter/4.

Thus the velocity varies as the square root of h or f.

The volume discharged varies with the value of the factor v × s where s = sectional area of stream.

If h remains constant, with a varying volume of s, then the volume discharged may remain constant. Thus h and v in a circular sewer are the same, whether the sewer runs full or half full. In a V-shaped channel the velocity remains the same whatever the depth of the stream, as its bed and area preserve the same proportions. An egg-shaped sewer approximates the V shape in form.

Similar volumes of sewage have velocities which vary not only with the amount of fall, but the size of the sewer. The friction, as represented by the wetted perimeter, would be much less with sewage half filling a circular sewer, than with the same amount of sewage forming a broad shallow stream on the invert of a large sewer.

175

CHAPTER XXVIII

THE DISPOSAL OF SEWAGE

The water-carriage system of sewage is, as the late Dr. Parkes put it, "the cleanest, the readiest, the quickest, and in many cases the most inexpensive method." But when the sewage is conveyed to the outfall of the sewer, its ultimate disposal is still one of the most difficult problems of the present day. Various plans have been adopted, of which the following are the chief:—

1. *Discharge into running water.*

2. *Discharge into the sea.*

3. *Separation of solid and liquid parts* $\begin{cases} By\ settlement. \\ By\ precipitation. \end{cases}$

4. *Filtration through various artificial media or through land.*

5. *Irrigation.*

6. *Bacterial methods.*

Discharge at once into running water was formerly the favourite plan, as it was certainly the most convenient. The sewage was turned into the nearest water-course, regardless of the facts that this might have to supply the drinking water of people at a lower point, that the mouth of the river tended to become obstructed by sewage mud, that valuable stocks of fish were destroyed, and that the river which had practically become a sewer was a source of annoyance and danger to all on it or near it. The enforcement of the Rivers Pollution Prevention Act of 1876 has not been followed by as great improvement as is desirable.

The sewage entering rivers undergoes considerable purification by subsidence, by oxidation, by the influence of water plants, and still more by the active work of microbes, causing nitrification of nitrogenous matter. The vitality of the typhoid bacillus and of the cholera vibrio when discharged by sewage into a large river is probably not very protracted; but water from such a river would form a very dangerous source of domestic supply.

Discharge into the Sea is resorted to in seaboard towns. The outfall must be carried well below the lowest low-water mark, and to such a point that the incoming tide or wind will not bring the sewage back upon the shore, or on the shore of neighbouring places.

Discharge into an Estuary is only justifiable when the flow of the river is rapid, when the volume of water passing out to sea is very greatly in excess of the volume of sewage, and when there is no possibility of contaminating oyster-layings or beds of mussels or other molluscs.

Objection has been taken to the above method on the ground of waste of manure; but modern sewage is so dilute that its profitable utilization on land still remains a dream.

For a single house or small village, the sewage may be stored in a tank, with an overflow-pipe, out of which the liquid parts escape, and are systematically used to irrigate land, while the solid parts are removed at intervals.

A similar subsidence system has been employed on a larger scale, the liquid parts being irrigated over land, while the solid parts are mixed with street sweepings, and sold as manure.

If the liquid parts in any such system as this are turned into a stream, they are as dangerous as the entire sewage, and the legal prohibition to discharging sewage into streams applies equally to them.

The precipitation of the solid parts of the sewage is rendered much more perfect by the use of chemical agents, and at the same time the dissolved matters are to some extent removed.

Milk of lime has been employed, 6 to 12 grains of quicklime being used for each gallon of sewage. Secondary decomposition is apt to occur in the effluent, causing an offensive smell. Salts of alumina, iron salts, and various combinations of these have also been employed, but with imperfect results.

The London sewage for some years has been treated by adding 2·5 grains of sulphate of iron and 3·7 grains of lime to every gallon of sewage; a reduction of 15 to 20 per cent. in the amount of dissolved organic matter being secured. Polarite or magnetic spongy carbon is used as a filter in certain places, the solid and some of the dissolved sewage being first precipitated by magnetic ferrous carbon (ferrozone). The Amines process consists in applying a mixture of herring brine and lime to the sewage. The sewage is stated to be sterilized by this means. Electrolysis has also been applied to the purification of sewage, as in the Hermite process. In this process sea-water is electrolysed, oxygen-yielding compounds and chlorine being produced.

With regard to all the chemical processes hitherto introduced, the following general statement appears to hold good: they are expensive and not thoroughly efficient.

Sewage sludge is deposited in the tanks in chemical processes and needs separate disposal. At Birmingham the amount of sludge produced daily from the sewage of a thousand persons is nearly a ton. This sludge has been run into rough filter beds and left to dry or carted away for manure, but in its crude state its manurial value is very slight. At Ealing it is mixed with house-refuse and burnt in a destructor. The more modern method is to pass it through a filter-press, thus compressing it into solid cakes which can be sold for manure.

Filtration of the sewage matter has been accomplished in various ways.

Intermittent downward filtration through a considerable depth of soil was stated by the Rivers Pollution Commission to be attended with good results. A porous soil is chosen, and the purified water is received in drains under it. A large part of the organic matter is removed by bacterial

177

agency. Frankland's experiments shewed that upward filtration through the same media did not purify.

Filtration through artificial media has not been successful with crude sewage. Precipitation by ferrozone followed by filtration through polarite is said to be satisfactory.

Broad Irrigation purifies the sewage efficiently under favourable conditions, the possible exceptions being during rainstorms and during frosty weather. The effluent into the river cannot, however, be regarded as certainly innocuous, though it is better than the effluent from most other processes. Sewage farms are not a commercial success. In such a farm liquid sewage is allowed to flow at intervals over the land, different fields being irrigated in rotation. Immense crops of grass are obtained, but the grass is coarse and rank.

The soil to be irrigated should have a gentle slope, and the effluent be conveyed by subsoil drains about 5 or 6 feet deep into the nearest water-course. The sewage should be delivered in as fresh condition as possible, and should be freed from its coarser portions by settlement or precipitation. The amount of land required is about 1 acre for the sewage of 100 persons. The irrigation must be on the intermittent plan, in order that the soil may undergo aeration; as it is only in this way that the best purifying results can be obtained. The sewage farm should be well drained by deep-laid agricultural drains. The chief purification of the sewage occurs in the superficial layers of the soil. Nitrification ceases at a depth of about 18 inches. The great point, therefore, is to keep the superficial soil in good condition. A similar nitrification occurs in earth-closets. No nuisance need arise in connection with a sewage-farm, and the supposition that milk and other products from such a farm are less wholesome than the same products from other farms has proved to be unbased.

Bacterial Methods of Treating Sewage.—Chemical precipitation of sewage is likely to be completely superseded by biological or bacterial methods of sewage disposal. When sewage is treated by filtering through land or by broad irrigation the process is bacterial, bacteria or microbes in the soil converting injurious organic matter into innocuous mineral products. The typical process is one of nitrification. The novelty of recent methods is in utilising bacteria for the whole process of purification, and not only for its final stages. The object is, in fact, not as in chemical processes to arrest, but by confining the sewage in tanks to aid and hasten decomposition or putrefaction. Two kinds of microbes serve in this process; those living in air, known as aerobic, and those living in other gases than air, called anaerobic.

Three biological methods of preliminary treatment of sewage are employed. (1) Mr. Scott Moncrieff passes the sewage slowly upwards through a filter 14 inches thick, consisting of successive layers of flint, coke, and gravel. This is called a "cultivation tank." The solid sewage becomes liquefied in passing through this medium, the microbes in the filter dissolving the sewage. (2) In the "septic tank method," introduced by Mr. Cameron at Exeter, a tank is employed which is covered in to exclude light, and to a large extent air. The tank is large enough to hold 24 hours' flow of sewage. The microbes in the sewage under these conditions multiply rapidly, attack, and liquefy the sewage. As in the first process little or no sludge is left. The ultimate products of the decomposition are water, ammonia, and carbonic acid, and other gases. The effluent from the tank is comparatively clear and inoffensive. (3) Aerobic biological filters are employed, as in Mr. Dibdin's installation at Sutton, where the filtering material is coke. The sewage slowly passing through the filtering medium becomes liquefied, the solid matter being peptonised. This action is in part at least due to anaerobic microbes. The filtering beds are used intermittently to allow of aeration, and the liquefaction of solid organic particles entangled in the filter probably chiefly occurs at this stage. It is desirable to have small subsidence tanks, for the removal of large suspended matters and of road debris, etc., before the sewage is spread over the filtering beds. The material used in the filter varies. Most commonly coke-breeze has been employed, but coal slack and other material have also been utilised.

After the preliminary treatment above described, the sewage requires to be passed over finer filtering beds, in which aerobic microbes complete the purification by changing the dissolved organic matter into inert inorganic compounds, by the process known as nitrification. The two processes run into one another, to some extent going on together.

Hitherto the Local Government Board have required filtration of sewage through land before any sewage effluent is allowed to pass into a stream. In view of the successful results now obtainable by bacterial processes this requirement will be occasionally waived. It is unsafe to assume, however, that the clear effluent obtained is free from all disease-producing microbes; and drinking water should not be obtained from even a very large river below the point of discharge of such an effluent, without the most efficient sand filtration.

CHAPTER XXIX

CONSERVANCY METHODS

The refuse to be removed from a house consists of fouled water, which is at least equal in quantity to the water-supply of the house; the excreta of the inhabitants; and "dust," which contains, besides ashes, considerable kitchen refuse; consisting of both vegetable and animal matters.

In dry methods of removing refuse, the "dust" is often added to the excreta, and the two removed together; or the "dust" may be separately removed. In either case the foul water, and to a large extent the urine, remain to be dealt with, and require special drains for their removal. Thus in large towns, whether dry or wet methods of removing sewage are adopted, drains for the removal of foul-water and rain-water will be required, and it is found that they are practically as foul as if they contained the solid excreta.

The dry methods of removing sewage involve a certain amount of retention about the house; hence the general name of conservancy methods. Of these the most important are—

1. The pail system.
2. The dry-earth system.
3. The midden or privy system.

The Pail System implies in reality the use of a movable cesspool. The pail may be used alone, or may contain ashes and house refuse, or some deodorant. Where the pail is used without any admixture of foreign matter, it should be emptied daily, and care should be taken that the pails for different houses are not exchanged.

In the Goux System the tubs are lined with a composition containing clay and furnished at the lowest part with some absorbent material such as chaff, straw, or hay, which serves to absorb the urine and retard putrefaction. This is, when well managed, somewhat less offensive than the ordinary pail system.

The pails may be supplied with a deodorant, such as sulphate of iron, as at Birmingham, Leeds, etc.; they may be packed with absorbent material, as in the Goux system (Halifax); the ashes and house-refuse may be deposited in the same pail (Edinburgh, Nottingham); or coal ashes may be scattered over the excreta (Manchester, Salford); but all these systems are rapidly being superseded.

Although the pail or tub system is an improvement on the midden system, it is necessarily a cause of considerable nuisance, and its replacement by water-closets should be recommended in towns. In detached country houses it may be retained without nuisance, if the pail or tub is emptied daily, and its contents at once placed in the garden beneath a shallow layer of earth. The pails in large towns are usually collected in specially-constructed closed wagons. In some towns the pail contents have been burnt in a "Destructor" after having been mixed with ashes. In other towns attempts have been made to utilise the excreta, either by selling in their crude condition or after drying and deodorising them by heat. None of these methods repays the cost of collection. Mixing ashes with the excreta diminishes any possible value they may possess as a manure.

The Dry-earth System is an important modification of the pail system. In it dry earth or some other material is added to the excreta, thus converting them immediately into an inodorous mass. Probably the best contrivances for thus deodorising the excreta, as soon as they fall into the receptacle, are Moule's or Moser's Earth-Closets.

It is found that 1½ lbs. of dry earth completely deodorise the closet each time it is used. Loamy earth is the most valuable material; a mixture of peat and earth or ashes is very good; sand, gravel, and chalk are practically useless. It is necessary that the earth should be very dry, and that it should be finely sifted. If the earth is damp, decomposition of the

180

excreta speedily occurs. The act of sitting and rising works a hopper which scatters a supply of earth.

Charcoal and sawdust have also been used in connection with Moule's or Moser's closet, and with good results. Charcoal has been obtained cheaply for the purpose from street sweepings, and from seaweed, as in Stanford's closet, in which ½ lb. of charcoal from seaweed is used each time. Mr. Stanford found that while dry clay absorbs only 4 to 5 per cent. of water, dry charcoal prepared from seaweed absorbs 14·7 per cent. The best material, however, is dry earth, but it must be thoroughly dry. The microbes in the earth disintegrate the excreta, converting them into mineral compounds, such as nitrates. Even the paper used disappears. Hence the same earth may be used over again after being stored dry for six weeks. Whether the excreta of an infectious patient are freed from infection by this process is doubtful; if not, the infection might be scattered by means of dust.

The dry earth system is more expensive in use than the pail system, and although applicable to villages and isolated houses, is quite unsuited to large towns, owing to the practical difficulties connected with the procuring and storing of dry earth. The dry earth closet requires frequent attention, in addition to not being so convenient as the pail closet; and there is much less manurial value in the contents of earth closets than in those of pail closets.

The advantages of the earth-closet as compared with the water-closet have been thus summarised by the late Sir Geo. Buchanan. "It is cheaper in the original cost, it is not injured by frost, it is not damaged by improper substances driven down it, and it very greatly diminishes the quantity of water required by each household." These advantages only accrue when the system is perfectly worked, and do not counterbalance the immense advantage and greater safety of the water-carriage system in towns.

The Privy or Midden System, involving the use of a fixed receptacle, is still prevalent in many towns as well as in innumerable villages. In its worst form, the receptacle consists of a pit with sides of porous materials, allowing percolation of filth in every direction; and in this pit the excreta of whole households are allowed to collect for months. It has been improved by providing a cover to keep out the rain, and thus retard decomposition; still more by providing a drain for the excess of liquid; and by making the sides and bottom of the pit impervious to moisture. The addition of dry ashes to the excreta tends still further to prevent any smell; and the greatest improvement of all consists in raising the receptacle above the ground level, and providing for easy cleaning from the back. The raising of the receptacle involves a diminution in its size, and so prevents the retention of putrefying matters near a house for a long time.

The model Bye-laws of the Local Government Board recommend a capacity for the privy not exceeding 8 cubic-feet, the provision of means for the frequent application of ashes, dust, or dry refuse; they forbid any connection between the privy and the drain; insist on its being at least 6 feet from a dwelling-house (too low a limit); and require a flagged or asphalted floor at least 3 inches above the level of the surrounding ground.

The Nottingham tub-closet forms a link between the pail and midden system. It is really a small movable middenstead, used for receiving excreta, vegetables and ashes.

Even when carefully supervised, middens are almost certain to be productive of evil. They possess two great disadvantages as compared with pails or dry closets. (1) The time between collections of excreta by the scavengers is much longer; and (2) the receptacle for the refuse is part of the structure of the building, and cannot easily be renewed when it has become saturated with excreta.

The use of pails or dry-earth closets is a great improvement on the old middens, but even these compare very unfavourably with water-closets in two respects. (1) The excreta require to be retained about the house for a longer or shorter period, whereas with an efficient water-carriage system, they are at once projected into the sewer. (2) In removing the excreta, the weight of the receptacle has to be added to that of the excreta, while in the water-carriage system, the water serves as the means of transport.

In villages and isolated houses, where no drains are provided for waste water, and the dry system of closets is adopted, the disposal of waste water requires special provision. Very commonly the slops are thrown out of the door, and soak into the ground about the house. They should be carried by means of a waste-pipe into a water-tight cesspool, remote from the house, whence they can be pumped into a field, or carried away by special conduits.

Relative Merits of Dry and Wet Methods. No absolute answer can be given in exclusive favour of either plan. Each is the best under different circumstances; the dry method being chiefly suitable for small villages, and for temporary collections of people, as in camps; and the wet method for towns. The question of value of manure does not enter into the problem, as it seldom repays for carriage.

The objections to the water-carriage system are really due to its not being carried out in an efficient manner. When sewers are properly laid; when they, as well as house-drains, are freely ventilated; when house-drains are efficiently trapped and ventilated near their junction with the sewer; when the drains are efficiently flushed, and the outflow from the sewer is unimpeded, the objections disappear.

These objections are that—(1) the sewers, as underground channels, transfer effluvia and the germs of disease from one place to another; (2) pipes become disjointed owing to being badly laid, and the ground is contaminated; (3) the water supply is in danger of receiving impurities from the sewers. These objections do not hold good in practice. The contamination of water-mains or of wells from sewers implies gross carelessness in the method of laying of sewers or pipes.

The only objections which are of any force, are (4) that water-closets require a large amount of water, and the sewage obtained is greatly diluted, and consequently diminished in value; while (5) the disposal of such an amount of water, in the case of a large inland town, is a problem of the utmost difficulty. Modern engineering enterprise by bringing water from a greater distance, and by aiding the discharge of sewage when necessary by pumping, has overcome these difficulties.

182

There are many objections to the dry methods of removing excreta. (1) Whatever dry method be adopted, the excreta are retained for some time in or about the house, instead of being immediately removed.

(2) Although the initial outlay in closets and sewers is less than with the water-carriage system, there is the constantly recurring expense of removing the excreta, as well as of cleansing the pails, etc.

(3) In the dry-earth closets, the provision of dry earth or other material involves some expense.

(4) Whatever dry method be adopted, sewers are always required to carry off the foul water, as well as liquid trade products, and a certain proportion at least of the urine. It is impossible to supply sufficient dry earth to absorb all the urine and slops of the population.

Thus, as the Indian Army Sanitary Commission said, speaking of barracks, "to have two systems of cleansing stations—a foul-water system, and a dry-earth system—would simply be paying double where one payment would answer; or, if all the excreta, solid and liquid, are to be carried away, this must be done at a cost ten times greater than that which would be necessary, if all the excreta were removed by drains."

With some of the dry methods, as where middens or cesspits are drained into the sewers, the sewer-water is more offensive than in towns supplied with water-closets. When a midden or cesspool is drained, the principle of conservation, which distinguishes the dry system from the wet, is practically abandoned; and not only so, but the solid matters still remain to be disposed of, by a tedious process.

(5) The dry systems, involving the retention of excreta about the house, poison the atmosphere. In all towns where the refuse matters are not removed immediately, there is a high mortality, especially among children.

On the other hand, the introduction of the water-carriage system into large towns, with the abolition of midden-heaps and cesspools, has been followed in nearly every case by a diminution in the death-rate, and especially a considerable diminution in that from such diseases as enteric fever. It has furthermore increased the comfort of life, and removed those serious nuisances which are inevitably associated with privies and pail closets, and to a less extent, when care is not exercised, with earth closets.

HOUSE REFUSE

In an ordinary household the disposal of ashes from fires, of broken pots and cans, of waste-paper, and of vegetable and animal debris form a serious difficulty. The difficulty is one that can be minimised by the careful housekeeper. Old newspapers, etc., may be sold, though their value is very small; other waste-paper should be burnt. All vegetable and animal debris should be burnt. This may be effected without nuisance if coal-fires are in use, by placing potato-peelings, cabbage leaves and similar substances under the fire until thoroughly dried, and then burning them. The careful housewife will not waste bones, but utilise them for soup. After being boiled they are much less liable to putrefy in the dust-bin; but should even now be burnt in the fire. If this plan be pursued, the contents of the dust-bin will be simply ashes, broken pots and cans, and a few cinders—here again a sifter is desirable—and no nuisance can arise. It is only organic refuse that smells. If only gas or paraffin stoves are in use, as during the summer months, any possible nuisance in connection with the dust-bin is minimised by allowing all refuse to dry before it is placed in the dust-bin, or by wrapping all putrefiable substance inside several layers of newspaper.

In emptying the dust-bin or ash pit, care must be taken that the bottom is thoroughly scraped out. It is well to keep some quicklime (thoroughly dry) for sprinkling on the bottom and sides of the receptacle each time after it is emptied. This greatly helps in keeping it dry and diminishing nuisance during summer.

In many households a separate receptacle is kept for what is known as "hog-wash," containing waste-food, often in a foul and putrefying condition. In well-ordered households, except in hotels and similar establishments, there is no necessity for a "hog-wash" tub, and its presence argues wastefulness and carelessness. Food which cannot be eaten because it has "gone bad" should be burnt.

Two forms of receptacle are used for house-refuse, an ash-pit or a dust-bin. An ash-pit is a fixed receptacle for the reception of house-refuse. In many towns the same receptacle is used for excreta. Then we have a privy or privy midden, according to size. Ash-pits for household refuse alone should be small, so as not to hold more than a week's refuse. No part should be below the ground level. The floor and walls should be lined with impervious smooth cement, and the ash-pit should have a hinged cover to keep out rain, and a door on one side to facilitate emptying. The ash-pit should be at least six feet distant from any wall of the house. Even the best constructed ash-pit is as much worse than a dust-bin, as a privy is worse than a pail closet. A fixed is always less easily cleansed than a movable receptacle.

A dust-bin is usually made of galvanized iron with a tight-fitting lid. This receptacle can be kept clean, and can be carried without any transference to another tub direct to the cart.

The removal of house refuse constitutes an important part of municipal work. In most towns it is carried out weekly, sometimes less frequently, while in some towns removal twice or three times a week is secured. A daily removal is carried out in a few towns, and this is by far the best plan, as decomposition and the dangers associated with it have then no chance of becoming serious. The house refuse should always be conveyed through the streets in covered carts.

The disposal of house refuse constitutes a problem of increasing difficulty. Unfortunately in the suburbs of many towns it is deposited on low-lying land in disused quarries and brickfields. When land has been thus levelled, it often next appears as "an eligible building site." A very common practice has been to excavate gravel and sand upon the site of proposed dwellings, and allow the excavation to be filled with dust-bin refuse. Before building on such a soil it is necessary to excavate down to the virgin earth, and to render it impervious by a layer of cement concrete.

A second method is to sift and sort the refuse, separating by means of sieves the finer ash and dust from the coarser parts. This is usually carried out in a large dust-yard adjoining a river or railway-siding. The "breeze," consisting of cinders and coals, along with the fine ash, are sold to brickmakers; the "hard core," consisting of clinkers, broken crockery, etc., is used for road making; and the "soft core," consisting of animal and vegetable refuse, to which is often added stable manure, is sold for manure. Iron, tin, paper, rags, bottles, and corks are separately collected and sold. This disgusting process, often carried on by women, is now gradually being disused.

A third method is to cremate the house refuse. This has been done to a large extent by burning the house refuse for making bricks. This method of slow and imperfect combustion necessarily involves a nuisance. A more elaborate means of securing the same end is by the modern Destructor, which has been gradually brought towards perfection. A destructor is a large furnace, in which, after the fire has been first lit, the combustible matter in the house refuse suffices to keep it alight. Various mechanical devices are in use for emptying the trucks of house refuse on to the fires without handling it, for clearing out of the fire the inorganic refuse, and for ensuring sufficiency of draught. The amount of draught has in the older destructors been dependent upon the height of the chimney. In some more recent destructors the same end has been more efficiently secured by injecting a steam blast into the furnaces. A temperature of about 2,000° F. is reached in certain parts of the destructor, the rapid draught ensuring enormous heat. In view of the possibility of a portion of the smoke not being completely burnt, a second "fume cremator" is often provided, through which the products of combustion in the furnace are passed. The fuel in the "fume cremator" is coke. Besides incomplete combustion of combustible material, which is rare when the fume cremator is provided, the escape of fine dust up the chimney requires to be guarded against. This is partially prevented by ledges near the bottom of the chimney. In a destructor the house refuse is reduced to about one-third of its original bulk, the residue being innocuous clinker, metallic refuse, and dust. This material can be utilised for making roads, and in the manufacture of mortar. The waste heat of the destructor has been partially utilised for various purposes. This method of disposal of house refuse is usually the best available for large towns, and offers the additional advantage that no nuisance is caused by the deposit of offensive material in neighbouring districts.

185

CHAPTER XXX

POSITION OF THE HOUSE

Lord Bacon said: He who builds a fair house upon an ill seat committeth himself to prison." The first considerations, therefore, in choosing a house are those of aspect, surrounding objects, and soil. On the first of these considerations, that of aspect, Thomas Fuller's quaint remarks give the essential points. He says:

"Light (God's eldest daughter) is a principal beauty in a building; yet it shines not alike from all parts of heaven. An east window welcomes the beams of the sun before they are of strength to do any harm, and is offensive to none but a sluggard. A south window in summer is a chimney with a fire in it, and needs the screen of a curtain. In a west window in summer towards night the sun grows low and even familiar, with more light than delight. A north window is best for butteries and cellars, where the beer will not be sour from the sun shining on it."

A workroom or study requiring steady light, should point north or some point between north-east and north-west. A breakfast room should face north-east to south; while one aspect of a drawing-room should be south-east to north-east. Store-rooms, dairies, larders, should have a northerly aspect. It is preferable, as a rule, for the house not to face in the direction of the four points of the compass, but diagonally to these.

Surrounding Objects of an objectionable character, as factories, noisy or offensive trades are to be avoided. The possibility of neighbouring cesspools contaminating the water supply must be considered. Trees close to a house are objectionable, rendering it damp, and preventing the free access of sun and air. More remote from the house they form a useful shelter, especially when to the north or east.

The banks of water courses are to be avoided for similar reasons. If there is a choice, the slope of a hill should be selected; and it is essential that no part of the dwelling should rest against sloping ground at a higher level. Rank vegetation indicates a damp clayey soil.

The main point is to secure that the house shall receive ample light and ventilation. In calculating the amount and intensity of sunshine which a house built on a given site will secure the variations according to season must be remembered. The direction (orientation) of the sun is the same all the year through; but the altitude of the sun varies with the latitude. Thus in a house facing directly south in the latitude of the south of England the sun's altitude at noon on the 21st of December is $15° 4'$, on the 21st of June $62° 4'$. A ray of light entering the highest point of a window facing south at each of these seasons will illuminate a much larger part of the room in summer than in winter. Not only so, but inasmuch as it enters the room more nearly vertically it is more powerful than when entering at an angle more nearly approximating a horizontal direction, in accordance with the general law that the intensity of illumination falling on a horizontal surface (as the floor of a room) is inversely as the square of the width of the area embraced within the same angle of incidence of light.

In houses in a street the angular aperture through which light enters is greatest in the upper stories. It may be increased (a) by increasing the height of rooms; (b) by carrying the window heads nearly to the level of the ceiling; and (c) by avoiding the proximity of other buildings which would impede the access of light. Fig. 36 shows the importance of the last consideration. This represents a three-storied house in a street, of which the opposite house L is of the same height. It will be observed that each room is divided into two regions of different degrees of illumination by a plane Lm, formed by a line connecting the ridge of the roofs of the houses on the opposite side of the street with the interior surface of the rooms and touching the uppermost point of the window in transit. Below this line there is "sky-light" sufficient in quantity; above this line light is insufficient in amount and is diffused and reflected. The area receiving sufficient light increases from the ground floor upwards. We have already seen that its intensity similarly increases in the higher stories, the rays of light being more nearly vertical in these.

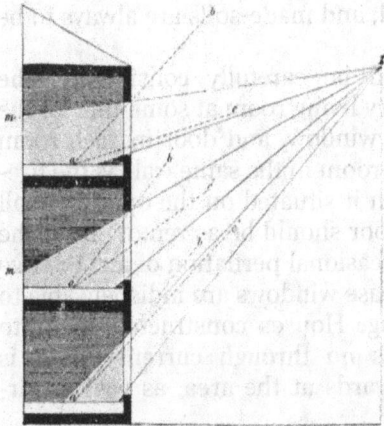

Fig.36.
Showing Variations of Illumination in Different Stories.

The amount of sky-light visible can be expressed in terms of the angle of aperture, i.e. the arc of sky visible at any given point a in the room. Thus in Fig. 36 the triangle of aperture bac is greater than b′a′c′, and this greater than b′′a′′c′′. The sides of the angle of aperture, it will be seen, are formed by drawing one line from the point a to c, which, if prolonged, would touch L, and another line to b, which passes through the highest point of the window.

The amount of light received in a dwelling-house is largely determined by the width of the street and the distance between the backs of the houses in adjacent streets. The model Bye-laws of the Local Government Board insist that no new street shall be less than 36 feet wide if it exceeds 100 yards in length or is intended to be a carriage road, not less than 24 feet in any case. Furthermore, a new house must have in the rear an open space exclusively belonging to the house, at least 150 square feet in area, and free from any erection above the ground level. This must extend along the entire width of the house, and must never measure less than 10 feet from every part of the back wall of the house; the distance must be at least 15 feet, if the house is 15 feet high; 20 feet if 25 feet high, and 25 feet if 35 feet high or more.

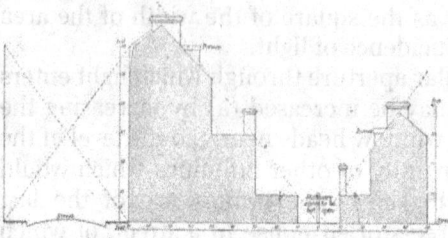

Fig.37.
Diagram Illustrating the Necessary Requirements as to Open Space in Front of and at the Rear of Dwelling-houses.

Streets should never be less in width than the height of the houses in them; and a line drawn from the ridge of the roof to the foot of the wall of the opposite houses (Fig. 37) or in the rear to the foot of the wall or fence dividing the back yards of contiguous houses, should not make an angle of more than 45° with the ground (Fig. 37). This is the angle required for new buildings in the residential parts of Liverpool, and was proposed for London, but unfortunately not made obligatory. The size of windows is discussed on page 198. The light received in a given house is often diminished at corners of streets by contiguous houses.

The Soil has an important influence on the healthiness of a site. The relative merits of the different kinds of soil are discussed on page 201. Undrained soils of whatever kind are bad, and made-soils are always to be regarded with profound distrust.

The planning of a house should be carefully considered. The principle is that the sun should enter every living room at some time of the day. The relative positions of fire-place, window, and door in each room are important. With the sole window of a room in the same wall as the fire-place the area ventilated is the least, with it situated on the opposite wall the area ventilated is the greatest. The door should be as remote from the window as possible, in order to secure occasional perflation of air; the two being preferably on opposite walls. Staircase windows are indispensable to secure through ventilation of a dwelling. Houses constructed "back to back" cannot be properly ventilated as no through current of air is possible. Hence the necessity for open yards at the area, as well as air-space in front of the house. (Fig. 37).

In the construction of a house, apart from access of light and air, the main problems are to secure dryness and equability of temperature. We shall consider in this connection the materials used in the construction of walls, floors, and roofs.

CHAPTER XXXI

THE MATERIALS USED IN THE CONSTRUCTION OF A HOUSE

In this country walls of houses are usually built of brick, stone, timber, or concrete, of which the first two are the most important. Timber is, owing to its inflammability, only allowed to be used in towns under special restrictions. Bricks and stones are bonded together and imbedded in mortar or cement.

There are several kinds of bonds in brickwork, of which the strongest is the English. This consists of alternate courses of "headers" and "stretchers," the former being bricks carried through the wall from face to back, the short end showing on the face, and the latter bricks laid lengthwise along the face of the wall. Hence the wall is held together in every direction. A Flemish bond consists of alternate headers and stretchers in the same course. It is used where a specially smooth wall is desired, but is not so strong as the English bond.

Bricks are generally of a uniform size, of 9 inches in length by 4½ in width and 2¾ inches in thickness. Those bricks which are heaviest and hardest are generally the most durable; bricks of good quality when knocked together give a clear ringing sound.

The relative conductivity for heat of brick as compared with other materials, is shown in the following table, from Galton, which gives the units of heat transmitted per square foot per hour by a plate 1 inch thick, the two surfaces differing in temperature 1° Fahr.:—

Stone—ordinary free stone	13·68
Glass	6·6
Brickwork	4·83
Plaster	3·86
Fir planks	1·37
Brick dust	1·33

It is evident that in this respect, brick walls compare very favourably with stone walls, and are much more economical of heat. Increased conductivity of a material may be counteracted by increased thickness.

Brick is very porous, as shewn by its power to absorb moisture. A good brick can absorb from 10 to 20 per cent. of its weight of water; while good granite only takes up ½ per cent., sandstone usually from 8 to 10 per cent., marble only a trace, and Portland limestone 13½ per cent.

Being porous, brick allows the passage of a considerable amount of air, unless its pores are occupied by moisture. The following table, from Galton, shews the number of cubic feet of air which every hour pass through a square yard of wall-surface of equal thicknesses, built of the following materials, there being a temperature of 72° Fahr. on one side the wall, and of 40° on the other:—

Wall built of brick		7·9	cubic feet.
„	quarried limestone	6·5	„
„	sandstone	4·7	„
„	limestone	10·1	„
„	mud	14·4	„

Mortar should consist of clean sharp sand and slaked lime, usually in the proportion of three of the former to one of the latter. Grouting, or liquid mortar, is merely ordinary mortar to which a larger quantity of water has been added. It is used for filling up the crevices between the brickwork about every fourth course, and is required to a greater extent in stone work, owing to the difficulty in filling up spaces left by inequalities in the stone.

The sand used in mortar should be free from small stones. It should not contain any earthy or clayey matters, as these greatly diminish the adhesive quality of the mortar, which depends on the combination of the sand and lime. All the sand used in a building should be washed, unless it is perfectly clean, in order to remove impurities. Many builders use an inferior mortar, in which other materials, such as "road scrapings," are substituted for sand. Sand taken from the sea-shore is unfit for making mortar, as the salt contained in it is apt to deliquesce and weaken the mortar.

Lime is obtained by burning chalk or limestone in a kiln. Thus $CaCO_3 = CaO + CO_2$. There are three kinds of lime: (1) Fat or quicklime, used for internal plastering, (2) stone lime, used for ordinary building work, and (3) hydraulic lime, used for building in damp situations. The last named contains a quantity of silicates, and sets under water.

Common mortar crumbles away, if laid under water before it has had time to harden.

Portland cement is an artificial cement, of a dark grey colour. It is made by grinding chalk, mixing it with blue clay or river-mud in certain proportions, and then burning it in a kiln and afterwards grinding it to a fine powder. It is used, mixed with sand, for external plastering ("compoing") of walls, for making concrete, or instead of lime for making mortar if extra strength is required.

Compo consists of Portland cement and sand, and is used for covering walls when an impervious smooth surface is required, and for keeping out rain. It is laid on in two coats. The first or rough coat ¾ inch thick, is composed of one part cement to 5 parts compo sand, i.e. coarse sand mixed with fine beach. The outer or fine coat is composed of two parts fine or washed sand to one part cement. To "render" or "compo" a wall is to cover it with this material. The internal plastering of a chimney flue is called "pargetting."

Concrete is of two kinds, lime or cement concrete. It is composed of three parts broken ballast or large beach, two parts of sand, and one part of lime or cement. Lime concrete has no resisting strength, and is only used for surrounding drain-pipes, or where no great strength is required.

Stone varies very greatly in character. It is uncommon for the whole thickness of the walls of a house to be built of stone; usually there is merely a facing of stone and a backing of brickwork. If good stone is not available, the less it is used the better.

The stone chosen should be durable, and able to resist the action of the sulphuric, sulphurous, and carbonic acids absorbed from the atmosphere, and brought in contact with it by means of rain. The stone of which a considerable part of the Houses of Parliament consists is dolomite, a double carbonate of lime and magnesia. The acid fumes in the air produce on its surface sulphate of magnesium, which is washed away in successive layers.

If the stone presents any stratification, it should be laid in the wall in the same position as that in which it was originally deposited in the quarry. Thus, any planes of stratification will be horizontal, and the scaling off by the action of frost and rain is minimised. Comparatively homogeneous stones, such as granite and millstone-grit, can be laid in any position. In testing the character of any stone, the least porous, densest, and most resistent to crushing, will as a rule be the most durable.

The chief difficulty in the use of stone for the walls of houses, is that of keeping out the wet. To obviate this, stone-houses are often built of great thickness, and are consequently cooler in summer and warmer in winter.

In and near large towns brick is chiefly used for walls of houses, and stone employed only for window-sills, columns, steps, etc. It is even more important in these cases to carefully select the stone, as the parts where it is placed are those most exposed to the weather. If a soft, friable freestone is used, after a sharp frost large scales are seen falling off in flakes, owing to the freezing and subsequent thawing of the moisture in the stone.

Portland stone is the best-wearing stone to be had in the neighbourhood of London. Bath stone is also considerably used, but it varies greatly in quality, and should be very carefully selected. For landing-steps and paving, Yorkshire stone is extensively used, but artificial cement pavings are replacing it to some extent. Most kinds of stone can only be economically used near the quarries from which they are derived.

The Slate used for roofs is an altered form of clay, possessing a laminated structure. The ease with which it splits along the planes, renders it peculiarly suitable for this purpose. The Welsh slates are considered the best.

Terra-cotta is made from certain kinds of clay, mixed with glass, pottery or sand; then ground up, strained, and kneaded; and lastly thrown into moulds and baked in a kiln.

Iron and Wood have occasionally been employed alone in building houses. The former, owing to its good conducting powers for heat, is cold in winter and hot in summer; while the latter becomes rotten from exposure to wet, and is also very combustible. Corrugated iron buildings lined with wood are also employed, but are not very satisfactory.

For roofs, slates or tiles are the materials most frequently employed; but occasionally lead and corrugated iron are used, also thatch in country places, and tarred felt for temporary buildings.

Lead is the most suitable metallic covering for roofs, as it is durable and easily worked. It is, however, heavy and demands considerable strength in the timbers by which it is supported. Galvanized iron has also been largely used. It is cheaper and lighter than lead. Both lead and zinc require very careful laying if they are to be weather-tight.

Thatch protects the interior of a house well from extremes of heat and cold.

CHAPTER XXXII

CONSTRUCTION OF THE HOUSE

In preparing to build a house, or in entering into a house already built, the following requisites should each receive careful attention:—

1. The site of the house should be healthy, and its relation to surrounding objects in accordance with the laws of health.

2. The house should be warm in winter, and cool in summer.

3. It should be always dry.

4. There should be an abundant and uninterrupted supply of air.

5. The water supply should be abundant, conveniently arranged, and pure.

6. The excreta and waste-water should be immediately removed from the house and its annexa.

The three last requisites have already received consideration. Of those still to be considered, dryness is the most important. A damp house is certain to be an unhealthy one. It is this for two reasons:—1st, it is a cold house, as damp walls, like damp clothes, conduct the heat of the body away much more rapidly than dry walls; 2nd, if the pores of the bricks are occupied by water, air cannot pass through, and thus the ventilation and purification of the house are greatly impeded. Damp may arise from the ground on which a house stands, or from the rain beating against the walls, or from a defective roof. Unless special means are taken to prevent it, moisture rises by capillary attraction through brick after brick.

The Foundation requires to be solid and substantial, otherwise sinking occurs, with cracking of the walls, resulting in an unsafe condition, and an exposure to rain and wind.

In making the foundation for a house, the ground should be excavated, so as to secure a solid bed of earth or rock not liable to be affected by the weather. A continuous bed of the best cement concrete should then be laid, not only under the walls, but covering the entire site of the house, and extending on every side at least 6 inches beyond the footings of the wall; and for footings it should never be less than 18 inches thick. The concrete serves two purposes: it, to a large extent, cuts off the entrance of the ground-air through the basement floor into the house; and prevents the entrance of damp into the house from below. To further ensure dryness where the floor is below the level of the adjacent ground, a dry area is frequently provided, that is, a closed chamber lined with stone or cement below the ground level of the house, and surrounding the underground part of its four walls, or a hollow wall is built below the ground-level, as shown in Fig. 38. Neither a dry area nor a hollow wall constitutes the best arrangement, as the cavity is usually inaccessible, and rather aids than hinders the entry of the ground air into the house. The best plan is to provide a solid wall, impervious to both moisture and air. A vertical layer of roofing slates is sometimes used for this purpose; or, still better, a narrow cavity about ½ to ¾-inch wide is provided in the body of the wall, and this is run full with molten asphalte.

The Walls of the house must be provided with a "damp-proof course" carried through their whole thickness, slightly above the highest point at which the ground is touched. It may be formed by (1) sheet lead, which possesses the disadvantage of being costly; (2) two layers of ordinary roofing slate, set in cement, with broken joints," i.e. the joints of the upper layer over the centre of the slates below them; (3) a layer of good asphalte, about ¾-inch thick; (4) perforated glazed stoneware slabs; or (5) two or three courses of hard blue Staffordshire bricks, laid without mortar. The use of asphalte is an excellent plan, and is now commonly adopted in good buildings.

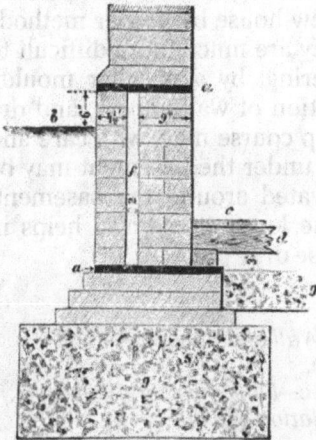

Fig. 38.
Double Damp-Proof Course and Hollow Wall. a, a—Damp-proof courses. b—Level of neighbouring ground. c—Floor-boards. d— Floor joist. f—Vertical space in wall. g— Concrete under foundation and over site of house.

(1) Rain falling on window-sills which do not project beyond the walls, and consequently do not throw the water clear of them. This is remedied by constructing the window-sills so as to project beyond the walls, and "throating" them to prevent rain from running along the bottom of the sill. The throat is shown at a, Fig. 39.

(2) Rain falling on cornices and other projecting portions of the wall itself. The evil from this source may be diminished by sloping the top of the projection, downwards from the face of the wall.

(3) Parapet walls, gables, etc., not being properly covered with coping. All such walls should be topped with a projecting slab of stone, or with a damp-proof course under the top course of bricks, which should be laid on edge.

193

(4) Overflow from defective roof-gutters or rain-water pipes. In this case, either clearing out, repairing, or renewing is required.

(5) Rain beating against the walls. This as a rule produces no great harm, if the walls are well constructed. Most of the water runs off as it falls on the surface. It is advisable, however, to protect a much exposed wall by a coating of Portland cement, or in extreme cases with slate. Various impervious paints have also been employed.

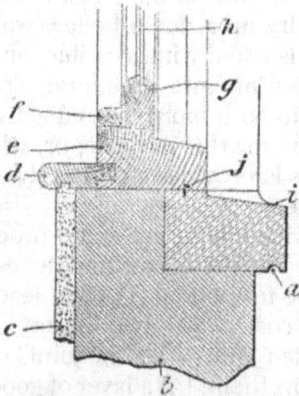

Fig. 39.
Section Through Window.
Showing stone sill "weathered" at i, and "throated" at a. b—Wall. c—Inside plaster of room. d—Window-board. e—Oak sill. f—Beading and g—bottom rail of window-sash. h—Window. j—Iron tongue let into slot in i and e to prevent rain driving in.

If it is not proposed to coat exposed surfaces of brickwork, the wall may be formed of two parallel walls, two inches apart, and tied together by a sufficient number of bonding-ties of iron or glazed stoneware, or some other non-absorbent material. This arrangement is shown in Fig. 40.

An excellent plan is to fill in the narrow space between two such walls, as the building proceeds, with asphalte or slab slate, thus forming a vertical damp course, in the same way as below the ground level. The evils arising from damp can be avoided in every new house by proper methods of construction. In an old house, however, they are much more difficult to remove. The dampness is indicated on entering, by a peculiar mouldy smell, and by the discolouration and destruction of wall-papers, and dry rotting of floor timbers. In such a case a damp course may, with care and patience, be inserted in the wall, and the soil under the basement may be covered with concrete, and a dry-area excavated around the basement. Free ventilation under the floor-boards of the lower floors also helps in keeping the house dry.

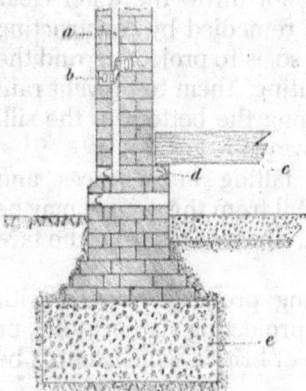

Fig. 40.
Showing Hollow Wall and Bonding-ties of Glazed Stoneware.
a—Cavity. b—Tie. c—Floor-joist. d—Wall-plate. e—Concrete foundation of wall.

The thickness of the walls of a house requires to be sufficient to ensure stability, to keep out the damp, and to prevent a too rapid loss of heat from the walls. The relative merits of the different materials employed for these purposes have been already considered. A thin-walled house is hot in summer, and cold in winter. The upper

194

stories of houses are often built with too thin walls, the result being chilly bedrooms. A single-brick wall (9 inches thick) will rarely keep out the weather effectually, and frequently a brick-and-a-half wall (14 inches thick) is insufficient for this purpose. The bricks should be so interlaced as to "bond" or tie the wall together in all directions. The strength of walls may be increased by the introduction of hoop-iron between the courses of brickwork.

In the construction of fire-places and chimneys, it is important to avoid the proximity of timber and wood-work to the inside of flues, as this is a common cause of fires.

Inside Coverings of Walls

Plaster is made of lime mortar, or cement mortar; the former is generally preferred for domestic dwellings because it remains porous and moisture does not condense on it.

In houses built by speculative builders, the plaster commonly used consists of a mixture of lime with road scrapings. The result is a composition which unless supported by the wall-papering, is soon damaged.

Ordinary plaster consists usually of three layers. The first is laid on with a mixture of about equal parts of lime and sand with long ox-hairs if required for ceilings. The second coat consists of slaked lime, mixed to the consistency of cream. The last or setting coat consists of a thin layer of slaked lime called plasterers' putty. Some plaster of Paris (gypsum) may be added, to ensure rapid setting, but it should only be used in small quantities. For the internal plastering of rooms serapite (a form of cement) is now commonly employed. This is not so absorbent as mortar, but is sufficiently so to prevent condensation of moisture on the walls. Its chief advantage over plaster is that it hardens quicker and is smoother, and can be used in a single thin layer. This, however, diminishes the impermeability of ceilings for sound.

Keene's cement and Parian cement are mixtures of calcined gypsum and other substances; Keene's cement being the hardest, and capable of receiving a high polish.

Selenitic cement contains a small proportion of plaster of Paris ground along with lime. Lime may also be selenised by the addition of any other sulphate, or of sulphuric acid. The presence of the sulphate causes the lime to set rapidly. Selenitic cement is useful in plastering, as a backing of cements, such as Parian.

The treatment of the internal wall-surface of a room differs according to circumstances. Lime-washing is suitable only for stables and other outbuildings. It is made by the addition of water to quicklime, no size being added. It is an excellent germicide and insecticide. Whitewashing is quite different from limewashing. "Whiting," i.e. finely-ground chalk, to which a certain proportion of size and alum had been added is mixed with water. The size and alum are added to prevent the whitewash from being rubbed off. Distempering is identical with whitewashing, except that pigments are added. It is distinguished from painting in oils, by the fact that the pigments are mixed with size, instead of with linseed-oil and turpentine. Painting in distemper is practically limited to plaster, which should first receive a coat of whitewash to diminish its porosity. Oil-paints are impervious, distemper is as absorbent as plaster or whitewash. Various washable distempers, as duresco, are made, which are more durable and non-absorbent. Water-glass consists of silicate of potash, which in the gelatinous form is soluble like size in hot-water, but when allowed to dry forms an impervious film. It can be used for protecting porous stone from the effects of weather; and renders internal surfaces of walls non-absorbent and washable.

Oil-painting renders wall-surfaces impervious, and enables them to be easily washed. The importance of this in the event of any infectious disease occurring, is obvious. The question arises whether distempered or papered walls, which are porous, or painted walls, which are non-porous, are preferable from the standpoint of health. The difference between the two is seen during damp weather, when moisture condenses and runs down the latter and is invisible in the former. In practice in domestic dwellings the former are preferred; but although some advantage is thus secured in ventilation through the wall-substance, there is the serious disadvantage that particles of dirt accumulate and may seriously interfere with the purity of the air of a room. Hence the importance of rubbing down the internal surface of a room, whether distempered or papered, at intervals with bread crumb or dough. This effectually removes all accumulations of dirt. A painted wall presents the enormous advantage that it can be frequently washed; while the loss of ventilation may be ignored, if windows and doors be properly utilised for this purpose. The presence of poisonous pigments in oil-paints is of importance to the workman, but not to the householder except during the painting, as paint, unlike distemper, does not rub off the wall. Lead is the chief poison present, as white lead (carbonate of lead). Various substitutes for lead paints have been introduced.

Painting wood or iron-work is valuable, not only as a preservative from the effects of the weather and the oxidising action of the air, but also because it tends, to a large extent, to prevent the absorption of organic matters; and its surface can be frequently cleansed.

Paper is the material most commonly employed for covering walls. It is more absorbent and retentive of moisture than distemper.

Light-coloured papers should be chosen, as they are more cheerful, and are not so likely to harbour dust. Glaring patterns are objectionable, as they tire the eyes. The paper should not present any surface-projection for the lodgment of dust.

In bathrooms and water-closets, the wall-surface should be non-absorbent. Paper, unless varnished, should therefore be avoided. The best covering for these places is glazed tiling, or painted cement.

Not uncommonly, a new paper is pasted over an old one; and this may be repeated several times. Under these circumstances dangerous dirt accumulates. Before new papering is put on, the walls should be cleared of

196

all vestiges of the old, thoroughly washed down, and subsequently coated with size (that is, "clear coloured"). The sizing diminishes the absorptive power of the wall, and gives a good surface for applying the paper.

Bed-room papers require to be more frequently changed than those of other rooms. Bed-rooms in regular use should be re-papered at least every two years. It is still better to use distemper for such rooms, as this can be washed off in a few hours with comparatively little expense, and can be made of any tint desired.

Rooms in the basement should not be papered, as the walls require frequent washing down and cleaning. Here also a washable distemper colour can be used.

Various kinds of sanitary paper are now sold which are washable, and relatively non-absorbent. Some of them require varnishing; others do not. Such papers are certainly cleaner than ordinary paper; but it would not be safe to trust to their non-absorptive character. Lincrusta Walton is non-absorbent, and can be scrubbed with soap and water; but it is expensive. Other cheaper materials possessing the same properties can now be bought.

Arsenic in Wall-Papers and Paints has until a few years ago been a not uncommon source of prolonged ill-health—the cause of which has possibly not been detected until the illness disappears, when the offending room is vacated for a period. Arsenical pigments are now only rarely used for wall-papers. The symptoms produced vary greatly, and may closely simulate those of different diseases. In some cases repeated attacks of diarrhœa and abdominal pain occur. Or there may be nausea, headache, frequent griping pains, and loss of appetite. In other cases restlessness, loss of sleep, and general malaise are the chief symptoms, with the occasional addition of conjunctivitis (superficial inflammation of the eye). Out of 100 cases collected and reported on by a Committee of the Medical Society of London, diarrhœa, nausea, and intestinal mischief occurred in 85; severe depression in 16; conjunctivitis in 19; and cough, asthma, etc., in 9.

The severity of the symptoms produced will vary with the amount of arsenic contained in the paper, and the length of time daily that the patient is exposed to the fumes.

Some persons again are much less susceptible to the influence of arsenic than others. This will explain why some escape while occupying the same room in which others suffer severely. More commonly, however, the exemption is due to shorter exposure.

The most dangerous preparation occasionally employed in wall paper printing is Scheele's green (arsenite of copper). Emerald-green—an aceto-arsenite of copper—is sometimes used to produce more delicate tints. Aniline dyes, especially the red, may contain much arsenious acid (white arsenic). The arsenic compound is made to adhere to the paper by size or some other material. When dry, it cracks and peels off, and minute particles get into the air as dust. In addition, arsenic compounds easily volatilise, and become diffused in a gaseous condition throughout the atmosphere of a room, even when its temperature is not greatly raised. The virulence of the arsenical colouring is in proportion to its volatility. Arsenic seems to be much more dangerous when associated with size. It has been shown that a mixture of white arsenic and starch paste, or other organic substance, leads to the formation of gaseous arseniuretted hydrogen, while this does not occur when no organic matter is present (Dr. Fleck). Distemper frequently contains arsenic, and as it also contains size, arseniurretted hydrogen is liable to be given off at any time. Size is largely used for fixing colour; thus, the proper conditions for the development of arseniurretted hydrogen—the most dangerous compound of arsenic—are present. As much as 17 grains of arsenic have been discovered in each square foot of a wall-paper. Now, arsenic is sometimes given internally for certain skin and other diseases, but the dose is only from 1/60 to 1/12 grain; the capacity for poisoning of such a paper as the above will therefore be evident.

Papers of other colours than green have been found to contain dangerous quantities of arsenic; thus blue, mauve, red, and brown may contain large quantities; the delicate greys often yield a considerable amount, and some white papers are heavily loaded with it. Arsenic is occasionally present in stockings and other wearing apparel, artificial flowers, toys, etc. In these cases, it may produce irritation of the skin, and even eczema.

The presence of arsenic may be detected by the following tests:—

(a) Reinsch's test. A portion of the suspected paper (two or three inches square) is cut into small pieces, and placed in a good-sized test tube; water is added until the tube is about a third full and then one or two teaspoonfuls of pure hydrochloric acid, and a small piece of pure copper foil. If the test tube is now heated for a few minutes over a spirit lamp, arsenic, if present, will be deposited as a black or dark steel-coloured coating on the copper. A mere tarnish of the copper must not be accepted as evidence of the presence of arsenic, but an almost complete obliteration of the colour of the copper.

(b) Take the copper covered with arsenic, dry it, and then heat it in a perfectly dry test tube. Crystals of white arsenic, which may be identified under the microscope, will be deposited higher up in the tube.

(c) Marsh's test. The ordinary apparatus for developing hydrogen by the action of diluted sulphuric acid on zinc is employed, the suspected paper being inserted in the bottle. The hydrogen coming off is burnt, and a clean porcelain surface is applied to the flame. If there is arsenic in it, it is deposited on the porcelain in a black patch.

Windows are required to open directly into the external air in every habitable room. The window area according to the model bye-laws of the Local Government Board and the London Buildings Act of 1894, must be at least one-tenth of the floor area, and half of this at least must be made to open. The following rules have also been given. (B = breadth, L = length and H = height of room.)

$$\text{Area of window} \begin{cases} (B \times L)/10 & \text{London Building Act} \\ (B \times L \times H)/100 & \text{Gwilt} \end{cases}$$

In a room measuring 15 × 20 × 12 feet, the preceding rules would give a superficial area of window space of 30, 36, and 60 square feet respectively. Plate glass dissipates heat less quickly than sheet glass.

Objection may be taken to plate glass windows, in passing, especially for shops, banks, etc., in view of the fact that they are commonly made without any arrangement for ventilation.

The hygienic necessities of Floors are that they shall be impervious to moisture and to dust. On the ground floor the ordinary arrangement is to provide a joisted and boarded floor raised about a foot above the ground. Dry rot is one of the dangers in connection with such boarded floors on the ground floor. The chief causes which tend to induce rotting, are damp walls, lack of ventilation, contact with mortar, damp earth, or vegetable mould, and worst of all, alternations of damp and dryness, or wet along with heat.

In order to avoid these dangers in connection with boarded floors, the ends of all timbers resting on walls should have a clear air-space around them, and communicate with the external air by means of perforated bricks. The larger timbers, girders, etc., should rest on stone templates, and the smaller joists on hoop-iron bonds. In all cases, the timber used should be well seasoned, and properly ventilated. The ends of oak posts, which are to be driven into the ground, should be charred, if the timber is old, or steeped in a solution of chloride of zinc.

The ends of the joists should be trimmed, so as not to come too near to chimney flues.

The best plan for flooring is to place an impervious flooring resting on the solid ground. This is more secure against rot than the boarded floor, and affords no space for dirt and vermin to lodge. Such an impervious floor may be formed of concrete over a layer of asphalte, as in the well-known terrazzo flooring. This is very suitable for corridors, pantries, etc. For living-rooms wood-block flooring is placed over the cement, molten pitch connecting the two. The blocks are 2 to 3 inches thick. If the wood is soft, as deal, it must be kept clean by washing; if hard, as oak or teak, it can be wax-polished. Parquetry consists of small pieces of hard woods carefully fixed and polished.

For upper floors the ordinary flooring is of floor-boards supported on wood joists, beneath which are wood laths and plaster. The floor-boards should be thoroughly seasoned, otherwise they will shrink, and the joints be filled with dirt. This dirt may accumulate for years between the floor and the ceiling of the room below, vitiating the air and helping to increase the stuffiness characteristic of dirty houses. Various plans are adopted for uniting the edges of floor-boards and preventing dust from dropping between the boards.

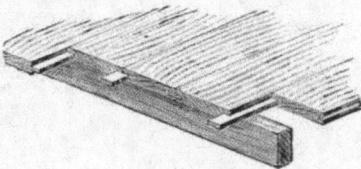

Fig. 41.
Tongued Floor.

The one most commonly employed is the ploughed and tongued floor (Fig. 41). In this, both edges of the floor are grooved so as to receive strips or tongues of iron or wood, an equal half of each strip being in the groove of each of two boards when they are in place. A less expensive method than the above is to splay the ends of the boards so that they slightly overlap each other. This is not so efficient as the above, but is much better than simply placing the boards side to side as is commonly done.

Solid wood floors resting on a bed of concrete are free from the risk of harbouring dust, and are relatively fire-proof.

Oak or teak in narrow boards, made with close joints, and then oiled and beeswaxed and rubbed to a polish, makes a good and almost non-absorptive floor. One of the best floors is made of concrete, with iron joists, and oak boards laid above this.

Carpets are commonly made to cover the entire floor of rooms. This cannot be too much deprecated. Carpets, like curtains, are mere dirt-traps, which become loaded with filth of every description. This is abundantly proved when a carpet is swept, and the dust allowed to settle on all the articles in the room. Such dust, if examined, will be found to consist not only of mineral matter, but also of every description of vegetable and animal impurities. The inhalation of such dust, which may contain particles of fæcal matter, as well as the dried expectoration from consumptive or other infectious patients, is a not infrequent cause of infection to healthy persons.

The substitution of a central carpet, for one covering the entire floor, is a great improvement.

The carpet should be easily removable, in order that it and the floor may be thoroughly cleaned at intervals.

In bedrooms, the less carpet the better. Good Chinese or Indian matting is serviceable, as it does not retain the dust and other impurities which are apt to become fixed in the woolly texture of the carpet. Oil-cloth, linoleum, and similar materials are in common use for covering halls, passages, etc. They are particularly useful in preventing dust from gaining access to the spaces between floor-boards.

The prevention of dust should be the great aim of the householder, as dirt frequently carries infection. Sweeping as ordinarily done scatters dirt over the room, and dusting with a dry cloth fails to remove it. Mechanical sweepers, in which the dirt is collected in a box are valuable. The best plan is to have movable carpets, roll them up for shaking or beating at a distance from any house, and wipe the boards with damp cloths. All wooden and leather furniture, picture frames, etc., should be wiped down with cloths rung out of water so as to be just damp.

CHAPTER XXXIII

THE SOIL

The Varieties of Soil.—The following facts summarise what is regarded as the relative healthiness of various sites for dwellings. The differences between different sites may, however, be reduced to a minimum by having the dwelling well above the ground-level and by protecting it from dampness.

1. Granitic, Metamorphic, and Trap Rocks usually form healthy sites for houses. The slope is generally great, and the ground consequently dry.

2. Clay Slate resembles the last in its effects on health. Water is, however, often scarce, owing to the impermeability of the rocks, and for the same reason occasional floods occur.

3. Limestone and Magnesian Limestone Rocks resemble the last in possessing considerable slope, so that the water passes away quickly. The hard oolite is the best formation under this head, and magnesian limestone the worst.

4. Chalk is a healthy soil when unmixed with clay, and permeable. Goitre is not so common as in limestone districts. If the chalk be mixed with clay, it is often damp and cold.

5. The Sandstones are healthy, soil and air being dry. If mixed with clay, or if clay lie under a shallow layer of sand-rock, the site may be damp. The hard millstone grit is a healthy formation.

6. Gravels of any depth are healthy, unless they are water-logged, as near rivers. Then a house on impervious clay may be drier than one on gravel.

7. Sands are healthy when of considerable depth; they may be unhealthy when shallow, and lying on a clay basis; or when the ground water rises through them from ground at a higher level.

8. Clay, Dense Marls, and Alluvial Soils generally, are apt to be cold and damp. Water is retained in them, and is often very impure. Thorough drainage improves a clay soil, and a house on a clay soil may be so constructed, as not to be damp.

9. Cultivated Soils are not necessarily unhealthy; but

10. Made Soils are always to be carefully avoided, as sites for houses. The materials with which inequalities have been filled up are commonly the contents of dust-bins, or some other refuse. The gradual putrefaction of organic matters renders the air about the houses impure. Such soils require free subsoil drainage, in order to keep them dry. It appears that the organic matters in soil are gradually removed by oxidation and bacterial purification. At least three years should be allowed before any such site is built on.

The following table places different geological formations in their order of healthiness for the purposes of a site (Parkes):—

	PERMEABILITY OF WATER	EMANATIONS INTO AIR
1. Primitive rocks, clay slate, millstone grit	Slight.	None.
2. Gravel and loose sands, with permeable subsoils	Great.	Slight.
3. Sandstones	Variable.	Slight.
4. Limestones	Moderate.	—
5. Sands with impermeable subsoils	Arrested by subsoils.	Considerable.
6. Clays, marls, alluvial soils	Slight.	Considerable.
7. Marshes, when not peaty	Slight.	Considerable.

The general geological conditions have an important bearing on the choice of a site for a house in so far as they affect the local climate, and the difficulty of keeping the house warm and dry. Pettenkofer expressed this in his dictum, that we take holiday for change of soil, rather than for change of air. The character of a soil has an important influence on humidity, radiation, evaporation, and in fact most of the factors going to make up "climate." The immediate local surroundings of a house have an even greater influence on its salubrity than the underlying geological formation.

The soil consists of mineral and organic matters. On the amount and character of the animal and vegetable matters (along with the condition of moisture and aeration), the healthiness of a given soil depends. The presence of vegetable matter, subject to alternate wettings and dryings, and to heat, has until recently been regarded as the condition on which malaria depends; but it is now known that malarial places owe their character to their being favourable to the growth of the larvæ of certain mosquitoes; and that drainage of the soil cures malaria by removing the ponds in which these develop. The two chief agencies at work to rid the soil of organic impurities, are nitrification and the influence of growing plants. The organic matters become oxidised into ammonia, nitrites, and nitrates, and these are eagerly assimilated by vegetation.

Nitrification is effected by micro-organisms in the soil. Ordinary garden mould and agricultural humus contain large numbers of micro-organisms. Their number diminishes with the depth of the soil, and below 12 to 15 feet there are few. Apart from the occasional presence of pathogenic (disease-producing) micro-organisms, the most important are those producing oxidation of organic matter, especially nitrification. This occurs at a less depth than 4 feet from the surface of the ground. The operation of these micro-organisms is necessary to convert sewage and other impurities into harmless nitrites and nitrates, and it is regularly going on in all normal soils. That the power of purification of sewage by soil is due to the micro-organisms in the latter, can be proved by the fact that when the soil is baked, it loses for a time its purifying power.

The Air contained in the Soil varies greatly in amount with the character of the soil, and with the level of the ground-water. As the ground-water rises, the ground-air is driven out. Thus, after a heavy rainfall a large proportion of this air will be displaced. Variations in barometric pressure, and a rise or fall of temperature, cause movements in ground-air. A house artificially warmed is liable to receive air from underground, unless means are adopted to make the floors impervious. The warmth of the house acts as an air-pump, aspirating the colder air into its interior. The air from cesspools or defective drains may be similarly aspirated into the house; and the same cause particularly explains the unhealthiness of houses built on "made soils". Coal gas has occasionally made its way into houses when not laid on to them, by the gas escaping from leaky pipes in the street often following the track of water or drain-pipes until it is aspirated from beneath the house into its interior. This has resulted in one instance in an explosion, and in others in poisoning by the gas.

Fig. 42.

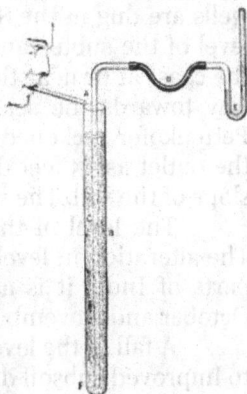

The occurrence of currents of air in soil may be illustrated by a simple experiment. In Fig. 42 B is filled with fine sand in which is imbedded the tube A with its open end F at the bottom of the sand C. The upper end of A is connected by the rubber tubing D with the U-shaped tube E, in which is inserted some coloured water. When the experimenter blows on the surface of the sand at A, the impulse passes through the sand up the tube from F, and deflects the water in the syphon bend at E.

The amount of ground-air varies greatly. Loose sands often contain 40 to 50 per cent., soft sandstone 20 to 40 per cent., and loose surface-soil many times its own volume.

The nature of the air is not accurately known. It is, however, extremely rich in carbonic acid, of which it contains from 1 to 10 per cent. or even more. The carbonic acid is derived from the organic matter in the soil, by the action of bacteria, in a manner analogous to nitrification.

The Water contained in the Soil is divided into moisture and ground or subsoil-water. When air is present in the soil as well as water, the soil is merely moist. Pettenkofer defines the ground-water as that condition in which all the interstices are filled with water, so that, except in so far as its particles are separated by solid portions of soil, there is a continuous sheet of water.

The Moisture in the soil varies in amount. Open gravel will absorb from 9 to 13 per cent. by weight of water; gravelly surface soil 48 per cent.; light sandy soils from 23 to 36 per cent.; loamy soil 43 per cent.; stiff land and clay soils from 43·3 to 57·6 per cent.; sandy and peaty soils from 61·5 to 80 per cent.; peat 103 per cent. (B. Latham). The moisture being derived from the rainfall on one side, and the ground-water on the other, will vary with the amount of these. Some soils are practically impermeable to water, such as trap or metamorphic rocks, unweathered granite, hard limestone, and dense clay; while others, such as chalk, sand, sandstone, vegetable soils are permeable. Commonly the metamorphic rocks and hard

203

limestones present fissures, which render them pervious. The rainfall which does not penetrate the soil flows into the streams and rivers at once, or is re-evaporated. The amount of percolation of rainfall is estimated by an artificial soil-gauge. Most percolation and least evaporation of rainfall occurs from October to March inclusive. The difference between the percolation and rainfall is the loss caused by evaporation and vegetation.

The Ground-water forms a subterranean sheet of water, which is in constant motion. There is first of all, an irregular rise and fall of the water, according as it receives new additions from the rainfall, or loses a certain amount of its substance by percolation and evaporation; and there is, secondly, a constant movement towards the nearest water-course or the sea. Many towns derive their drinking-water from the ground-water, especially that in the chalk. Thus in Brighton there are no streams; but wells are dug in the South Downs about 150 to 180 feet deep down to the level of the subterranean water. Then long adits are tunnelled, parallel to the coast at or near the level of this water, which is thus intercepted on its way towards the sea, and pumped up to supply the town. In Munich, Pettenkofer reckoned the rate of movement of the ground water towards the outlet as 15 feet daily. It is impeded by impermeability, or a deficient slope of the soil. The roots of trees also greatly impede its flow.

The level of the ground-water is constantly changing (see Fig. 7). The alteration in level may be only a few inches either way, while in some parts of India it is as much as 16 feet. The level is generally lowest in October and November, highest in February and March.

A fall in the level of the ground-water may be due to a dry season, or to improved subsoil drainage. A rise in its level is due to an increase in the rainfall, or some obstruction in the outflow, as from a swollen river. The tide may influence the level of the ground-water at a great distance. A sudden alteration in the level of the ground-water is a common cause of floods in mines.

The distance of the ground-water from the surface may be only two or three feet, or several hundred feet, the difference being due to the varying level of the nearest impervious stratum of soil. Its distance below the surface of the soil can easily be measured by ascertaining that of the water of a shallow well in the neighbourhood. It should preferably not be nearer the surface than five or six feet. Sudden changes in the level of the ground-water from inundations render any soil unhealthy, and are even more objectionable than a persistently high level. This is especially true in the case of permeable soils. A sudden rising of ground-water expels the air in the soil, together possibly with particles which may comprise infectious material; it also washes similar impurities out of the subsoil, and carries them into neighbouring wells. Numerous epidemics have been traced to this source.

The Temperature of the Soil varies greatly with its geological character, as well as with the temperature of the atmosphere. The daily changes in the temperature of the atmosphere do not affect the soil beyond a depth of about three feet. The annual changes in the atmosphere will affect the soil in a varying degree, the amount being dependent on the character of the soil as regards conductivity and retentiveness for heat. Such annual variations do not penetrate below forty feet, and are very small below twenty-four feet. The temperature of the earth increases with its depth, the rate of increase in England being stated to be about 1° Fahr. for every 54½ feet.

In England the water of permanent springs has a fairly constant temperature of 49° to 51° Fahr., which is the temperature of the deeper part of the subsoil. The method of taking the daily temperature of the subsoil at a depth of 4 feet is described on page 220.

Although the average temperature of any soil depends on the climate, soils conduct heat in a very varying degree, and therefore absorb unequal quantities. This has an important bearing on the comfort of those living on a particular soil. Schübler's experiments give the absorbing power of the chief kinds of soil, 100 being taken as the standard.

Sand, with some lime	100·0
Pure sand	95·6
Light clay	76·9
Gypsum	73·2
Heavy clay	71·1
Clayey earth	68·4
Pure clay	66·7
Fine chalk	61·8
Humus	49·0

It is evident from this table that sand is very retentive of heat, while clays and humus are very cold. Green vegetation lessens the absorbing power of the soil, and radiation of heat is more rapid, evaporation occurring constantly from the herbage.

Damp soils are colder than dry soils because of the evaporation going on. Buchan finds as the result of drainage of the soil, that (1) the mean temperature of arable land is raised 0·8° Fahr.; (2) cold is propagated more quickly through undrained land; (3) drained land loses less heat by evaporation; (4) the temperature of drained land is more equable, and (5) in summer is often 1·5° to 3° above that of undrained land.

DISEASES ARISING FROM THE SOIL.—The soil may be a cause of disease: (a) indirectly and (b) directly.

Indirectly a damp soil may cause disease by acting as a means of lowering the vitality of man and diminishing his resistance to disease. It is in this way that it has been credited with causing such diseases as neuralgia, catarrhs, and rheumatism. It is one of the elements in producing a climate unfavourable to health.

Directly the soil may transmit the actual contagia (micro-organisms) of disease either by means of the subsoil water or its air. In the former case the disease-causing material gains access to the drinking water of wells, springs, or rivers; in the latter case it may be borne to the surface of the soil by currents of the ground-air or by insects, and then inhaled as dust, or gain access to food.

Certain disease-producing micro-organisms have been proved to be

205

capable of living for some time in the soil. The chief of these found in the soil are the bacilli of tetanus (lockjaw), of anthrax, of malignant oedema, and of enteric (typhoid) fever. There are reasons for thinking also that the micro-organisms causing diphtheria, rheumatic fever, and epidemic diarrhœa, and possibly some other diseases, may occasionally live in the soil. In some diseases as enteric fever, cholera, dysentery and anthrax, the contamination of the soil can be shown to be derived from a patient suffering from the same diseases. In others, and particularly in tetanus, the same chain of evidence is obtainable.

(1) The conditions favourable to the production of malarial diseases have been generally considered to be the presence of a certain proportion of dead organic matter, the exposure of the soil to alternations of heat and moisture, with a limited access of air, and a temperature of at least 65°F. Though most common in marshy districts, and in recent alluvial soils, malaria may develop in connection with any geological formation. That it may be removed by drainage of the subsoil, is well known.

(2) According to observations made by Pettenkofer in Munich, attacks of enteric (typhoid) fever are connected with fluctuations of the subsoil-water. He states his conclusions as follows:—

"Between the fluctuations of subsoil water and the amount and severity of enteric fever there is an unmistakable connection in this wise, that the total number of cases of and deaths from enteric fever falls with a rise of the subsoil water, and rises with fall of it; that the level reached by the disease is not in proportion, however, to the then level of the subsoil water, but only to the variation in it on each occasion; or in other words, that it is not the high or low level of the subsoil water that is decisive, but only the range of fluctuation."

His observations have not been confirmed in this country; and the coincidence between excess of enteric fever and lowness of ground-water has been explained by the fact that under these circumstances the water in wells is low, and the area of drainage and the consequent risk of contamination are proportionately increased. There can be no doubt that the most common origin of enteric fever is from the infection of water or milk by infective matter from a recent case of the disease. This does not exclude the fact that enteric fever in this country is more prevalent in hot dry autumns, in which the ground water is low. Probably under such conditions the contagium of the disease multiples more rapidly in the soil, in privies and other polluted places, and consequently the risks of infection of water and food as well of infection by dust carried from the contaminated spot are greatly increased.

(3) In regard to cholera, Pettenkofer holds similar views. He believes that the contagium of cholera can only be developed when there is a damp porous subsoil to receive the infected stools from a cholera patient; the damp porous subsoil forming a second host in which the poison of cholera must pass through one stage of its existence, before it is again capable of producing the disease. Such an essential relationship of the soil is not borne out by observations in India; and in England cholera has been repeatedly shown to be due to contamination of food (e.g. oysters) or water

by the stools of preceding cholera patients, without the intervention of any agency of the soil.

(4) It has been repeatedly stated that a damp soil favours the prevalence of diphtheria. I have shown elsewhere, however, that this is not true, and that the greatest epidemics of diphtheria have occurred in exceptionally dry years, especially when several years of exceptionally small rainfall have succeeded each other; and have suggested that this may be associated with an intermediate stage in the life-history of the diphtheria-bacillus in the soil. A low ground-water and a comparatively high temperature of the soil go along with deficient rainfall, and would probably favour the multiplication of this bacillus in the soil.

(5) In rheumatic fever I have similarly shown that the supposed connection between damp soil and this disease is erroneous, the disease being most prevalent, both in this and other countries, in years of exceptional drought.

(6) Epidemic or Summer Diarrhœa has been supposed to have a special relationship with soil-temperature, Ballard having found that the summer rise in the mortality from this disease does not commence until the mean temperature recorded by the four-foot earth thermometer has attained somewhere about 56°F. The soil-temperature may be accepted as a convenient index of the conditions causing this disease. The disease I have elsewhere shown occurs most severely with a high temperature of the air and a deficient rainfall, and its fundamental cause is an unclean soil, the particulate poison from which infects the air, and is swallowed most commonly with food, especially milk.

(7) The close connection of consumption (phthisis) with a damp soil has been independently stated by Drs. Buchanan and Bowditch. Buchanan found that in the districts where improved sanitary arrangements had led to a drying of the soil, the death-rate from phthisis diminished; but where with sanitary improvements the soil was not dried, the death-rate from phthisis remained in one or two instances almost stationary. In Salisbury, Ely, Rugby, and Banbury, the death-rate from phthisis fell from 141 to 49 per cent. The amount of reduction in the death-rate from phthisis did not appear to be consistently proportional to the amount of drying of the subsoil. In a later investigation into the incidence of deaths from phthisis in the south-east of England, Buchanan came to the further conclusions that (a) there was less phthisis among populations living on pervious soils than among populations living in impervious soils; (b) less phthisis among populations living on high-lying pervious soils than among populations living on low-lying pervious soils; and (c) less phthisis among populations living on sloping impervious soils than among populations living on flat impervious soils. He, therefore, concluded that wetness of soil is a cause of phthisis to the population living upon it.

Drainage of the Soil.—There are two chief plans for rendering the soil drier—deep drainage and opening the outflow.

Subsoil Drainage should always be carried out by drains, separate from those for sewage. If the sewers are utilised for this purpose, their contents when full contaminate the surrounding soil. The subsoil drains should be composed of agricultural, i.e. unglazed, drain-pipes laid in towns in the same trench, but above the sewers, and they should discharge into the nearest water-course. If it is necessary to join them with a sewer, they should not pass directly into it, but into a disconnecting man-hole.

Opening the Outflow, in order that water may not remain stagnant in the soil, is occasionally required. This may be done by clearing water-courses, removing obstructions, and forming fresh channels.

The provision of sufficient surface-drains to carry off ordinary water and storm-water helps in drying the soil of urban districts.

Vegetation tends to diminish dampness of soil by causing rapid evaporation, and at the same time uses up the organic matter in the soil. Certain plants are more active in producing these effects than others: the Eucalyptus genus, including many species, and represented by the well-known blue-gum tree of Australia, is noted for its power in this respect; and the common sun-flower, which is very easy of cultivation, has a powerful influence in the same direction.

CHAPTER XXXIV

CLIMATE AND WEATHER

The Climate of a country has an important influence on the health and character of its inhabitants. The character of a climate depends on four main conditions:—

    1. The distance from the equator.
    2. The height above the sea.
    3. The distance from the sea.
    4. The prevailing winds.

There are other conditions which are of subsidiary importance, but which have great influence in modifying the climate of any given locality. Thus:—

    5. The nature of a surface—its aspect, shelter, slope; the colour of the soil or rock, the reflection from rocks or sheets of water, and the influence of vegetation.
    6. The cultivation of the soil.
    7. The drainage of marshes and damp soils.
    8. The planting and clearing away of forests.

The Distance from the Equator is the most important factor in relation to climate. The sun's rays become less powerful as they fall more obliquely, in travelling from the equator. This primary factor in producing climate is largely modified, however, by the relative distribution of land and water, and by the character of the prevailing winds of a district.

The Elevation of a locality affects the temperature and the barometric pressure, both falling as the height is increased. The amount of fall varies with the latitude of the place, with its situation in regard to surrounding districts, the degree of moisture of the air, the presence of winds, the hour of day, and the season of the year. It is usual to allow 1° Fahr. for every 300 feet of ascent above the level of the sea, and one-thousandth part of an inch depression of the barometer for every increase of one foot in height.

Hills, Plain and Valley.—The law of decrease of temperature with increase of altitude, is liable to great modifications, and even subversions, from various causes. The chief cause producing such modification of the law is the elevation in relation to the surrounding district. Thus, in the case of rising ground, the higher parts become rapidly cooled by radiation. The air here is likewise cooled by contact, and becoming heavier in consequence, flows down to low-lying ground. Hence places on rising ground are not so fully exposed to the intensity of frosts at night as places in the valley.

Valleys surrounded by hills and high grounds, not only retain their own cold and heavy air, but serve as reservoirs for the cold air falling from neighbouring heights. One finds, in consequence, mists in low situations, while adjoining eminences are quite clear.

The air of mountains is (1) cooler than that of lower districts with the exception already named. (2) It is less dense in proportion to the altitude; its pressure at the height of 16,000 feet being only half that at the sea level. (3) Its absolute humidity is decidedly diminished; there is some difference of opinion as to the relative humidity. (4) The air is as a rule purer. It is generally free from dust, and to a large extent aseptic (that is, free from microbes). (5) The amount of ozone is commonly greater than in lower regions. In addition to these characters, (6) the light is intense, and (7) the direct heat of the sun is greater, and the difference between sun and shade greater than in lower regions.

Owing to these peculiarities of mountain air, it is of great value as a restorative. The circulation of blood is increased, nutrition is improved, the chest expands, and the increase in its size may be permanent.

The presence of forests and sheets of water counteracts the effects of radiation from the earth. Thus if a deep lake fills the basin of a valley, the cold air descending from higher levels cools the surface water, which sinks and is replaced by warmer water from below. In this way deep lakes are sources of heat in winter, and places on their shores are free from the severe frosts which are peculiar to other low-lying situations.

If the slopes of a hill are covered with trees the temperature of its sides and base are considerably increased, as the trees obstruct the descending currents of cold air. The frosts of winter are felt most severely in localities where the slopes above them are destitute of vegetation, and especially of trees. It follows that in any given locality, the best protection against the winter cold is ensured by a dwelling situated on a slope a little

209

above the plain or valley from which it rises, with a southern exposure, and sheltered by trees planted above it. Such local conditions should always be carefully enquired into, when a choice of site is possible, as the temperature of one part of a neighbourhood may differ by several degrees from that of another part near at hand. This is particularly important in the case of invalids.

Forests tend to modify a climate, and mitigate its extremes, whether situated on the slopes of mountains or on plains. In America, as elsewhere, the effect of destruction of forests has been to produce greater variation in the annual rainfall, to lengthen periods of drought, and to increase the power of floods and cloud bursts. Trees are heated and cooled by radiation like other bodies, but from their slow conducting power, the periods of their maximum and minimum temperatures are not reached for some hours after the same phases of the temperature of the air, and the effects of radiation are not confined to a small surface on the soil, but distributed to the level of the tree-tops. For these reasons, trees make night warmer and day cooler, thus giving to forest districts something of the character of an island climate. Evaporation occurs slowly from the damp soil beneath trees, as it is screened from the sun, and the trees prevent a free circulation of wind. Hence the relative humidity and rainfall are increased. At the same time forests mitigate the disintegrating effect of the rainfall on the soil.

Ground covered with Vegetation has a more uniform temperature than bare soil, the effect being much the same as that of forests, though on a smaller scale.

All growing vegetation evaporates a large quantity of water. A plant evaporates 200 pounds of water while it forms one pound of woody fibre; the effect of a forest must, therefore, be enormous. At the same time, vegetation, and especially trees, retain moisture in the soil. The water-supply of barren regions may be greatly increased by planting trees.

The absence of vegetation leads to extreme fluctuations of temperature. An extent of sand, for instance, raises the temperature of the air greatly during the day, as it is a bad conductor; but at night, radiation is very great, and the temperature falls accordingly.

Relation of Sea to Climate.—Water has the greatest specific heat of any known substance, being four times greater than that of the earth's crust. On this account it takes longer to heat and to cool than the earth. Unlike the earth, likewise, it allows free penetration of the sun's rays,—in clear water probably to a depth of at least 600 feet; consequently, the surface of the water becomes less rapidly heated. The freezing point of fresh water is 32°, while that of sea-water is 27·5°-28·4°. Thus, the sea remains open at a temperature at which inland lakes freeze, and has, therefore, a greater influence in moderating winter cold and summer heat. Another factor rendering it more competent to mitigate extremes of temperature than lakes, is the presence of currents, causing admixture of the water of different climates. Of these currents the most important for this country is the Gulf Stream, an immense stream of water which, when it leaves the Gulf of Mexico, is travelling at the rate of four to five miles an hour, and has a surface temperature of 88° F.

It is important to distinguish between the surface temperature and the deep-sea temperature, the latter being fairly constant. The whole of the depths of the sea is filled with water at or near 32° Fahr., which in the tropics is 40°-50° below the temperature of the surface-water.

The influence of seas on climate is so great as to lead to a classification of climates into oceanic, insular, and continental.

An oceanic climate is least liable to violent changes of temperature. It can only be obtained by a sea-voyage.

An insular climate presents smaller differences between the temperature of summer and winter than the interior of great continents, especially when the island is small and in the midst of the ocean. In the British Islands, the prevailing winds being westerly, places on the east coast are less truly insular than similarly situated ones on the west coast; and their climate approaches more nearly that of inland countries.

A continental climate is drier and more subject to extreme alternations of temperature than insular and oceanic climates.

Isothermal lines (lines of equal mean temperature) around the world bend up and down, the bendings being determined by the relative position of continents and oceans. New York has the same mean temperature as London, though New York is as far south of London as Madrid. This fact illustrates the fallacy in judging of the climate of a locality by the annual mean temperature. Means, it has been well said, are general truths but particular fallacies. One should know the extremes of temperature, and the extremes for each month of the year, as well as the amount and distribution of the rainfall, and the amount of sunshine, before judging of a local climate.

Winds are due to differences in atmospheric pressure caused by changes in temperature and moisture. Inasmuch as the temperature and degree of moisture of air vary with the prevailing winds, their consideration becomes very important. Winds bring with them the temperature of the air they have traversed: thus, in England, south winds are warm, while north winds are cold. Winds coming over an ocean cause less variation in temperature than those which have passed over an extensive tract of country. Thus, moist ocean winds are accompanied by a mild winter and cool summer, while dry continental winds cause the reverse conditions. The amount of moisture capable of being carried by a current of air increases with its temperature; therefore, equatorial winds become moister as they proceed, while north winds become drier. The south-west winds, in the British Isles, being both oceanic and equatorial, are very moist, while the north-east winds, being both northerly and continental, are peculiarly dry and parching.

Owing to the atmospheric pressure diminishing from the south of Europe northwards to Iceland, south-west winds are the most prevalent in Great Britain; and as this diminution of atmospheric pressure is greatest in the winter months, south-west winds are most common at this season. The result is that the temperature of these islands is higher than that due to mere latitude, and the temperature on the west coast is fairly uniform from Shetland to Wales.

211

Mountain ranges have an important bearing in determining the character of the prevailing winds. If the range is perpendicular to the direction of the winds, the latter lose the greater part of their moisture, and the places to leeward being exposed more completely to solar and terrestrial radiation (from comparative absence of aqueous vapour), winter becomes colder and summer hotter. The difference between the climates of the west and east parts of Great Britain is largely due to this cause. In Ireland, the mountains are not grouped in ranges running north and south, but in isolated masses, and the difference in climate between the east and west coasts is consequently less marked.

The prevailing winds have a great influence on the rainfall. (1) Thus if the wind has traversed a considerable extent of ocean, the rainfall is moderately large. (2) If a wind reaches into a colder region, its saturation point is lowered, and the rainfall is greatly increased; and if a range of mountains lies across its path, the rainfall on the side facing the wind is greatly increased, but diminished on the opposite side of the range. (3) If a wind after reaching land proceeds into lower latitudes or warmer regions, the rainfall is small, or absent. This accounts for the rainless summers of California, North Africa, and South Europe.

The Barometric Pressure varies daily, being at its maximum at about 9 a.m. and 9 p.m. The average range in the tropics amounts to 0·1 inch, but in this country does not usually exceed 0·02 inches. During the year the minimum barometric pressure usually occurs about the end of October, while the maximum is usually at the end of May or early in June. The ordinary variations in barometric pressure with changes of weather have little apparent effect on health; but more extreme changes produce marked effect. In mountain-climbing faintness and nausea may be caused at great altitudes. At the opposite extreme, in pier-driving and laying the foundations of bridges, men have to work in air-chambers at a pressure of from three to four atmospheres. Then what is known as "caisson disease" may be produced. The usual symptoms are discomfort or pain in the ears, giddiness, bleeding at the nose, vomiting, or even temporary paralysis. In such occupations it is most important that on leaving the air-chambers the atmospheric pressure should be gradually lowered.

The use of the barometer as a weather indicator is based on the fact that moist air is lighter than dry air. Hence, if the air is moist and rain imminent, the barometer falls rapidly. The maximum daily range in this country is rarely greater than 3 inches. Weather observations can be based on records kept at one spot. Their value is greatly enhanced, when such observations are compared with others distributed over a wide area. The wider the area from which such observations are collated, the more accurate the deductions that can be secured. If observations of places at which the barometrical pressure is identical be recorded on a map, we have a synoptic map, and the lines of equal barometrical pressure connecting these points are called isobars. The modern development of meteorology, enabling forecasts of weather to be made with approximate accuracy, is based chiefly on telegraphic communication of information, enabling isobars to be constructed.

It is found that isobars arrange themselves into seven chief forms (1) Cyclones. (2) Secondary cyclones. (3) V-shaped depressions. (4) Anticyclones. (5) Wedge-shaped isobars. (6) Cols. (7) Straight isobars.

Each of these varieties is shown in Fig. 43, which embraces the conditions in Europe, the eastern part of the United States, and over the North Atlantic on a certain day.

The closeness of the isobars, i.e. the rapidity of changes in atmospheric pressure determines the barometric gradient. The steeper this gradient, the greater the velocity of the wind in any given place. The distance between two isobars is equal to a change of a tenth of an inch in the mercury in the barometer. The direction of the wind in a given place is from the higher to the lower isobars. This is expressed in Buys Ballot's law, which states that in the northern hemisphere, if you stand with your back to the wind, the lowest pressure is to your left and in front.

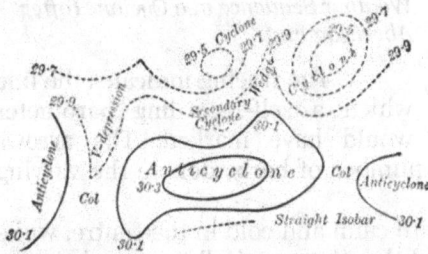

Fig. 43.
The Seven Fundamental Shapes of Isobars (*after Abercrombie*).

Cyclones or depressions are areas of low barometric pressure. A cyclonic system (Fig. 43) is formed by circles of concentric isobars. The differences between cyclones and anti-cyclones are as follows:—

Cyclones.	Anti-cyclones.
Wind moves in the opposite direction to the hands of a watch.	Wind moves in same direction as the hands of a watch.
Barometer is lowest in the centre.	Barometer is highest in the centre.
Area comparatively small.	Area comparatively large.
Gradient from centre to circumference steep.	Gradient not steep.
Short duration.	Long duration.
Velocity of wind great.	Air comparatively quiet.
Weather bad; much rainfall.	Weather fine.
Cool in summer; warm in winter.	Hot in summer; cold and frosty in winter.

Cyclones usually travel from west to east, and are always associated with bad weather. The essential point in determining the character of the weather, both in cyclones and anti-cyclones, is the barometric gradient. Thus, according to the gradient, a cyclone may mean mild wet weather, a gale, or a hurricane. The turning point of a cyclone, just before the barometer begins to rise again, is called the trough. Cyclones are usually oval in shape, except in the tropics, where they are smaller and circular. The ordinary course of events in a cyclone is shown in Fig. 44, reading it from left to right.

213

In Secondary Cyclones, bad weather is usually associated with a stationary barometer and no wind. They are incompletely circular looped concentric isobars, with the lowest pressure in the centre. They frequently follow primary cyclones.

V-shaped Depressions are angular areas, with the lowest pressure in the centre, frequently forming between adjoining anti-cyclones (Fig. 43). In the northern hemisphere the tip usually points south. They usually move with great rapidity from east to west, and are always associated with squalls or thunderstorms. Their movement is very uncertain, and their forecast therefore more difficult than that of cyclones and anti-cyclones.

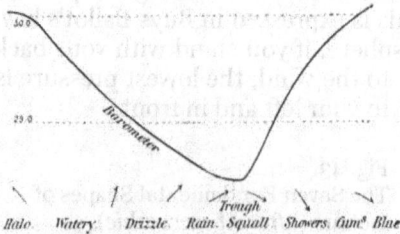

Fig. 44.
Weather Sequence in a Cyclone (after Abercrombie).

The tracing indicates the line which a self-recording barometer would have marked. The arrows mark the shift of the wind, and the number of barbs denote the varying force of the wind.

Anti-cyclones are associated with calm and cold in the centre, while on the borders the wind blows around the centre, spirally outwards in the direction of the hands of a clock. An anti-cyclone is usually accompanied by a blue sky, dry cold air, a hot sun, a hazy horizon, and little or no wind.

Wedge-shaped Isobars, unlike V's, usually point north. They are areas of high pressure moving along between two cyclones, being really projecting parts of an anti-cyclone. The fine weather accompanying them is only temporary, because they are never stationary, and are generally followed by cyclonic disturbances. At the narrow end of the wedge thunderstorms or showers often occur, and at the wide end fog is common.

Cols or necks of relatively low barometric pressure occur between two anticyclonic areas. Like straight isobars they are intermediate systems. Over cols the weather is dull and gloomy; in summer they may be associated with thunderstorms.

Straight Isobars obviously do not enclose any area of high or low pressure. They form an intermediate condition, preceding the formation of a cyclone; and are usually associated with a blustering wind and hard sky.

Weather forecasting is necessarily somewhat difficult and uncertain. If one is dependent on observations at a single point the following rules are useful:—

(a) If the barometer falls slowly and steadily bad weather will follow.
(b) The barometer falls for rain with S.W., S.E., and W. winds.
(c) When the barometer falls rapidly, heavy storms may be expected.
(d) The barometer rises rapidly for unsettled weather.
(e) The barometer rises gradually for fine, settled weather.

The Thermometer also is of great value as a weather indicator,

214

especially if one knows what is the average temperature at the place of observation for each day of the year. Thus:—

(a) A temperature continued for some time above or below the average, indicates a probable change.

(b) Electric storms follow unusual warmth in summer.

(c) A low thermometer and almost steady barometer are succeeded in winter by gales from N.N.W. or N.E.

The veering of the wind in England is also useful as an indicator. Thus:—

(a) When the wind, in shifting, goes round in the same direction as the hands of a clock—i.e., from N. by E. to S., or from S. by W. to N.,—favourable changes of weather may be looked for.

(b) When the wind backs—that is, veers round in the opposite direction—bad weather generally follows.

The direction of the wind is an important factor. Thus:

(a) Settled N.W. winds bring cold and fine weather.

(b) Continued W. and S.W. winds are followed by rain.

Clouds give useful indications. Thus:—

A mackerel sky, that is, one covered with lines of cirrus clouds, causing halos around the sun and moon, presages rain in summer and thaw in winter. By degrees the light clouds descend and pass into either masses of cumulus, or into dense, horizontal stratus, which form at sunset and disappear at sunrise. Both these kinds pass into the grey, shapeless nimbus, which soon covers the entire sky and is followed by rain.

When numerous observations can be synoptically studied, forecasting becomes much more nearly certain. For this purpose telegraphic communications are indispensable. The continent of Europe is better placed than England for accurate forecasting. Areas of high pressure coincide usually with large areas of land, of low pressure with large surfaces of water. Thus England is placed near the boundary of the usual anticyclonic and cyclonic systems, and its chief disturbances come from the Atlantic from which early communication is impracticable. Furthermore cyclonic disturbances may be diverted from their course by a coastline or mountains or by the formation of an anticyclonic area. In view of these uncertainties, the large proportion of correct forecasts is somewhat surprising.

The Moisture of the Air depends upon the amount of vapour present in it, and the ratio of this to the amount which would saturate the air at the actual temperature. The former is called the absolute humidity, the latter the relative humidity. The dew point is the point at which condensation of some of the vapour in the atmosphere occurs, either as dew, rain, snow, or hoar-frost. The amount of moisture which the atmosphere can retain before such condensation occurs, varies with the temperature. Thus the air is drier at noon than at midnight, though the amount of vapour present in the two cases be the same; and it is for the most part drier in summer than in winter. This refers to the relative humidity, which is highest in cold weather. The absolute humidity is higher in summer than in winter; it varies more in continental than in maritime and insular climates; and there are daily variations according to the state of the sky, the movements of air, etc. The relative humidity is expressed as a percentage of what would be required to produce saturation at the given temperature. The usual relative humidity is 50 to 75 per cent. A moist air prevents excessive changes of temperature due to radiation. It protects the earth from too great intensity of the solar rays by day and from too rapid loss of heat by radiation at night. The inhalation of a dry air plays an important part in the cure of consumption. When the air is almost saturated with moisture, evaporation from the skin and lungs is diminished, and there is a feeling of oppression and disinclination to work caused by the interference with the tissue changes of the system.

Rainfall is caused by over-saturation of a column of moist air. This may be due to the contact of the air with a cold surface, as the ridge of a mountain or a large surface of water, or to the impact of a colder wind.

The amount of rainfall varies greatly. In some parts there is no rain, as in the desert of Sahara; while on the south-east slopes of the Himalayas, which are exposed to winds laden with moisture, it may be several hundred inches.

The latitude of a place has a great influence. As a rule the rainfall decreases with increasing distance from the equator; but local conditions may produce great modification, or even alterations of this law.

The elevation above the sea-level has a varying influence. In the Swiss Alps it is said that the rainfall increases with the elevation; but this rule does not hold good in America.

The nearness of large surfaces of water in summer tends to increase the rainfall, when water is colder than its surroundings, while in winter it has the opposite effect. The neighbourhood of the sea is for the west of England and islands adjacent, a cause of increased rainfall.

The influence of winds on the rainfall has been already considered. In Great Britain south-west winds more especially increase the rainfall. In their course they have travelled over the Gulf Stream and the general equatorial current, and have thus received warmth and moisture. The condensation of their moisture liberates a large amount of latent heat, thus raising the temperature of this country. In summer, however, south-west winds are cool and moist, as the Atlantic is not so hot as the continents of Asia and Europe over which other winds have travelled.

In England the average rainfall is about 33 inches, in Scotland 46, and in Ireland 38 inches. In the east of Great Britain, the rainfall is from twenty to twenty-eight inches. On the west coasts of Scotland and Ireland it is from 60 to 80 inches; and in some parts of Cumberland may be about 150 inches per annum. The annual rainfall varies greatly from the average for a number of years. In this country it has been estimated that the maximum annual rainfall exceeds by one-third, and the minimum annual rainfall is less by one-third than the average rainfall of a series of years.

The number of rainy days by no means corresponds with the amount of rainfall. There are fewest rainy days at the equator, where the

216

rainfall is greatest. The rain diminishes the relative humidity of the air, and purifies it from dust.

CHAPTER XXXV

METEOROLOGICAL OBSERVATIONS

The Royal Meteorological Society recognises stations for the making and recording of observations of three kinds: (1) Second Order Stations, at which observations are taken twice daily at 9 a.m. and 9 p.m.; (2) Climatological Stations, at which the observations are taken once daily, at 9 a.m.; (3) Stations at which one or more elements only, e.g. rainfall, are observed. All instruments used should have been previously verified at Kew Observatory, so that the corrections for index error may be known.

The Barometer used should be of a standard kind. Five chief kinds of barometer are in use, only the last two of which are sufficiently accurate for scientific purposes.

1. The Dial or wheel barometer consists of a bent tube A B, the open end of which supports an ivory float B. This, as it rises and falls with the mercury, by means of the rack C turns a wheel, in the axle of which a needle is fixed. The needle turns in one direction, or the other as the mercury rises or falls (Fig. 45); the dial is divided by comparing it with a standard barometer. As the ordinary variations of the barometer are from 28 to 31 inches, the circumference of the wheel is made exactly 1½ inches, and thus the float B will rise or fall 1½ inches for a rise or fall of 3 inches in the barometer.

1. The Dial or wheel barometer consists of a bent tube A B, the open end of which supports an ivory float B. This, as it rises and falls with the mercury, by means of the rack C turns a wheel, in the axle of which a needle is fixed. The needle turns in one direction, or the other as the mercury rises or falls (Fig. 45); the dial is divided by comparing it with a standard barometer. As the ordinary variations of the barometer are from 28 to 31 inches, the circumference of the wheel is made exactly 1½ inches, and thus the float B will rise or fall 1½ inches for a rise or fall of 3 inches in the barometer.

2. The ordinary *syphon barometer* (Fig. 46) consists of a bent tube attached to a piece of wood, and furnished with a screw *v*. The atmospheric pressure acts on the mercury at *d*, and the difference between the level of the mercury in the two arms of the syphon is the height of the barometer. To find the true height of the barometer the screw is turned till the shorter column stands at *a* opposite zero.

217

3. The aneroid barometer is made by exhausting the air from a small round metal box. This box is closed by a flexible lid of metal which, being elastic, yields to changes in the atmospheric pressure. To the lower end of the lid a spring is attached which runs downwards to the floor of the box and resists the atmospheric pressure. The movements thus produced by variations in pressure are magnified by a rack and pinion, and so communicated to a long index which moves over a graduated scale.

Fig. 46

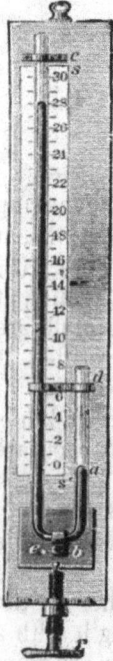

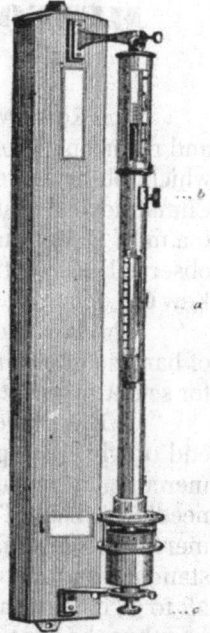

Fig. 47.
Fortin Barometer.
a—Attached thermometer. b—Screw of vernier. c—Screw for setting level of cistern.

The standard Kew and Fortin barometers are both cistern barometers, the mercury in the inverted tube communicating with the mercury in a cistern below.

4. The *Kew pattern barometer* has a closed cistern below, the area of which being accurately known, the inches on the scale are not real inches, but inches of pressure, *i.e.* inches so shortened as to compensate for the rise of the mercury in the cistern. This compensation is necessary inasmuch as changes in atmospheric pressure affect the level of the mercury in the cistern as well as of that in the tube.

5. In the *Fortin barometer* (Fig. 47) the cistern has a pliable base of leather, which can be raised or lowered by means of a screw. The upper part of the cistern is made of glass, a piece of ivory indicating the zero of the scale. Before taking a reading, the level of the mercury must always be set exactly to this point by means of the screw. The Fortin is the most sensitive form of barometer, and the adjustment required in order to take a reading is easily performed.

To ensure more accurate reading of the barometer, a secondary scale or **vernier** is used, which slides upon the principal scale. This vernier is so graduated that 25 of its divisions correspond to 24 of the divisions on the fixed scale. The fixed scale is divided into inches, tenths (·1), and half-tenths (·05). Each division of the movable scale or vernier is therefore shorter than each division of the scale by $1/25$ of ·05, *i.e.* ·002 inch. Consequently the vernier shows differences of two thousands of an inch.

Method of reading Fortin's Barometer.—First note the reading of the attached thermometer; next turn the screw at the bottom of the cistern, so that the ivory point just touches the surface of the mercury. Next adjust the vernier by means of the rack and pinion at the side of the barometer (Fig. 47) so as to bring its two lower edges exactly on a level with the convex surface of the mercury. In reading the barometer, first read off the division next below the lower edge of the vernier. In Fig. 48 this is 29·05. Then the true reading is 29·05 *plus* the vernier indication. Next look along the vernier until one of its lines is found to agree with a line on the scale. In Fig. 48 this is at the fourth division on the vernier. But each of the figures marked on the vernier counts as $1/100$ (·01), and each intermediate division as $2/1000$ (·002); hence the reading of the vernier will be ·008 inch, and239 the reading of the barometer 29·05 + ·008 = 29·058 inch. If two lines on the vernier are in equally near agreement with two on the scale, the intermediate value should be adopted.

Certain *corrections* are required in the actual reading for (1) index error; (2) temperature; and (3) height above sea-level.

The *index error* is found by comparison with a recognised standard at Kew. Correction for *temperature* is required. Every barometer has a thermometer attached, and the reading is reduced to the standard temperature of 32° F, by means of tables such as are given on page 29 of Marriott's *Hints to Meteorological Observers*.

The height of the *cistern* of the barometer above *sea-level* should always be exactly obtained.

The correction necessary to reduce observations to sea-level (*i.e.* mean half-tide level at Liverpool), depends on the temperature and pressure of the air, as well as on the altitude. The data for this correction are given in Table III. of Marriott's *Hints*.

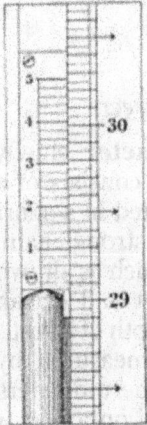

Fig. 48.
Scale of Barometer (to Right) and of Vernier (to Left).

Thermometers.—The **maximum thermometer** may be on Negretti and Zambra's, or on Phillips' principle. In the former (Fig. 49) the bore of the tube is reduced in section near the bulb (A) in such a way that while the expanding mercury forces its way into the tube, the column of mercury breaks off on contraction, so that its upper limit shows the highest temperature that has been reached. The thermometer is set by holding it bulb downwards and shaking to make the mercurial column continuous. It is mounted in the screen horizontally (Fig. 51).

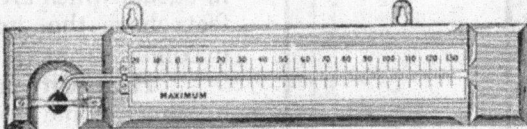

Fig. 49
Negretti and Zambra's Maximum Thermometer.

The **minimum thermometer** chiefly used is Rutherford's. It contains spirit in which is an immersed index (A, Fig. 50). With a falling temperature the spirit draws the index along with it; but on rising again, the spirit passes the index, leaving it at the lowest point to which it has been drawn. Thus the end farthest from the bulb registers the minimum temperature. The instrument is set by raising the bulb and allowing the index to slide to the end of the column of spirit. The thermometer must be firmly fixed and mounted quite horizontally.

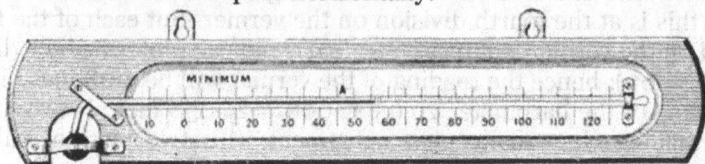

Fig. 50.
Minimum Thermometer.

Thermometer Screen.—The above thermometers, as well as the dry and wet bulb thermometers are mounted in a Stevenson's screen (Fig. 51). This is a doubled-louvred box through which the air can pass freely, but the sun cannot enter. The horizontal position of the maximum and minimum and the vertical position of the dry and wet bulb thermometers are shown in Fig. 51.

Three additional thermometers are usually included in a well-organised meteorological station.

A **minimum thermometer** placed on the grass gives the lowest temperature on the grass, which is often considerably lower than that of the neighbouring gravel walk. This record is chiefly useful for agricultural purposes.

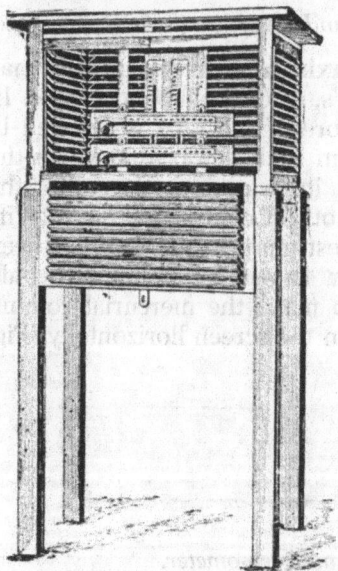

Fig. 51.
Stevenson's Thermometer Screen.

The **earth thermometer** chiefly used is shown in Fig. 52. It consists of a sluggish thermometer mounted in a short weighted stick attached to a strong chain, and of a stout iron pipe which is drawn out at the bottom to a point and driven into the earth, usually to a depth of 4 feet.

Solar radiation is measured by black-bulb and light-bulb thermometers in *vacuo*, which are mounted on a post 4 feet above the ground and record the maximum temperature.

Humidity in the air is measured by direct or indirect hygrometers. Of the former Dines', Daniell's, and Regnault's are the best known, but as they are not used in observations acknowledged by the Royal Meteorological Society, the reader may be referred to their description in books on physics. The indirect hygrometer which is universally employed in this country is that furnished by the **dry and wet bulb thermometers**. In frosty weather they require much attention, and then a Saussure's hair hygrometer may be used as supplementary. The general arrangement of the dry and wet bulb thermometers is shown in Fig. 53.

The wet bulb is covered with a single layer of soft muslin, while a noose of six to eight strands of darning cotton connects the neck of the wet bulb with a covered water receptacle 2 to 3 inches distant, below and at its side. This receptacle is kept filled with rain-water.

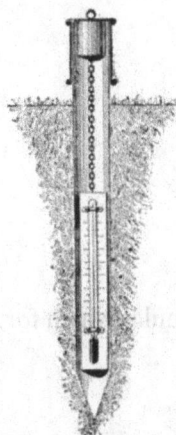

Fig. 52.
Symons' Earth Thermometer.

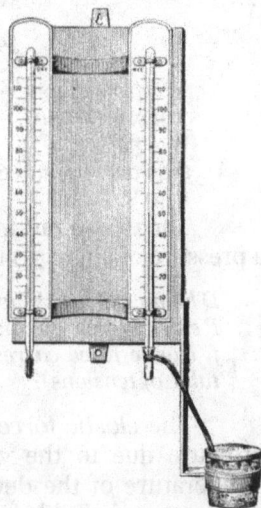

Fig. 53.
Dry and Wet Bulb Thermometers.

From the readings of the dry and wet bulb thermometers three deductions can be made:

1. The temperature of the dew point.
2. The elastic force of aqueous vapour.
3. The relative humidity.

The **dew point temperature** is that temperature at which the outside air at the time the observation is taken will deposit the moisture contained in it. It is the temperature at which the air is saturated with moisture. It is calculated from the readings of the wet and dry bulb thermometers

(*a*) by Glaisher's tables; (*b*) by Apjohn's formula.

Glaisher's tables are based on a series of numbers called Greenwich or Glaisher's factors, which he determined by comparison between

221

observations made with the dry and wet bulb thermometers and with Daniell's hygrometer. The formula for using the factors is as follows:—

$$d = D - \{(D - W) \times f\}$$

where d = dew point, D = dry bulb temperatures, W = wet bulb temperature, and f = factor.

The following examples are from Glaisher's table of factors.

READING OF DRY BULB THERMOMETER FAHR.	FACTOR.
55°	1·96
56°	1·94
57°	1·92
58°	1·90
59°	1·89
60°	1·88

Thus, if D = 60°,
W = 55°,
then dew point = 60 - {(60 - 55) 1·96}
= 50°·2.

The dew-point may also be obtained by Apjohn's formula; which for a pressure of about 30 inches is $F = f - (D - W)/87$

D being dry and W wet bulb temperature,
F elastic force of vapour corresponding to dew-point, and
f, elastic force corresponding to wet bulb temperature (ascertained from a table of tensions).

The *elastic force of aqueous vapour, i.e.* the amount of barometric pressure due to the vapour present in the air is dependent upon the temperature of the dew-point. It is given for every tenth of a degree of temperature in Table VI. (p. 42) of Marriott's *Hints.*

The *relative humidity* is a term expressing the percentage of saturation of the air with water vapour. It is obtained from Table VI. (above) as follows:—

$$\left. \begin{array}{l} \textit{Relative} \\ \textit{Humidity} \end{array} \right\} = \frac{\textit{Elastic force of water vapour at the temperature of the dew-point}}{\textit{Elastic force of water vapour at the temperature of the air (i.e. the dry-bulb reading.)}}$$

Thus elastic force with dry bulb = 55° is ·433 in. in the table.
Thus elastic force with dew-point = 46°·5 is ·317 in.,,
·317/·433 = ·73.
If saturation = 100, relative humidity is 73.

In Table VII. of Marriott's *Hints,* a table is given which enables the relative humidity to be found by mere inspection. Thus if the dry bulb temperature is 58°·5, wet-bulb 51°·7, and the difference 6°·8, the relative humidity given in the table is 62.

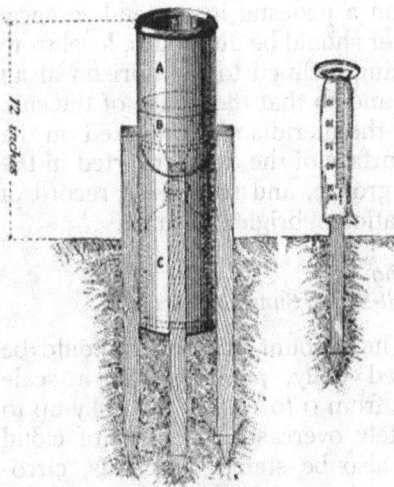

Fig. 54.
Snowdon Pattern Rain-Gauge.
A. Copper Upper Part of Gauge. B.
Funnel. C. Bottle. To the right is shown the
glass measure inverted.

12 inches

The **Rain-Gauge** is best made of copper in the shape of a circular funnel, usually 5 or 8 inches in diameter, leading into a bottle underneath. It must always be set in an open situation away from trees, walls, and buildings. According to Scott no object ought to subtend a greater angle with the horizon than 20° in any direction from the gauge. The rain is measured by pouring the contents of the bottle into a glass measure, which is graduated to represent tenths and hundredths of an inch on the area of the gauge, the measure holding half an inch of rain on this area. Snow is melted before being measured.

Observations of **wind** should include its direction and force. The direction is observed by means of a well-oiled and freely exposed vane. There are 32 points to the compass, but a reading to eight points suffices. The force of the wind should be estimated by Beaufort's scale, from 0 to 12. Thus:—

FORCE	MILES PER HOUR
0. Calm	3
1. Light air	8
2. Light breeze	13
3. Gentle	18
4. Moderate	23
5. Fresh	28
6. Strong	34
7. Moderate gale	40
8. Fresh	48
9. Strong	56
10. Whole	65
11. Storm	57
12. Hurricane	90

Robinson's anemometer is also employed, but it is not altogether trustworthy.

Sunshine is recorded by the Campbell-Stokes burning recorder, and the Jordan photographic recorder. Of these the former is the more easily worked and gives more uniform results. It consists of a sphere of

223

glass 4 inches in diameter, supported on a pedestal in a metal zodiacal frame (Fig. 55). The setting of the recorder should be due south, level from east to west, and with the axis of the ring inclined to the horizon at an angle equal to the latitude of the place, and so that the image of the sun, when the sun is due south, shall fall on the meridian line marked on the ring. The sun burns away or chars the surface of the cards inserted in the proper groove, and so gives a record of the duration of bright sunshine.

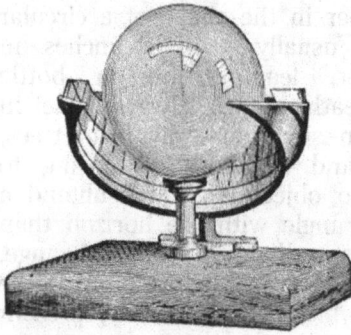

Fig. 55.
Campbell-Stokes Sunshine Recorder.

The amount of **Cloud** should be estimated daily, according to a scale ranging from 0 to 10, *i.e.* clear sky up to completely overcast. The form of cloud should also be stated, as cirrus, cirro-cumulus, cirro-stratus, cumulus, cumulo-stratus, stratus, and nimbus.

CHAPTER XXXVI

PERSONAL HYGIENE

Certain personal factors are very important in relation to health. The chief of these are constitution, temperament, heredity, idiosyncrasy, age, sex, and habits.

Constitution.—Health may vary in degree without the presence of actual disease. This fact is expressed by the use of such terms as "perfect," "strong," "feeble," "delicate," in speaking of the health of the same person at different times, and also as distinguishing one person from another. The constitution is an important factor in resisting disease, and a robust constitution may determine recovery from a severe illness, while the patient with a feeble constitution falls a victim to it.

The constitution of an individual is partly acquired, partly inherited. A feeble or delicate constitution may be acquired by unhygienic conditions, such as deficient exercise, the prolonged breathing of impure air, unhealthy occupations, some imperfection in diet, or dissipation.

But while many a robust constitution is enfeebled by such conditions, a weak constitution may happily be strengthened by careful and prolonged attention to the laws of health. This is especially well seen in the case of those who strengthen their muscular system by carefully-graduated and not excessive exercise.

224

Heredity has a great influence on health. As a rule the children of healthy parents are robust, and on the contrary, any "weak point" in the parents' constitutions is liable to be participated in by their children. Both mental and physical conditions may be inherited. A peculiar habit of mind, as well as the same expression of features, may be inherited.

As regards physical diseases, the influence of parents is not less remarkable. The son of a gouty father requires to be particularly abstemious in order to avoid his father's disease. Certain specific febrile diseases, e.g., enteric fever, diphtheria, and still more rheumatic fever, are hereditary in the sense that the members of certain families are more prone to them than others. Insanity, epilepsy, asthma, neuralgia, and hysteria are also hereditary in the same sense, and it is noticed that they occasionally alternate in different generations. Cancer, consumption, certain skin diseases, and a tendency to the early onset of degenerative diseases, appear also to occur more often in certain families than in others.

In most cases it is the tendency to disease which is transmitted, and not the disease itself. When an actual disease is inherited, as happens very rarely in tuberculosis and often in syphilis, the actual infection is transmitted before birth from the parent.

A peculiarity of form, character, or tendency to disease has been known to disappear in one generation and re-appear in the next; this variety of heredity is termed atavism. The evidence showing the inheritance of acquired characters, i.e. those which arise in consequence of the effect of external forces on the organism is not conclusive. Weismann believes that only those forces that influence the germ-plasm are inherited. It must be admitted that the instances of inheritance of acquired characters can be better explained otherwise. Thus the long neck of the giraffe was formerly explained on the supposition that the neck became gradually lengthened owing to the efforts made generation after generation in reaching food; but is better explained by Weismann on the supposition that those giraffes which, during times of famine were able to reach higher and obtain food from the twigs of trees would survive and pass on their characteristics to their young, while shorter necked giraffes would be exterminated.

The inheritance of proclivity to or immunity from attacks of infectious diseases is a problem of great difficulty; but there is no substantial reason for thinking that the efforts being made to diminish the prevalence of these diseases (including consumption) are likely to produce a weaker race or one more likely to suffer with excessive severity from these diseases should they be introduced after a long absence.

Temperament indicates a peculiarity in constitution, causing a liability to particular diseases, or to a special character in any disease to which a person becomes subject. Four temperaments are usually recognized—the sanguine, phlegmatic, bilious, and nervous, but unmixed specimens of these temperaments are rarely seen.

By idiosyncrasy is understood a peculiarity limited to a comparatively small number of individuals. Four varieties of idiosyncrasy may be described.

The first consists in an extreme susceptibility to the action of certain things, or an extreme lack of susceptibility. Thus most people at some time or other inhale the pollen of grasses, but only in a few cases does it produce that troublesome and distressing complaint—hay asthma. In certain persons a very minute dose of iodide of potassium produces distressing symptoms; in most cases these symptoms arise if the drug is taken for a prolonged period; but in a few cases it may be taken for an indefinite period without troublesome result. The case of a physician at Bath is very curious. The smell of hyacinths in bloom always made him faint away; so constant was this result, that before entering a room during the hyacinth season, he always asked the servant if there were any hyacinths in it.

The second form of idiosyncrasy consists in the production of poisonous results by common articles of diet. Thus some people cannot partake of shell-fish or lobsters without having severe nettlerash. In rare instances the smallest amount of egg, or in other cases mutton, or pepper, or some other substance will produce severe indigestion or nettlerash.

The third form consists in an inversion of the usual effects of certain substances, especially drugs. Thus opium in rare cases produces convulsions; while the aperient Epsom salts have been known to produce constipation.

A fourth form, that of mental idiosyncrasies, may be added, as where there is a strange preference or aversion for objects usually regarded as indifferent. Many cases of mental peculiarity, short of actual insanity, will come under this head; as will instances of depraved appetite for food, etc.

Age and Sex.—According to the period of life, danger arises from different sources. In infancy and old age extreme changes of temperature are especially dangerous, and additional protection is required. Thousands of deaths occur in the first year of life, from substituting starchy foods for milk, the natural food for infancy and childhood. In childhood the danger from bad feeding is still present, and is evidenced by the frequency of rickets; infectious diseases claim their thousands; and the disorders associated with dentition are common. In youth rapid growth is proceeding, and so the food must be abundant and nutritious. A proportionately larger amount is required than by an adult, as the functions of the body not only require to be carried on, but material is necessary to build up the growing tissues.

Manhood is the period of greatest stability of health. The health now depends on the use made of the previous periods of life, and on the habits acquired.

With the onset of old age come various degenerative diseases. The tendency is to death by gradual decay—a euthanasia or easy death, which is too seldom seen. Commonly, bronchitis or apoplexy or kidney diseases bring the scene to a somewhat premature end.

The mortality of man is greater than that of woman at all ages except 5—20.

Habits.—The immense power of habits in the formation of character is perhaps duly appreciated; but their influence on physical health is not so

226

well appreciated; though it would be difficult to exaggerate it. The laws of health are as inexorable and unaltering as all other laws of nature; and whether broken through carelessness or ignorance, the Nemesis of disease inevitably follows. Whatever a man sows he reaps, in health as in other matters.

Habits are easily formed; but, when once formed, not so easily broken. They ought to be our servants; very commonly they become our masters.

In reference to eating and drinking, habits regular as to time and moderate as to quantity are especially important. The habit of eating hastily and masticating the food imperfectly, is certain, sooner or later, to produce disease. Over-eating, again, is a fertile source of disease, especially when the excess is in animal food. The amount of stimulation produced by a given dose of alcohol, gradually diminishes with its repetition; the consequence is, that in order to produce the amount of stimulation to which the system has become habituated, the stimulant requires to be gradually increased. The craving for stimulants is often a sign of ill-health, owing to disregard of hygienic laws or actual disease. Not infrequently it is due to badly-ventilated rooms or long hours of work without food, producing a sense of depression which food does not immediately allay. When the cause is unknown, recourse should be had to competent medical advice, and not to the brandy bottle.

Attention to the Action of the Bowels is a matter which is commonly neglected. The importance of a regular habit in this respect cannot be exaggerated; the bowels should always be relieved at a particular time each day. Where this does not occur the condition of constipation results. Owing to the retention of the fæces in the intestines beyond the normal period, the stomach and higher parts of the intestines do not perform their functions normally; indigestion and "dyspepsia," accompanied by headache, flatulence, and other symptoms follow. Hæmorrhoids (piles) are another frequent consequence. At the junction of the small and large intestines is a dilated sac (in the cæcum). This becomes distended when constipation occurs; inflammation may be set up, and an operation required, or the condition is fatal. Powerful purgative medicines are injurious to the bowels, and they tend afterwards to increase constipation. It is better to take slow-acting aperient remedies, and better still not to take any at all, but relieve the condition by means of such articles of diet as stewed fruit, pears, figs, olive oil, or brown bread. As a rule more exercise is required in this condition, and always a prompt attention to the calls of nature.

CHAPTER XXXVII

PERSONAL HYGIENE—EXERCISE

Physiological Considerations.—In the strict sense of the word, exercise signifies the performance of its functions by any part of the body; thus, digestion is exercise of the stomach, respiration is exercise of the lungs, thinking is an exercise of the brain. But the term is usually applied chiefly to muscular contraction, and restricted to contraction of voluntary muscles. Involuntary muscles, which are concerned in the carrying on of the unconscious organic functions of life, are not directly controllable, and so their growth and state of nutrition cannot be regulated. There are two sets of involuntary muscle, which are of special importance—the heart and the muscles of respiration. The heart contracts at least sixty times per minute; the respiratory muscles contract about seventeen times per minute; and this amount of exercise goes on throughout the whole day. But although we cannot make our hearts beat quicker by a direct volition, and cannot breathe more rapidly than usual beyond a few seconds, yet a brisk walk will cause increased action of the heart and respiratory muscles, as well as a vigorous contraction of the muscles directly concerned in walking. Going uphill is a valuable exercise for the heart. The vermicular contractions of the intestines are to some extent also increased by voluntary exercise, through the indirect excitation of the whole system; thus, exercise is an important element in the treatment of constipation.

The muscles contain about a fourth of the whole blood of the body, and a very large share of the metabolism of the body occurs in them.

Hence the importance of keeping them in a healthy condition by exercise. The great danger is of not equilibrating the muscular and nervous functions. The ideal condition is where neither mental nor muscular culture is neglected, but both are co-ordinated to the production of a healthy man.

Effects of Healthy Exercise.—1. The Nutrition of the Muscles is improved. The volume, density, and energy of the muscles are increased.

2. The action of the lungs is increased. Dr. E. Smith found that if the air inspired while lying down be represented by unity, the amount inspired when erect is 1·33; when walking at the rate of one mile per hour, 1·9; at four miles per hour, 5; at six miles per hour, 7; riding on horseback, 4·05; swimming, 4·33. Or, putting it in another way, under ordinary circumstances a man inspires 480 cubic inches per minute; if he walks four miles per hour, he inspires 2,400 cubic inches; if six miles an hour, 3,260 cubic inches.

At the same time the amount of carbonic acid expired is increased. Its amount bears a nearly constant relation to the amount of muscular exercise, and consequently the amount of carbonic acid eliminated in various forms of exercise affords a just estimate of their relative value. The increased elimination of carbonic acid, the corresponding increased absorption of oxygen, and the absence of increase of elimination of urea are shown in the following summary of observations by Pettenkofer and Voit:—

	ABSORPTION OF OXYGEN IN GRAMMES	ELIMINATION IN GRAMMES OF CARBONIC ACID	WATER	UREA
Work day	955	1284	2042	37·0
Rest day	709	912	828	37·2

The above amounts are for the entire day. During actual exercise the excess of elimination of carbonic acid is much greater. Thus, Dr. E. Smith experimentally found that if the amount of carbonic acid eliminated during rest be represented by one, the amount walking at two miles an hour and carrying 7 lbs = 1·85, the amount walking at three miles an hour = 2·64.

Alcohol diminishes the excretion of carbonic acid, and should therefore be avoided during muscular training.

By muscular exercise the size of the lungs is increased, and their vital capacity, that is, the amount of air capable of being expired after a forced inspiration, is considerably increased. Corresponding with this increase of vital capacity, exercise, especially that in which the arm and chest muscles are systematically developed, increases the size of the chest. A perceptible difference in the circumference of the chest may be noticed after only a few weeks' methodical exercise.

3. The action of the skin is increased.—Sensible perspiration is commonly induced, but less readily in those habituated to hard work. Insensible perspiration is always increased.

4. The temperature of the body is not increased, so long as perspiration occurs. Every muscular contraction involves the production of heat; but this is counteracted by increased evaporation from the skin, and by the circulatory current carrying the hotter blood to every part of the body, and so rapidly equalising its temperature. Chilblains are due to the defective circulation of the blood, and can in most cases be cured by active exercise aided by warmer clothing and an abundant supply of oxidisable food.

5. The Heart and Blood-vessels.—By exercise the heart's action is increased in frequency and force. The pulse usually increases from ten to thirty beats per minute above the rate while at rest. After prolonged exercise it may temporarily fall below the normal standard.

6. The Digestion and assimilation of food are aided by exercise, especially when taken in the open air.

7. The nervous system is improved in nutrition and power by a moderate amount of exercise. In fact, a certain amount of muscular exercise is essential for a healthy mind.

8. The elimination of urea is not increased by exercise. Evidently then it is not the metabolism of the nitrogenous substance of the muscles which supplies the energy for muscular contraction; but of the other oxidisable and non-nitrogenous substances (such as glycogen and sugar) contained in them.

229

In practice it is found that with exercise more nitrogenous and non-nitrogenous food are both required.

Effects of Excessive Exercise.—After prolonged exertion muscles become exhausted. This is associated with an accumulation in the muscles of the products of their action (especially sarcolactic acid). Then rest becomes necessary, in order that the effete products may be removed, and the nutrition of the muscles restored.

Long-continued over-exertion produces chronic exhaustion, which may, if excessive, cause wasting of muscles. Exhaustion is much more liable to occur when a small group of muscles are exercised out of all proportion to others. Thus, in clerks, we have what is known as the writer's or scrivener's palsy. The muscles of the hand, and especially of the thumb, cease to respond to the volition of the writer, but are seized with spasm every time writing is attempted; and the muscles of the thumb tend to waste. A similar condition sometimes arises in violinists, tailors, etc. The practical inference from these facts is, that one group of muscles should not be exercised disproportionately to the muscles of the rest of the body, and that proper intervals of rest should be allowed.

Excessive exercise of the whole muscular system is very apt to harm those of previously sedentary habits. A walking tour entered on with more zeal than discretion, and not taken by easy stages for the first few days, is often productive of more harm than good.

In the intervals of great mental labour, as with students, the amount of exercise should not be suddenly increased, but should be regular and moderate in amount.

Competitive exercise should be strictly regulated. The Oxford and Cambridge crews have been said to acquire heart-disease more commonly than the average, but this is not correct. Hypertrophy of the heart may occur as the result of severe exercise, and this within certain limits is not an abnormal condition. Occasionally dilatation of the heart has been produced in weakly lads.

Amount of Exercise Desirable.—According to Parkes, the average daily work of a man engaged in manual labour in the open air is equivalent to the work involved in lifting 250 to 350 tons one foot high; this is a moderate amount, 400 tons being a heavy day's work. The amount of muscular exercise involved in this may be easily known by remembering that a walk of 20 miles on a level road is equivalent to about 353⅔ tons lifted 1 foot; and that a walk of 10 miles while carrying 60 lbs. is equivalent to 247½ tons lifted 1 foot. (Haughton).

The amount of work done by a healthy adult per diem is stated by M. Foster to be about 150,000 metre-kilogrammes (i.e., 150,000 kilogrammes lifted 1 metre). Metre-kilogrammes can be converted into foot-pounds by multiplying by 7·233; into foot-tons by multiplying by ·003229; 150,000 metre-kilogrammes therefore equal 484·35 foot-tons. This is considerably in excess of Parkes' estimate, but in certain laborious occupations this high amount is reached.

In addition to this amount of external work, there is the internal work of the heart, muscles of respiration, digestion, etc. This is estimated by Parkes at about 260 foot-tons.

The internal and external muscular work of the body together amount to about 1/7th to 1/8th of the total force obtainable from the food.

Every healthy man probably ought to take an amount of exercise represented by 150 tons raised 1 foot, which is equal to the work done in walking 8½ to 9 miles on a level road. A certain amount of this exercise is taken in performing one's daily work; but apart from this, out-door exercise should be taken equivalent in amount to a walk of five or six miles. It is impossible to lay down rules to suit all cases, but a less amount of exercise than that named is probably incompatible with perfect health.

Effects of Deficient Exercise.—The muscles themselves become enfeebled and wasted. Some wasting of muscle occurs after a few days' confinement to bed; and a limb confined in a splint speedily loses its healthy, rounded contour. Oxidation processes are diminished; less carbonic acid is eliminated, and it tends to accumulate in the system, owing to the diminished activity of respiration. In consequence of the diminished oxidation, the temperature of the body is not well maintained, and the heat is not uniformly distributed. Cold feet are a common complaint of those who lead sedentary lives, though seldom complained of by others.

Along with the other muscles, the heart becomes enfeebled and the circulation less perfect. Digestion is enfeebled; the appetite is poor. The nervous system also suffers; nervous irritability is a common result, while sleeplessness—a thing almost unknown among those who live by the sweat of their brow—is becoming much more common among the worried and ill-exercised inhabitants of our towns.

Many diseases are favoured by deficient exercise, and can be averted by systematic exercises and the concomitant increased supply of pure air. It is often difficult to appraise the relative merits of exercise and pure air; but there can be no doubt that both are of extreme importance.

The prevention of consumption, even in those with a strong hereditary tendency, is greatly helped by systematic exercises, especially those directed to the expansion of the chest cavity. In cases of consumption there is commonly a history of deficient exercise or an occupation involving a cramped position, as well as of living in an impure air.

Various deformities are induced by defective exercise of particular groups of muscles. Thus drooping shoulders may be caused by shoulder-straps confining the action of the shoulder-muscles in the earlier years of life. Stooping is favoured by sitting in cramped positions in school, and by the use of desks not inclined at the proper angle. Lateral curvature of the spine is due to weakness of the muscles of the back, and is best treated in its earlier stages by gymnastic exercises specially directed to strengthening these muscles. The tendency to such curvatures is greatly increased in girls by the fact that their trunks are imprisoned in corsets as if in splints, and so exercise of the trunk muscles is reduced to a minimum.

Rules respecting Exercise. 1. The clothing during exercise should not be excessive, and should not interfere with the free play of the limbs, nor with full expansion of the chest. Flannel is the best material to wear next the skin, as it absorbs perspiration without becoming non-porous.

231

2. Avoid chill after exercise. It is well, if there has been any perspiration during exercise, to strip and scrub the skin, particularly about the chest and arm-pits, with a rough towel.

3. Exercise should be systematic and regular. It is important to avoid sudden, violent, and competitive exercise. No severe exercise ought to be undertaken without a gradual training.

4. The amount of exercise must be regulated by individual fitness. A chain is no stronger than its weakest link. The muscles may be stronger than the heart or lungs, and the latter may be fatally injured by an amount of exercise which the muscles can well bear. Hence the importance of ascertaining the condition of the vital organs before entering on a course of training.

Another important bearing of this rule is in relation to the exercise of growing boys and girls. When we remember that a boy at school will sometimes grow six to eight inches in a year, it is evident that much energy is being expended in this direction, and that excessive gymnastic exercise can only do harm. Between the ages of fifteen and seventeen there is usually the greatest amount of physical development, and if there is great muscular strain at this period, growth is interfered with, and the power of resistance to disease may be seriously lowered.

5. Every part of the body ought to be exercised. This is done spontaneously by the infant. Every muscle of his body acts in sheer delight. The evils of exercise confined to particular groups of muscles have been already described. Lawn tennis is very valuable as affording exercise for both limb and trunk muscles.

6. Exercise should not be taken immediately after meals, as thus digestion is interfered with.

7. Exercise should be taken, as far as possible, in the open air. A small amount of exercise out of doors is much more invigorating than a large amount indoors.

The Forms of Exercise taken may be divided into recreative and educational, though both of course may be recreative under many circumstances.

The primarily recreative exercises, such as rowing, cricket, football, tennis, hockey, will, it may be hoped, be never replaced by educational gymnastics, though the latter possess a high value. The recreative influence as well as the influence on the power of self-control of such games as cricket and football render them of national importance.

Educational gymnastics can be applied to exercise the muscles of any part of the body, and can be exactly graduated to individual requirements. Singing, speaking, and reading aloud, are forms of muscular exercise very much neglected, and they are particularly important, as the lungs and voice are by these means greatly strengthened, and rendered much less liable to the inroads of disease.

Professor Haughton has shown that the work done by a man walking on a level surface at the rate of three miles an hour is equivalent to raising his own weight, plus the weight he carries through 1/20 of the distance walked.

Thus, if W = weight of the man,

W^1 = weight carried by him,
D = distance walked in feet,
C = co-efficient of traction ($^1/_{20}$, at three miles an hour),

then we obtain by the following formula the amount of work done, the co-efficient of traction being multiplied by 2,240 (the number of pounds in a ton) to obtain the result in foot-tons.

$$(W + W1) \times D/(C \times 2{,}240)$$

In ascending a height, a man raises his whole weight through the height ascended.

A regiment of soldiers marches ten miles, each carrying a weight of 60 lbs. What amount of work is performed by each soldier?

If we assume the average weight of each soldier to be 150 lbs., and that the march was at the rate of three miles an hour, then—

$$(150 + 60) \times 10 \times 5{,}280/(20 \times 2{,}240) = 247 \cdot 5 \text{ foot-tons.}$$

In this example it is assumed that the march is on entirely level ground that all weights are carried in the most convenient manner, and that the rate of travel is three miles an hour. Velocity is gained at the expense of carrying power. It has been found that the amount of work is generally inversely as the square of the velocity. Haughton has determined from Weber's calculations the co-efficient of resistance for three velocities.

VELOCITY.	CO-EFFICIENT OF TRACTION OR RESISTANCE.
1·818 miles per hour	$^1/_{28 \cdot 27}$
4·353 miles per hour	$^1/_{13 \cdot 70}$
10·577 miles per hour	$^1/_{7 \cdot 51}$

Parkes has extended these calculations to show the distance in miles required to be travelled at various velocities to do work equal to 300 foot-tons, and the time required in each instance.

VELOCITY IN MILES PER HOUR	CO-EFFICIENT OF RESISTANCE	DISTANCE FOR MEN OF 156 LBS TO EQUAL 300 FOOT-TONS	TIME REQUIRED IN HOURS AND MINUTES	
			hrs.	mins.
2	$^1/_{26 \cdot 74}$	12·2	10	36
3	$^1/_{20 \cdot 59}$	16·3	5	24
4	$^1/_{16 \cdot 74}$	13·3	3	18
6	$^1/_{12 \cdot 18}$	9·6	1	36
8	$^1/_{9 \cdot 60}$	7·6	0	57
10	$^1/_{7 \cdot 89}$	6·3	0	38

The co-efficient 1/20, corresponds very nearly to 3·1 miles per hour, and it appears that at this rate of travel the greatest amount of work can be done with the least expenditure of energy.

How much work is done by a man weighing 150 lbs. who walks 15 miles up an incline 1 in 200?

The number of feet ascended in 15 miles

$$= 5{,}280 \times 15/200 = 396.$$

233

The amount of work done by the man in raising his own weight 396 feet high

$$= 396 \times 150/2,240 = 26{\cdot}5 \text{ foot-tons.}$$

The amount of work done in walking 15 horizontal miles at the rate of 3 miles an hour

$$= 150 \times 15 \times 5,280/(20 \times 2,240) = 265.2 \text{ foot-tons.}$$
Total amount of work done = 265.2 + 26.5 = 291.7 foot-tons.

Eight palanquin bearers carry an officer weighing 180 lbs. and a palanquin weighing 250 lbs., a distance of 25 miles. Assuming that each man weighs 150 lbs., what amount of work was done by each man? (Parkes.)

$$250 + 180 = 430$$
$$150 \times 8 = 1,200$$
$$\overline{}$$
$$W + W_1 = 1,630$$
$$1,630 \times 25 \times 5,280/(20 \times 2,240) = 4,802{\cdot}7 \text{ foot-tons.}$$

This being the total work done, the work per man = nearly 600.3 foot-tons.

A hill-coolie weighing 150 lbs. goes 30 miles with an ascent of 5,500 feet in three days, carrying 80 lbs. in weight. What is the work per day? (Parkes.)

Work of the ascent = (150 + 80) × 5,500 / 2,240 = 564·7 foot-tons.
Work of 30 miles walk = 230 × 30 × 5,280/ (20 × 2,240) = 813·2 foot-tons.
Total work = 564·7 + 813·2 = 1,377·9.
Total work per day = 1,377·9 / 3 = 459·3 foot-tons.

Suppose a man weighing 150 lbs. in his clothes, carries a load of bricks weighing 35 lbs. up a perpendicular ladder 30 feet high, 100 times daily, what amount of work does he do; and what will it equal in miles walked upon a flat road at the rate of 3 miles an hour?

(150 + 35) × 30 × 100/2,240 = 247·8 foot-tons
(185 × D)/(20 × 2,240) = 247·8.
Therefore D = 60,056 feet>
= about 11·4 miles.

Suppose a man strikes 12,000 strokes in 5 hours with a 14-lb. hammer, raising it at each stroke 4 feet, how much work does he do? Compare this with a walk of 15 miles on a level ground at 3 miles an hour, the weight of the man and what he carries being 180 lbs.

(a) 12,000 × 14 × 4 = 672,000 foot-lbs. of work
= 300 foot-tons.
(b) (180 × 15 × 5,280)/(20 × 2,240) = 318·2 foot-tons.

The two amounts of work are related as 300 : 318·2.

234

CHAPTER XXXVIII

PERSONAL HYGIENE (continued)—REST AND SLEEP

Physiological Considerations.—Life is made up of alternations of rest and action. The exercise of any organ is followed by a necessary period of repose, during which the oxidised materials produced by functional activity are removed by the blood, and carried to the excretory organs; while at the same time fresh nutritive material is supplied by the blood to make good the losses thus sustained.

The only apparent exceptions to this rule of alternation of rest and exercise are the heart and lungs, and some less important organs acting out of the control of personal volition. But even these organs obey the universal law. The difference is that their rest is very frequent and momentary; the heart having to contract sixty or seventy times per minute, rests 6/11 of a second each second, or more than thirteen hours in the twenty-four. The lungs and respiratory muscles rest a shorter time than this, but probably about three hours per day.

The necessity for rest is well shown by the sense of taste. If salt is kept in the mouth for a considerable time, the power of tasting it disappears, and only returns in its original strength after several hours. The gustatory nerve has been exhausted.

The other sense-organs illustrate the same principle. Persons are not uncommonly made deaf by the sounds of machinery. After looking at a particular colour for some time, the nerves receiving impressions from this colour are exhausted, and only its complementary colour is visible.

Rest may be either partial or general.

The principle of partial rest has very useful practical bearings. Such rest is illustrated by the student who takes a walk, or uses methodical gymnastic exercises; a concert may provide agreeable exercise for the auditory nerves and the part of the brain connected with them, while allowing the over-tired intellectual part of the brain to rest in peace; similarly, light literature may prove a pleasing rest after severer studies.

Walking is more especially the exercise of the brain-worker.

Partial rest is the same thing as change of occupation, and by a careful regulation of the relative amount of cerebral and muscular work, energy can be largely economised. The horse, which exercises chiefly his muscles, requires only five or six hours to recuperate his energy; and our muscles require less sleep than our brain.

Sleep is the only form of complete and general rest. In attaining this condition, the muscles sleep first, then the eyes close (owing to muscular rest), and the thoughts wander; hearing is the last sense to lose cognizance of the surrounding world; dreaming succeeds wandering thoughts, and even dreaming may cease if the brain repose is complete.

During sleep the brain diminishes in size, and becomes paler; the amount of blood in the brain being diminished. Probably the cerebral anæmia is rather a consequence of the functional inactivity of the brain during sleep than a cause of the sleep.

During sleep the heart and lungs continue their work; the blood is circulated and purified, the intestines continue their vermicular contractions, and absorb food from the alimentary canal, and the organs nourish themselves at leisure.

Two facts relating to sleep have important practical bearings. First, during sleep metabolism is less active, and so the temperature of the body tends to be somewhat lowered. Secondly, assimilation is more energetic; this favours the absorption of noxious vapours, if any are present. There is probably, therefore, slightly less danger of remaining in a stuffy, impure atmosphere during the day than at night.

Practical Rules Concerning Sleep.—1. Amount of sleep required. It is impossible to lay down any fixed rule applicable to all persons and circumstances. The amount of sleep required, like the amount of food, varies greatly.

Habitual deficiency of sleep produces a condition of wretchedness and prostration, with great restlessness. Prolonged watching inevitably breaks down the constitution. Not the least evil consequence of irregular and deficient sleep is, that sleep, when desired, is often courted in vain.

Habitual excess of sleep produces a condition of brain less active than usual, and less favourable for thought and action. Impressions are received less readily, and the power of will is correspondingly diminished.

The amount of sleep required varies with—

(1) Age.—The infant, if healthy, spends the larger part of his existence in sleep; gradually the amount required diminishes until, for the adult, seven or eight hours suffice. Children over two or three years old require sleep only during the night. In advanced life there is a tendency to revert to infantile habits, sleep occurring in frequent short snatches.

(2) Sex.—Women have been stated to require rather more sleep than men, but this is doubtful. The hours of sleep required have in accordance with this view been stated to be, "Six for a man, seven for a woman, and eight for a fool." A reversal of this order would more nearly approximate to the requirements of town life.

(3) Temperament.—Those of a cold lymphatic temperament require more sleep than sanguine or nervous people, though the latter sleep more deeply. Frederick the Great, John Hunter, and Napoleon I. are said to have required only five hours' sleep per day; but the last of these had the faculty of taking short naps at a few moments' notice.

(4) The sick and convalescent require much more sleep than those who are healthy.

(5) Habit has a very important influence. Many people appear to sleep too much, and thus dull to some extent their mental faculties; but on the other hand, modern life, with its nervous strain, keen competition, and constant hurry and worry may make a larger amount of sleep necessary than that required by our forefathers, who invented the foregoing proverb.

236

(6) Occupation.—Mental work requires more repose than physical.

2. Relation of sleep to food.—The molecular life of the tissues—that is, the processes of nutrition—ought to be undisturbed. These go on most perfectly when no active function, such as that of digestion, is being performed. But while the stomach carries on the digestive functions to only a small extent during sleep, the intestines continue still to digest and absorb food. In accordance with these facts, it is advisable to allow at least two hours between the last meal of the day and sleep, especially if animal food has been taken.

3. As absorption is increased and the temperature is lowered during sleep, it is important to sleep in pure air, and to have warm coverings, especially about the shoulders and arms. Many an obstinate cough might be cured by the simple expedient of wearing a flannel jacket at night.

4. Sleep during the night and not during the day. It should hardly be necessary to say this, as the universal instinct of animals shows its advisability; but, unfortunately, the habits of mankind have commonly led to a partial reversal of the natural arrangement.

5. The room should be dark; light, like sound, is inimical to sleep. The head should be moderately raised. The temperature of the room for robust persons need not be artificially raised.

Sleeplessness, as a rule, occurs only when some physiological law has been broken. To relieve it, it is essential to equilibrate muscular and mental functions. Increase of muscular exercise is an important element in its treatment. In addition it is advisable not to have any severe mental work during the evening, nor to indulge in late suppers. Sleeplessness is the bane of many men of a nervous temperament, and chiefly attacks those of sedentary habits. It is apt to recur, and for this reason, if for no other, narcotics ought to be scrupulously avoided. The habit of taking such soporifics is unfortunately becoming much more common, and is productive of many evils. Death from accidental overdose is a frequent calamity; and, apart from this possibility, the invalid's nervous system is completely ruined by persistence in the habit, his power of will is annihilated, and he becomes the miserable slave of an evil habit, whose end is death.

237

CHAPTER XXXIX

PERSONAL HYGIENE (continued)— CLEANLINESS

Physiological Considerations.—The skin consists of a superficial part or epidermis, and a deeper part called the dermis or cutis.

Tubes of two kinds open on the surface of the skin, penetrating at their deeper ends into the cutis, viz. sweat or sudoriparous glands and sebaceous glands. The sudoriparous glands are simple tubes, the lower ends of which lie coiled up in the dermis. Each tube when straightened out is about a quarter of an inch long. It has been estimated that in the palm of the hand there are 3,528 orifices of sudoriparous and sebaceous glands on a square inch of surface; reckoning each gland at ¼; inch long, this means 73½ feet of tubes in this small space. Assuming that there are 2,800 tubes to every square inch, and that the amount of surface in a man of ordinary height and bulk is 2,500 square inches, it follows that there are seven million pores in a man—that is, 1,750,000 inches, or nearly twenty-eight miles.

The perspiration secreted by the sudoriparous glands is constantly evaporating from the surface of the body. It is very important that the orifices of these glands should be kept open in order that the secretion may not be interfered with. Animals have been killed by covering their skin with gelatine, and so preventing the escape of perspiration.

The sebaceous glands are shorter than the sudoriparous, and commonly end alongside the hairs before the latter issue from the skin. They secrete an oily material which serves the purpose of a natural pomade. The sebaceous secretion also keeps the general surface of the skin unctuous and supple. The smell of the sebaceous secretion may be unpleasant, especially in the arm-pits and some other parts. Frequent washing is therefore desirable.

The Conditions Due to Uncleanliness are due to obstruction of the excretory ducts, to accumulation of débris on the general surface of the skin, and to the consequent interference with the circulation.

1. The obstruction of the sudoriparous pores of the skin interferes with the elimination of waste products by the perspiration; these are re-absorbed or retained in the system; consequently more work is thrown on the lungs and kidneys, and the equilibrium of health is destroyed.

Sebaceous obstruction causes an accumulation of oily secretion in the ducts. The black spots so commonly seen about the nose, are the blocked up orifices of sebaceous glands, and by squeezing the nose tiny threads of fatty matter are forced out from the interior of these glands. Pimples on the face are usually due to obstruction of the sebaceous glands; sometimes the obstruction leads to inflammation around the sebaceous gland (acne) which often permanently injures the skin.

238

2. Accumulation of effete matter on the skin occurs, unless frequent ablutions are performed. The epidermis is constantly shedding its older and more superficial parts, in the form of minute scales or "scurf." In the absence of frequent washing, the scales of epithelium tend to accumulate, the sebaceous secretion matting the scales together, and rendering them more adhesive. The saline matters of the perspiration also accumulate along with the scales and sebaceous secretion, and in virtue of their hygroscopic properties tend to keep the skin clammy and cold.

The obstruction of excretions and the accumulation of débris lead to other consequences. Thus:—3. The sensibility of the skin is dulled when the sensory papillæ are covered with dirt. The sensations received by the skin are important in regulating the temperature of the body. A cold external temperature should cause a reflex contraction of the small arteries bringing blood to the skin, thus diminishing the flow of blood and preventing undue loss of heat. Similarly, if the external temperature is high, or the internal development of heat is too great, these arteries dilate, and sending more blood to the skin, cause a greater loss of heat by radiation and conduction. Impaired sensibility of the skin leads to imperfect action of the reflex nervous mechanism to which the above effects are due, and consequently the dangers resulting from sudden alterations of temperature are greatly increased.

4. The tendency to chills is increased, not only by deficiency of the nervous tone of the skin, but also by obstruction of the pores of the skin, and by the hygrometric action of the saline matter collected on it.

5. Cutaneous diseases are due to, or favoured by, uncleanliness. These are of two kinds—parasitic and non-parasitic. Acne, which is the chief non-parasitic disease favoured by uncleanliness, has been already mentioned.

Parasitic skin diseases are greatly favoured by the presence of a dirty skin, which affords a suitable soil for the development of the parasites.

Uses of Soap.—Soap is produced by an action of an alkali on an oil. The alkali displaces glycerine from the oil, and forms an alkaline stearate, which is soap. Soft soap is chiefly stearate of potassium; hard soap is stearate of sodium. There may also be present the alkaline salts of oleic and palmitic acid. Soft soap is not used for washing the skin, as it is too irritating. All soaps contain a slight excess of soda; the greater this excess, the more irritating is the soap to delicate skins. Hard soaps may be also made with potash, if the fat employed be a solid one; but such soaps are rather softer than ordinary hard soaps, and more caustic. Cocoa-nut oil is used in making marine soaps, because, unlike all other kinds, it is not rendered insoluble by brine, and so will form a lather with sea-water. Normal soaps contain from 15 to 35 per cent. of water. "Liquoring" a soap consists in adding 5 to 25 per cent. of soluble silicates. By this means the soap may be made to hold 70 per cent. of water, which is obviously very wasteful.

In washing the skin, the water washes away a considerable amount of epidermis, and the saline matters which have collected. For the oily sebaceous secretion soap is required. The alkali in soap combines with the oily matter, forming an emulsion which carries away with it a quantity of the dirt which previously blocked the orifices of the sebaceous and sweat ducts. When the skin is rubbed by the towel after washing, the softened epithelium, and with it any remaining dirt, are rubbed off, leaving the skin clean, and able to perform its normal functions.

The Use of Baths.—The primary object of bathing is cleanliness. A secondary consideration is the pleasure derived from bathing. Baths are especially necessary for those persons who lead sedentary lives. When the skin is kept in an active condition by exercise, it to some extent cleanses itself. Thus, a farm labourer who has a weekly bath, may be really cleaner than a person of sedentary habits, who has two baths per week.

Baths are classified according to temperature as follows:—Below 70° Fahr. they are described as cold; tepid up to 85°; warm up to 97°; and hot over this temperature. It is important in deciding the temperature of a bath not to trust to one's sensations; the only accurate measure is by the thermometer. A cold morning tub in the summer will commonly contain water at 55° to 60°; while the same in winter will be down to 40°, or occasionally to 32°.

For purposes of cleanliness the warm bath is the most efficient, combined with the free use of soap. The chief objection to it is that it produces an increased flow of blood to the skin, by relaxing the cutaneous blood-vessels, thus increasing the danger of chills if there is subsequent exposure. The increased sensibility to cold resulting from a warm bath may be obviated by afterwards rapidly sponging the body all over with cold water, and then drying the body quickly, and using the friction of a moderately rough towel. It is desirable for both cold and warm baths to have a "bath-sheet," in which the person may be completely enclosed on coming out of the bath. Drying is thus much more quickly accomplished, and the danger of chill is minimised.

A daily morning cold bath is a most important agent in the maintenance of robust health. The first sensation on entering a cold bath is of shock, due to the cooling of the surface of the body. This is followed in a few seconds by a glow, due to the blood returning with considerable force to the skin. A cold bath ought to be taken as rapidly as possible. If soaping the body is desired, it should be done before entering the bath, and the stay in the latter should be little more than momentary. In this way the best reaction or "glow" is obtained.

If a feeling of cold and chilliness remains after a cold bath, it has done more harm than good. This condition may often be avoided by quick drying and brisk friction; if after this a good reaction is not obtained, the temperature of the water should be increased. For those who are not very robust, the "cold tub" in winter is to be deprecated. If the water be raised to 60° by the addition of warm water, or in some cases even to 70°, a good reaction may be obtained. In other cases, in which a reaction is not experienced even after a bath of the latter temperature, a tepid bath may be taken, and then the body rapidly sponged with colder water.

Cold baths increase the tone of the skin, rendering it less susceptible to changes of temperature. The tendency to "catch cold" is diminished, the blood-vessels and nerves of the skin both responding more readily to any stimuli.

Swimming is a valuable combination of bathing and exercise. A sudden plunge into cold water for swimming purposes is dangerous to those who are not hardened to it, and especially so in the case of running water, as in rivers or the sea. Here the water around the swimmer is constantly being changed, and each layer of water coming in contact with him abstracts a considerable amount of heat. Many of the cases of so-called death from "cramp" are really due to the benumbing and depressing influence of continued cold on the vital organs.

Swimming, under proper superintendence, ought to be universally enforced. The exercise accompanying it serves in most cases to counteract the depressing action of the cold water; but it is important in all cases to attend to certain rules. The immersion should not be prolonged; the body should be warm at the time of entering the water; and the bath should not be taken until about two hours after a meal; nor after prolonged fasting, as before breakfast.

Personal Cleanliness.—Personal cleanliness involves not only attention to the skin, which we have already considered, but to the hair, nails, mouth, and other parts of the body.

The hair ought to be carefully brushed and combed, but it is not desirable to use soap to it as often as to the skin. Soap removes the sebaceous secretion from the hairs, and renders them dry and brittle. Artificial pomades are, as a rule, unnecessary.

The nails should be cut square, and not down at the sides. It is hardly necessary to say that they should be kept clean: they may convey serious infection.

The mouth and all mucous orifices should be kept scrupulously clean. A fœtid breath is not uncommonly due to the discharges from carious teeth, or to the decomposition of food which has been allowed to accumulate in the cavities of teeth. Such decomposing matters when swallowed, are apt to produce indigestion; and this also occurs from imperfect mastication of food by the bad teeth. It is important that the teeth should be frequently cleansed, and that all carious teeth should be "stopped" at an early period, and tartar and other accumulations removed. Whether bad teeth, which are so extremely common, are due to the drinking of very hot liquids, or to the fact that the more perfect cooking of food gives less healthy friction to the teeth, is doubtful. Whatever the cause, by keeping the mouth thoroughly sweet and clean, and by having the carious teeth stopped as soon as discovered, their vitality may be greatly prolonged. Teeth should be periodically inspected by a competent dentist. Irregularities of the teeth may be corrected, if they receive early attention. Carious "milk-teeth" should receive attention from a dentist, as well as the permanent teeth.

General Cleanliness.—Next to cleanliness of the skin, that of the apparel is most important.

There is a general preference for colours "that do not show the dirt"; the fact that it is still there, though not seen, being partially ignored.

Changing of apparel is commonly confined to underclothing. It is forgotten that vests, trousers, dresses, etc., acquire a large amount of dirt and organic matter, and ought to be changed and well aired at intervals.

Cleanliness in respect to bedclothes is very important. Organic matters evolved from the skin, lungs, etc., hang about the bed-linen, and give the bedroom the "close smell" which can be perceived on entering it in the morning straight from the fresh air. The beds should not be made directly after being evacuated, but the clothes should be thrown over the bottom of the bed, the bolsters and mattress well shaken, and every part exposed to a free current of air during the greater part of the morning, before re-arranging the clothes. Eider-down quilts, unless frequently ventilated by exposure to outside air, are unwholesome. Superfluous bedroom furniture should be avoided, as it all takes away from the breathing-space. Bed-hangings should be reduced to a minimum, and all excretory matters covered up during their stay in the room, and removed as early as possible.

Cleanliness of the house is also very important as a means of health. Dust, in however obscure a corner it rests, attracts to itself organic matters, and forms a soil in which disease germs may grow. Besides this, it devitalises the air, depriving it of its active oxygen.

Dust in the streets serves to carry about various diseases, besides mechanically irritating any part it comes in contact with, producing bronchitis, etc.

CHAPTER XL

CLOTHING

Physiological Considerations.—The average temperature of the surface of the body in man is 98·4 to 98·6°. The maintenance of a tolerably uniform temperature is an essential condition of life. The factors governing the temperature of the body are the amount of heat produced and the amount lost. If more heat escapes, more has to be generated; and the source of all the heat produced in the body is the food taken. This becomes changed by the metabolic processes occurring in the body which produce heat.

Heat is lost, (1) by the skin; (2) in respiration, the expired air having been heated during its stay in the lungs; (3) with the food and drink taken, if not at the temperature of the body; (4) with the excreta; and (5) by transformation of heat into mechanical energy. Of the whole loss by these different channels, probably eighty to ninety per cent. is through the skin.

The Loss of Heat by the Skin is in three different ways. First, by conduction, when the skin comes in contact with anything cooler than itself; secondly, by radiation into space; and thirdly, by evaporation of the perspiration. The last cause produces a considerable reduction of temperature, even when the perspiration is not so abundant as to be visible, but is in the form of insensible perspiration. The losses by these different sources vary in amount; when one is increased, another is diminished, by way of compensation. Thus, in very cold weather, the amount of radiation and conduction of heat are increased; but evaporation greatly decreases, and the diminished loss of heat in this respect counterbalances in some degree the increased loss by radiation and conduction.

When the external warmth is considerable, increased evaporation occurs; while when the weather is cold, the cutaneous arteries contract, and less blood goes to the skin, and so the loss of heat is diminished. In most climates, however, this action of the skin requires to be supplemented by some kind of clothing.

Requisites of Dress.—1. The first and most important requirement is that clothing should maintain a uniform and equable temperature in all parts of the body.

In hot climates clothes are required in order to protect the body from external heat. In this country, they are required to prevent the too rapid escape of heat from the body. For both these purposes, dress must be of a non-conducting material, in order not to encourage transfer of heat into or from the surrounding atmosphere.

The loss of heat by the skin may be prevented by interfering with radiation or conduction of heat, or with evaporation from its surface. Radiation of heat from the skin is prevented by clothing, the dress taking the place of the skin as a radiating surface. The amount of radiation from the dress will depend on the rapidity of conduction of heat from the skin. The amount of conduction and of radiation of heat will vary considerably with the material and colour of the dress.

As regards conductivity, the two extremes are represented by linen and fur. It is found that if the conducting power for heat of linen = 100, then that of wool = 50 to 70. This partly explains why woollen goods are so much warmer than linen. We shall find that there is another explanation in the relative hygroscopic properties of the two materials.

As regards radiation of heat, in one experiment it was found that while a piece of linen took 10½ minutes to cool, a corresponding piece of flannel took 11½ minutes.

Apart from the material, the colour of dress has some influence in regulating the loss of heat. Dark-coloured materials absorb more light and heat than lighter coloured materials; they may be good or bad conductors of heat, according to the nature of the material. White reflects the rays of light and heat; hence it is a poor absorber. In summer it prevents the passage of heat inwards, and, in winter, may prevent its passage from the body. It is thus well adapted for both winter and summer clothing, and has the additional advantage of being the cleanest colour.

Franklin placed a number of squares of different coloured cloths of the same material on snow, and found after a time that the snow covered

243

by the black piece was most, and by the white piece least melted. In another set of experiments, shirting materials dyed various colours were taken, and it was found that if the rays of heat received by white were represented as 100, pale straw received 102, dark yellow 140, light green 155, Turkey red 165, dark green 168, light blue 198, black.

The influence of colour is antagonised to a large extent by the nature of the material; the increased heat absorbed by a dark material may be counterbalanced by the material being a good conductor. Also the influence of colour is only exerted superficially; hence, although it produces considerable effect in thin textures, as gauze, it has little influence on thick materials.

2. The dress should not interfere with perspiration. In order that it may not do this, it should be competent to absorb moisture easily, without its surface becoming wetted. Materials like linen which lose their porosity and rapidly become wetted by perspiration, cause rapid loss of heat from the body, inasmuch as water is a better conductor of heat than air. Pettenkofer found that while the maximum hygroscopic power of wool (flannel) is 174 and the minimum 111; the maximum of linen is 75 and the minimum 41. Hence, with a flannel vest next the skin, the liability to chill is much less than with a linen one. There is one slightly counterbalancing drawback; hygroscopic materials absorb moisture from the air, as well as from the skin. A woollen coat during a damp day, without rain, increases considerably in weight.

Waterproof clothing is injurious when worn beyond a short period, on account of its being non-porous and consequently keeping the body enveloped in a vapour bath composed of its own perspiration. For a similar reason India-rubber boots are objectionable, except for short periods; they make the feet damp, and even sodden. Sealskin jackets are objectionable for walking, not only because of their weight, but because they are not porous.

3. The warmth of clothing should be uniformly distributed throughout the body. This principle is very frequently departed from; and consequently one part may be chilled while another is over-heated. This is seen especially in female apparel. The same evil is seen in the short sleeves, and short and low-necked dresses of young children. "Combination" garments for women, and sleeves and leggings for young children are happily becoming more generally adopted, and will diminish the diseases due to exposure to cold.

4. The clothing should not be tight; and this for three reasons. First, because loose clothing is warmer than tight; this everyone has experienced in the case of gloves. The retention of air in the meshes of clothing is one of the main causes of its warmth, air being a bad conductor of heat. The imprisonment of air in the meshes of the material largely explains the warmth of eider-down quilts, furs, and flannels as contrasted with linen.

Secondly, clothing should not be tight, in order to avoid interference with the action of the muscles. Tight sleeves prevent the muscles of the arms and chest from being exercised. Tightly laced corsets imprison the trunk muscles, prevent their contractions, and so lead to muscular weakness and occasionally spinal curvature. Tight skirts similarly prevent free play of the lower limbs, leading to a halting gait, a diminished amount of exercise, with all the evils following deficient exercise. Tight clothing is not confined to one sex, and in all cases leads to hampered movements and deficient muscularity.

Thirdly, tight clothing tends to impede the functions of circulation, respiration, and digestion. The fashion which more than any other interferes with important functions is tight-lacing. This produces (1) compression and displacement of the viscera; the liver and the stomach especially suffer. (2) Respiration and circulation are impeded, the action of the diaphragm being impeded. (3) The muscles of the trunk being tightly encased, are incapable of movement, and consequently tend to waste and atrophy. The general outline of the body is altered. Instead of the waist being elliptical, as it naturally is, it becomes nearly circular; and instead of its circumference averaging twenty-six to twenty-seven inches, it may be eighteen to twenty-one inches. Tight garters tend to produce varicose veins.

Tight boots are injurious, as they tend to destroy the natural elasticity of the movements, and confine them within narrow limits. They act to some extent the part of splints. By interfering with the circulation of blood through the feet, they cause cold feet, and not uncommonly chilblains. High-heeled boots do not allow the natural elasticity of the foot to come into action. They distort the movements of the body and cause corns and bunions. Similar effects are produced by boots which are too narrow and have pointed toes, thus not allowing free movement of the toes.

5. The weight of the clothing should be the smallest amount consistent with warmth, and it should be evenly distributed. The chief weight should not be suspended from the waist, as here the parts are not well supported by bones. The shoulders and hips should share in the suspension of clothing, thus diminishing the danger of compression and displacement of internal organs. In order that garments may be as light as possible, they should be made to fit to each limb separately, thus diminishing the amount of material required.

6. The materials of dress should be as far as possible non-inflammable. This may sometimes be disregarded, but is often important, as in the nursery. In this respect, as in many others, wool possesses great advantages. Woollen fabrics smoulder rather than burst into flames, and thus the injury resulting from any accident is limited. Cotton is more inflammable than linen, linen than silk, and silk than wool. A closely woven cloth is less inflammable than one with open meshes.

Dress materials, and more particularly muslin, have been rendered non-inflammable by treating with a solution of ammonic phosphate, or ammonic phosphate and ammonic chloride mixed. The best material, however, is sodic tungstate, which, unlike the others, is not affected by ironing. Sodic molybdate is used in arsenals to render the workmen's clothing non-inflammable. All the above plans are objectionable, as the weight of the material is increased 18 to 29 per cent., and they all wash out.

To remedy this, a "fire-proof starch," containing sodic tungstate has been devised.

Perfect non-inflammability is only required in certain dangerous occupations. The plans hitherto mentioned simply prevent the fabric breaking out into flame. The only cloth absolutely unaffected by fire is asbestos cloth.

7. Elegance of dress, although not so important as utility, is not to be neglected, and the two are perfectly compatible. In fact, elegance is indirectly associated with utility, for nothing which is awkward, or leads to obstructed movements or distortions of the body, is really elegant. A sudden constriction, as in a very tight waist, is not only bad from a hygienic point of view, but is also ugly.

Materials for Clothing.—The materials used are derived partly from the vegetable world, as hemp, flax, cotton; and partly from the animal world, as silk, wool, hair, feathers. The most important materials are wool, silk, cotton, and flax.

1. Wool varies somewhat in character, according to the animal from which it is derived. In all its varieties, however, it preserves the character of a bad conducting and porous substance, the two most important requisites in a dress material.

(1) Wool from the sheep is really a soft and elastic hair, composed of fibres three to eight inches long, and about 1/1000 inch thick. The finer and shorter wools are used for fine cloth, the longer and coarser for "poplins," "worsted pieces," etc. Flannel is a woollen stuff of rather open and slight fabric. Wool is irritating to delicate skins, and may be so much so, that it cannot be worn next the skin, whether as flannel, worsted, or merino. In these cases, it may be worn outside a linen or gauze vest, and so all its advantages secured. It is one of the worst conductors of heat, and ought always to be worn in winter; while even in summer, it ensures a greater immunity from chill after perspiration than any other material.

(2) Cashmere is made from the down found about the roots of the hair of the Thibet goat. Imitation cashmere is made of various materials mixed together.

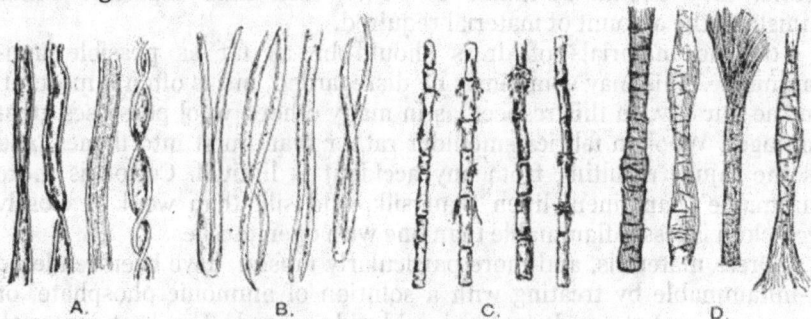

Fig. 56.
Microscopical Appearance of Fibres of
A—Cotton. B—Silk. C—Linen. D—Wool.

(3) Alpaca is obtained from the fleece of the llama, alpaca, and

vicuna. It is longer than the fleece of the sheep, the fibres, which are soft and strong, averaging six inches in length. It is commonly made up with cotton or silk.

(4) Mohair is the hair of a goat inhabiting the mountains near Angora. It is woven into an almost waterproof cloth, and used in making plush, braid, etc.

2. Hair derived from the horse or cow differs from the hair usually called wool, in the greater solidity of its structure, which makes it ill adapted for clothing. Its chief use is in the manufacture of felts, of which hats are made.

3. Leather is a kind of natural felt, very close and firm in its texture. It is used in this country chiefly for boots, but in some colder climates also for coats, etc. It is impervious to moisture, like sealskin, and is consequently not very healthy. The same objection applies to chamois-leather underclothing, which is non-porous, and consequently keeps the skin hot and clammy; also, it cannot be washed without becoming stiff on drying. This necessitates wearing the material after it has become impregnated with perspiration.

4. Silk. The thread spun by the silk-worm is composed of filaments 1/2000 inch wide, and is the strongest and most tenacious of textile fabrics. Its thread is three times as strong as a thread of flax of the same thickness, and twice as strong as a thread of hemp.

Its fibres are round like those of linen, but softer and smaller; it gives an agreeable sensation of freshness to the skin even more than linen. It is a worse conductor of heat than cotton or linen. Its great disadvantage for wearing next the skin, apart from its expense, is that it irritates delicate skins. Satin is silk so prepared as to form a smooth, polished surface.

Velvet is a silk fabric of which the pile is due to the insertion of short pieces of silk thread under the weft or cross-thread. Cheaper kinds are made, containing a certain proportion of cotton.

Crape is made of raw silk gummed and twisted to form a gauze-like fabric. Taffety, moire, brocade, and plush are made of silk alone or combined with cotton.

5. Cotton consists of the downy hairs investing the seeds of the gossypium plant. The threads of which it is composed are flat, ribbon-like, and twisted, about 1/800 to 1/2000 inch wide. Owing to its flat fibres with sharp edges, it is apt to irritate delicate skins; linen is preferable for dressing wounds for a similar reason. Cotton is warmer than linen, being a worse conductor of heat. It also absorbs moisture better, not becoming wet so soon; but it lacks the "freshness" which makes linen materials pleasant to wear. Calico, fustian, jean, velveteen, and muslin are the chief cotton fabrics.

6. Flax is formed from the fibres of the flax plant. Linen is made from it. Cambric and lawn are very fine and thin linen materials. The fibres of linen are round and pliable; thus it is smooth and soft, and peculiarly agreeable to the skin. It is, however, a good conductor of heat, and consequently "it feels cold" to the skin. Furthermore its pores quickly become filled with perspiration, which escapes rapidly, thus chilling the body.

247

7. Mackintoshes are valuable as a temporary protection against external wet. Worn for more than a short period, they produce great heat and a sense of closeness, owing to retention of the perspiration. The best form of mackintosh is one having a cape, with a space for evaporation between it and the rest of the garment.

The Amount of Clothing required varies with circumstances. 1. Health; those of robust constitution require less than the feeble. The more active are digestion and assimilation, the less is the amount of clothing required. If heat is preserved by clothing, less food is required. Thus a distinct saving of food is effected by warm clothes. Warm clothes are the equivalent of so much food that would have been required to keep up the temperature of the body, if the clothes had not been worn. Thinly clad persons under conditions of starvation die more quickly than those who are better protected.

2. Clothing requires to be adapted to climate and season. In winter and in cold climates the amount of clothing must be increased, and warmer materials chosen. In the changeable climate of Great Britain, it is difficult to adapt the character of one's dress to the requirements of the weather. Clothing ought, however, not to be changed according to the calendar, but according to the weather. The tendency is to assume summer clothing too early in the spring, and to continue it too far into the autumn. According to Boërhave, winter clothing should be put off on Midsummer day, and resumed the day after. This, although rather exaggerated, may serve to impress the caution required. The same authority says that only fools and beggars suffer from cold, the latter not being able to procure sufficient clothes, the former not having the sense to wear them.

3. Age. Those at the two extremes of life are specially susceptible to cold. The mortality of infants during the first three months of life is nearly doubled in winter. Bronchitis and pneumonia prove fatal chiefly at the two extremes of age.

The younger a child the larger is its surface as compared with its bulk, inasmuch as the area of a body varies as the square of its dimensions, while its mass varies as their cube. Thus a cube 1 inch each side has 6 square inches of surface to 1 cubic inch of bulk, while a cube 10 inches each side has 600 square inches of surface to 1000 cubic inches in bulk. Similarly a child 1/10 the size of its mother, besides its feebler powers of producing heat, has ten times as much surface in proportion to its size by which heat is lost.

After the age of thirty-five, it is better to exceed than to be deficient in clothing. A degree of cold that would act as a useful tonic to the robust and middle-aged, produces serious and even fatal depression of the vital powers in children or aged people. For the same reason it is advisable to discontinue cold baths as age advances.

A very pernicious delusion is prevalent, that children ought to be "hardened" to the influences of cold, and that too much clothing "makes them tender." Excessive clothing may possibly increase the tendency to "catch cold," owing to its exciting perspiration, or owing to the fact that the extra clothing is commonly thrown off at irregular intervals—witness the effects of wearing a scarf round the neck occasionally. But to suppose that children can be hardened by exposure of arms and legs, and other parts of their bodies, is irrational. A large amount of heat is lost from these bare surfaces, and apart altogether from the danger of chill, more food must be taken to compensate for this loss of heat, and keep up an equable temperature. Also if the food taken is expended in preserving the warmth of the unprotected body, less material is left for the purpose of growth. From these causes it frequently happens that children remain stunted in growth, even if latent disease is not actually developed by the extra strain on their resources.

The children of the very poor are often pointed to as demonstrating the power of hardening. It is forgotten how many of these poor children have perished under the hardening system, and that the good health of those remaining is in spite of the hardening.

Poisonous Dyes in Clothing.—These, like poisonous wall-papers, were formerly much more common than at present, and, as in wall-papers, the poisonous agent has most frequently been arsenic, large quantities of which were formerly used in the preparation of certain dyes. Occasionally such poisonous pigments are still employed.

CHAPTER XLI

PARASITES

Parasites (Greek, para, upon, and siteo, I feed), in the broadest sense of the word, are living organisms, which derive their nourishment from other living organisms. They may belong to the vegetable or animal kingdoms, and may live on the skin, in the alimentary canal, or in some one of the internal organs. Some, like the fungus causing ringworm, feed on the living tissues of the animal infested; others, like tape-worms, on the partly digested food; while other parasites, like fleas, only pay temporary visits to the surface of the body, for the purpose of obtaining food.

Vegetable Parasites.—Vegetable parasites all belong to the class of fungi, and more accurately to the two lowest divisions of this class which have been provisionally formed, viz.—Schizophyta, and Zygophyta. The Schizophyta include two orders, Schizomycetes and Saccharomycetes.

BACTERIA

Bacterium is the generic name given to the micro-organisms belonging to the schizomycetes, whether a bacillus (rod-shaped), coccus (rounded), spiral-formed (spirillum or vibrio), or filamentous (leptothrix and spirochœta). All these are destitute of chlorophyll and multiply by fission.[8] They are all extremely small, the width usually not exceeding 1 μ = 1/25000 inch. Various names are given to them, which are synonymous, thus: germs,

microbes,
micro-organisms,
microzymes,
bacteria (singular bacterium).

When they cause disease they are called contagia. They multiply rapidly, and may reach maturity in 20 to 30 minutes. One bacterium may, under favourable conditions, become 16,000,000 in 24 hours.

Methods of Examination.—Until Koch discovered the method of cultivating bacteria on solid media, the science of bacteriology remained in its infancy, as it was impracticable to obtain pure, i.e. unmixed cultures of a given bacterium. Koch hit on the idea of mixing minute portions of cultivations of bacteria which were growing in liquid broth with liquefied gelatine, and then spreading the mixture on glass plates, and allowing it to solidify under cover, so that no atmospheric bacteria could contaminate the growth. When this was done, individual bacteria formed individual "colonies" scattered over the gelatine, and these could be identified by sub-culturing and other methods, for the details of which books on bacteriology must be consulted.

The food supply of most bacteria is vegetable or animal refuse. Some of them have a most useful purpose in nature, that of breaking down complex organic substances and reducing them to a simpler form. Thus bacteria play an essential part in purifying the soil, and in the operations in sewage tanks and on sewage farms. A thimbleful of ordinary garden soil which has received a periodical manurial dressing contains one to three million bacteria. Certain bacteria have been found to be capable of exercising an opposite effect, i.e. fixing the atmospheric nitrogen and building it up into the nitrogenous tissues of plants. Thus the nodules on the roots of leguminous plants consist of bacteria living in symbiosis with the protoplasm of the plant and supplying it with nitrogen in an assimilable condition. Pure cultures of these bacteria have been put on the market as nitragin, for enriching land poor in nitrogen. Thus a fairly complete cycle of nature is secured, and by rotation of plants (legumes alternating with other seeds), manures, especially nitrogenous manures, may be partially saved.

The souring of milk is caused by the bacillus lactis. This souring is an indispensable preliminary to the making of cheese, and the bacillus can now be used in pure culture to hasten the natural process. The peculiar aroma of good butter is due to a bacterium which has been isolated; and it can now be supplied in pure culture for butter-making, thus obviating bad butter.

---

[8] Some bacteria form in their interior minute spores, by means of which they are able to resist ordinary destructive agents. These spores again develope into bacteria.

Certain bacteria are disease-producing or pathogenic. The largest of these is the Bacillus of Anthrax, a disease common in sheep and oxen, and sometimes communicated to man. This bacillus is 1·2 μ thick and 6 to 8 μ long. When an animal dies of this disease it should be buried without cutting the skin. When exposed to the air this bacillus forms minute spores, very difficult to destroy. They may live for several years in pits in which animals dying from anthrax have been buried. Butchers have died when inoculated through cracked fingers when dressing the carcase of a cow which has had anthrax. Similarly men handling the hides of such animals may be inoculated, either with a form of disease in which rapid blood-poisoning is produced, or with a malignant carbuncle, from which recovery is possible if it be treated promptly. Wool sorters of mohair wool are very liable to suffer from a fatal form of pneumonia due to the dust from wool derived from animals which have died from anthrax (page 107). This disease gives a good instance of possible attenuation of virus, of which another example is seen in small pox. Pasteur grew anthrax bacilli in broth at a temperature of 110° Fahr. At this temperature the bacilli multiplied by division, and no spores were formed. By repeatedly sub-culturing after the bacilli had become old (i.e. by putting minute quantities of the growth into fresh broth) and exposing to air, he obtained anthrax bacilli which were only slightly virulent, only producing slight constitutional disturbance when inoculated, i.e. injected under the skin of sheep, and yet protected them against ordinary infection by anthrax. Other methods of attenuation of virus have been discovered. For instance the growth of the bacillus in the presence of a feeble antiseptic, or passing it through the circulation of an animal which is relatively insusceptible to the particular bacillus has this effect.

Other important pathogenic bacteria will be considered later. It is only necessary here to mention that suppuration, erysipelas, puerperal fever, and a number of forms of blood-poisoning are due to the invasion of the system by cocci. A single round cell (commonly not more than 1/25000 inch in diameter) is called a micrococcus. When in pairs as in the micro-organism causing pneumonia they are called diplococci; when in chains, streptococci (i.e. twisted); when in masses, staphylococci. When cocci and other micro-organisms are kept out of wounds, healing occurs without suppuration; this is the principle of the antiseptic and aseptic methods of treating wounds.

Saccharomycetes occur in fermenting substances, as in the fermentation of saccharine solutions. The only organism belonging to this order, which is associated with diseased conditions, is the Sarcina Ventriculi. This is found occasionally in the vomit or even in the urine of some persons.

The Zygophyta occur as thread-like growths, forming a mycelium. This is composed of jointed branching tubular cells, in which minute spores are produced. Each spore, when liberated from its tube, is capable of producing another mycelium, and thus the growth spreads. The spores may be carried through the atmosphere, thus producing infection at a distance. They have an average diameter of 6 μ = about 1/4000 inch.

251

The following are the chief Zygophytous parasitic diseases:—Thrush is associated with the growth of a minute filamentous fungus, the oidium albicans. It is common in babies, who are improperly fed, and in old people, or in persons exhausted by any chronic disease. Small white patches collect on the tongue and neighbouring parts, and these are often followed by the formation of minute ulcers. When it occurs in children, the food must be carefully attended to, and feeding bottles frequently scalded, etc.

Ringworm is due to the growth of a large spored or a small spored fungus (known under the names of Microsporon Audouini; Trichophyton megalosporon endothrix, Trichophyton megalosporon ectothrix) which attacks the skin. It is most difficult to eradicate when it occurs in hairy parts, as the growth penetrates to the roots of the hairs, and continues to live here long after it has been destroyed on the general surface of the skin. The fungus spreads on the skin in gradually enlarging circles, forming rings with a slightly raised margin. It is extremely contagious, being especially apt to spread in schools. The spores may be carried about by means of hats or bonnets, by gloves, towels, razors, and other means. The disease often remains undetected for some time; and many cases, especially where the scalp is affected, remain contagious after they have been apparently cured.

The removal of ringworm, as of all other skin parasites, is effected by some local parasiticide. Prolonged treatment, including the pulling out of diseased hairs, is required for ringworm of the scalp. A special cap should be worn, when the patient mixes with others.

Favus, or "scald-head," is due to the growth in the skin of a minute fungus called the Achorion Schönleinii, which invades the same parts as those affected by ringworm, but differs in its mode of formation of spores; yellow cupped discs from ¼; to 1/3 inch in diameter being produced. It is very rare in England, and almost confined to persons (especially children) who are kept in a filthy condition. It is a common and fatal disease in mice. The treatment is similar to that of ringworm.

Tinea versicolor is caused by the growth in the epithelial cells of the skin, of a fungus called the microsporon furfur, which, unlike the two last, does not invade the hair or nails. It forms light brown patches covered with a horny scurf, which gradually spread, until nearly the whole trunk may be covered. It does not attack children, and never affects uncovered parts of the body. It chiefly occurs in those who do not take frequent baths, and who perspire freely. It can be removed by daily washing with soap and water and rubbing with a rough towel, followed by the application of a weak carbolic lotion.

Animal Parasites.—Animal parasites are found on the skin or in internal organs or in the blood or lymphatic vessels. The following are the most common:—

The Acarus Scabiei is a minute animal not unlike a cheese mite, which causes the disease known as scabies or the itch. It is probably never more than 1/77 of an inch in length. The female has eight legs, with terminal suckers on the four front legs and hairs on the hind legs. The male is smaller than the female, and in the adult condition the two hindmost legs have suckers, as well as the four anterior. It remains on the surface of the skin, while the female burrows deeply in the substance of the epidermis. At the bottom of the oblique burrow it deposits ten to fifteen or more eggs, which hatch in a fortnight and then commence similar operations on their own account. Scabies generally starts between the fingers, whence it rapidly spreads. The disease is acquired from some patient suffering from the disease, or by contact with his apparel. It may become very severe when suspicion as to its parasitic character has not been entertained. Formerly it was called "the seven years' itch," from the great difficulty in curing it before its true cause was discovered.

The irritation caused by the insect produces eczema, and this may be thought to be the only disease present, unless careful examination is made for the burrows of the insect.

To remove this parasite, first the skin is softened, the superficial epidermis is removed, and the burrows are laid bare, by the daily use of hot baths with soft soap, and subsequent rubbing with flesh towels. Then some parasiticide, such as the well known sulphur ointment, is rubbed into all the affected parts of the skin. A few days' perseverance in this treatment usually suffices for a cure. The patient's clothes and bed clothes ought also to be thoroughly purified by boiling or by steam disinfection or by baking in an oven; otherwise he may become re-infected.

The Larvæ of several insects have been found embedded in the skin. In the ox, the larva or bot of the gadfly produces a troublesome disease, a large boil being formed under the skin as the larva grows. This larva has, on rare occasions, attacked human beings. Rare cases are recorded where other larvæ have become developed in men, in all upwards of twenty separate kinds of insects having been recognized. The treatment consists in removing the parasite.

The Chigoe, commonly known as the jigger or sand-flea, is a minute parasitic insect, found in the West Indies and northern parts of South America. It is so small as to be scarcely visible; but the impregnated female possesses a proboscis, by means of which it penetrates the skin generally near the nails and there develops a bladder the size of a pea, which sets up severe inflammation. To get rid of the intruder, the orifice by which it entered must be dilated with a needle, until large enough to admit of its extraction, without rupturing the cyst.

Several species of Fleas infest the human frame. They are propagated by means of eggs, the worms from which enclose themselves in a tiny cocoon before assuming the adult form.

Three varieties of Lice occur on the human skin. The first (pediculus capitis) infests the head, especially of children, and multiplies with astonishing rapidity, the female laying altogether about fifty eggs. The other two varieties are the body louse (pediculus corporis) and the crab louse (pediculus pubis).

Strict attention to cleanliness is the best means of getting rid of fleas and bugs. A wash made of carbolic acid and vinegar painted over bed crevices is very efficient. Lice may be removed from the head by cutting the hair short, and carefully cutting out any hairs to which nits are attached. The nits are cemented to the shafts of hairs. Washing the hair with methylated spirit or paraffin is also helpful in removing them. Afterwards the use of white precipitate ointment will prevent their re-appearance.

The Trematoda or Flukes furnish two human parasites, viz. the liver-fluke (Distoma hepatis), and the Bilharzia hæmatobia. The liver-fluke occasionally produces jaundice in man. In sheep it is the cause of the disease known as the "rot." The Bilharzia hœmatobia is chiefly found in Egypt, and the Cape Colony. It is about a quarter of an inch long, and infests the blood vessels, more particularly of the kidneys; setting up severe irritation and the discharge of blood. It is probable that the eggs of this parasite are received in drinking water or on salads, though occasionally inoculation may occur through the skin when bathing.

The family of Nematoda possesses numerous parasitic members. The common thread worm (Oxyuris Vermicularis) is one of the most common of these. The female is 1/3 to 1/2 inch in length, and inhabits chiefly the lower bowel. The ova, which are from 1/490 to 1/1100 inch in diameter, often gain access to drinking water, or are carried by flies, or received on salads, etc. The injection of salt and water into the bowel, and treatment tending to improve the general health, are the proper remedies.

The round worm (Ascaris Lumbricoides) inhabits chiefly the small intestine; hence medicines for its removal require to be given by the mouth. The female is from 10 to 14 inches long; the ova, of which each female discharges on an average 160,000 daily, are from 1/340 to 1/440 inch in diameter.

The whip-worm (Trichocephalus Dispar) is a smaller nematode, which is rarely met with in this country. The Dochmius Duodenalis is met with chiefly in Italy and Egypt. It sucks the blood in the intestine, causing dangerous anæmia. The Strongylus Gigas is chiefly found in the kidneys of the ox, dog, etc., and is very rare in man. It resembles a very large round worm. In the kidney it produces severe disorders. How it gets there is not known.

The Filaria Dracunculus (Guinea Worm) seems to gain access into the stomach along with water, or possibly in some cases, by perforating the skin. It burrows among the tissues, especially of the legs, and attains a length of several feet. It causes large boils and sores, and through these the eggs escape and pass into water. Here the embryo which has escaped from the egg meets with a fresh water crustacean (cyclops), enters its body, undergoes larval growth, and is swallowed with its host by a man, in whom it burrows and undergoes its next stage of life.

The embryos of three species of Filaria infest the blood of man, chiefly in the tropics. One embryonic species is found in the blood of infested patients by day, one by night, and one during both day and night. The length of the embryos varies from 1/75 to 1/125 inch, and its width from 1/3000 to 1/3500 inch. The night embryo, which is the most common, is produced by the Filaria Bancrofti. This adult worm infests the lymphatic system of man, sometimes reaching a length of three to four inches. Its embryos may obstruct lymphatic vessels, causing obstruction of

254

the flow of chyle (hence originates chyluria), and elephantiasis, in which enormous swelling of the legs and other parts ensues.

The nocturnal migration into the lymphatic vessels, and thence into the blood of the embryo of the F. Bancrofti, is an adaptation to the nocturnal habits of a particular mosquito (culex pipiens or ciliaris). When the mosquito bites an infested person, his proboscis removes some embryo filariæ, which are quickly transferred to its stomach. Some of these escape digestion, develop within the mosquito, and when the mosquito dies in water they bore their way out, and are subsequently swallowed by man.

It is essential, therefore, in order to prevent this disease to boil or efficiently filter all drinking water, and to prevent the access of mosquitoes to water. Persons infested with filariæ should sleep inside mosquito nets, in order that they may not, when bitten by mosquitoes, spread the disease.

Tape-worms are found infesting the alimentary canal of man. Each has a double phase of existence. In the first, the characteristic head, or scolex, along with a bladder-like body, lies embedded in the solid tissues of an animal; in the second, the strobilus or tape-worm, occupies the alimentary canal of another animal. The tape-worm consists of a number of flat segments, each of which is capable of producing a large number of eggs, from each of which a six-hooked embryo is developed. The segments escape from the alimentary canal, and their ova are discharged and scattered broad-cast. These eggs are swallowed by another animal, the hooked embryo escapes from its case, migrates into the solid tissues, and there produces a scolex. When the host is eaten by another animal or by man, the scolex enters the alimentary canal, loses its bladder-like body, and developes a chain of segments. It follows from the above that two distinct hosts are necessary to complete the cycle of existence of these creatures, one being commonly a herbivorous, and the other a carnivorous animal. Thus:—

Cystic Form.		Tape-worm Form.
Cysticercus Cellulosæ in the muscles of the pig	becomes	*Tænia Soluim in the alimentary canal of man.*
Cysticercus Bovis in the muscles of the ox	”	*Tænia Mediocanellata in the alimentary canal of man.*
Cænurus Cerebralis of the sheep's brain	”	*Tænia Cænurus in the alimentary canal of the dog.*
Echinococcus of man, etc.	”	*Tænia Echinococcus in the alimentary canal of the dog.*

The cystic form of the dog's tape-worm (echinococcus) is a most dangerous parasite for man. When the egg of the dog's tape-worm is swallowed by man, the embryo escaping from this egg burrows from the alimentary canal, and forms large cysts, chiefly in the liver, but occasionally in the lungs, brain, and other organs. For the removal of these, surgical interference is required. This form of cyst is commonly known as a hydatid. It is most frequently seen in Iceland and Australia, though not uncommon in this country. Its frequency depends largely on the number of dogs, and on the facility with which the ova of their tape-worms can gain access to water.

The adult Tape-worms are usually derived in man from eating meat containing the cystic form. The cysticercus of the pig produces Tænia Solium; that of the ox, the Tænia Mediocanellata.

These are the two most common forms of tape-worm in man. The minute head of T. Solium has four suckers and a double row of hooklets, 28 in number; while the head of T. Mediocanellata has four suckers but no hooklets. The segments of T. Solium are smaller than of T. Medioc., and the structure of the segments of the two is somewhat different.

Preventive Measures.—In avoiding the various Entozoa described, it is important (1) to carefully avoid all underdone meat. The eating of smoked sausages, or of meat which is not cooked throughout, is a common source of tape-worm and of trichinosis.

(2) All vegetables should be thoroughly washed: this is especially important in the case of water-cress, lettuce, etc., which are eaten raw.

(3) If the purity of the water is not ensured, it should be boiled or filtered through a Pasteur-Chamberland filter (page 91), especially in tropical climates, and where many dogs are kept. Dogs should be kept out of the kitchen, lest ova accidentally gain access to articles of food.

(4) The possibility of flies and mosquitoes acting as carriers of parasitic disease must be remembered, and precautions taken.

CHAPTER XLII

THE RÔLE OF INSECTS IN SPREADING DISEASE

Insects are now known to be important agents, (a) as carriers and (b) as intermediate hosts of disease-agents.

The common domestic fly (Musca domestica) is the unwelcome companion of man in nearly every country. The eggs are usually laid and the larvæ undergo their development in excrement, but the female sometimes selects meal, bread, or fruit for the purpose. In practice, however, one of the best means of diminishing the number of domestic flies is to insist on the daily removal of all manure, especially horse manure, and to sprinkle the manure receptacle in the interval with lime. The fly may obviously be the means of conveying infected material from place to place. Anthrax has been ascribed to this cause. Nuttall has proved experimentally that flies are able to carry the infection of plague, and that they die of the disease. The presence of enormous numbers of flies in cholera times has been noted. Experimentally, flies caught in cholera wards have been found to harbour the cholera spirillum. It is probable that they play a serious rôle in spreading the infection of cholera. Hence all infectious dejecta (stools and urine) should be covered until finally disposed of, and food should be protected against flies. The same remarks apply for enteric fever. Flies fed with pure cultures of the bacillus of enteric fever pass these bacilli in their dejecta in a still virulent condition. In camps, especially in connection with large armies, there is the strongest reason for believing that flies carry infection from latrines to food. Flies have been known to feed on the expectoration of consumptive patients and it is possible therefore that they may thus infect food.

The bed bug (Cimex lectularius) has been stated to be capable of conveying by its bite the infection of plague and other diseases from an infected to a healthy person; but Nuttall's experimental results were entirely negative.

Fleas (pulex) probably do not play any part in spreading anthrax. Experimentally, anthrax bacilli die off rapidly in fleas. In India, persons who had handled rats dead of plague frequently acquired the disease. This was explained by Simond on the supposition that the fleas abandoned the dead rat for the human subject. The rats which appeared to have caused plague in man were stated to have died but a short time before; and the handling on the day after their death of rats dead of plague was stated to be safe because the rats' fleas had then deserted the dead rat. It is assumed that the flea injects the poison of plague under the skin. On the contrary it is to be remembered that the fleas infesting rats and mice belong to a different family from that which attacks man. Whether this is a usual means of conveying plague may therefore be regarded as still doubtful. That rats convey plague to man is certain; whether fleas act as an intermediary remains somewhat uncertain.

The Mosquito family (Culicidæ) has been found to be an important if not the sole means of spreading certain serious diseases to man. To this family belong all true gnats or mosquitoes; but the only two genera which have been proved to be able to cause disease are Culex and Anopheles. The culex may usually be distinguished by the fact that when alive and at rest its head is below the level of the thorax and abdomen, thus giving the insect a hump-backed appearance, while the body of the anopheles under the same circumstances is all in a line.[9] The anopheles is more slender and its head smaller than that of the culex. The anopheles usually confines its blood-sucking operations to the evening and night. During the day it remains in dark corners. It lays its eggs usually in a natural pool or pond on the ground, on the surface of the water. In about two days a minute larva is hatched out. This grows rapidly, assumes the pupa form, from which the perfect insect emerges. The female insect alone is blood-sucking.

---

[9] Furthermore, it is stated that when at rest on a plane surface the Culex assumes a position with the axis of the body more or less parallel to the surface; while the Anopheles, under the same circumstances, has the axis of its body more or less at right angles to the surface.

In about 20 days after birth, it lays from 150 to 200 eggs. Its relation to malaria may be gathered from the following historical sketch. In 1880 Laveran found in the red blood corpuscles of malarious patients minute bodies which he regarded as not bacteria, but a very low form of animal life, possessing amœboid movements. These grew at the expense of the blood corpuscles, deposited a dark pigment, and often assumed the appearance of a "rosace," a rounded body with little spherules at its circumference. Golgi in 1889 observed differences between the rosaces of tertian and quartan fever, and found that the periods of occurrences of the fever corresponded with the times of maturation of the rosaces. It was concluded therefore, that the rosaces caused the fever by shedding their sporules into the blood. These sporules when thus shed were found to attach themselves to, and grow in, other red blood corpuscles. It is now known that there are three species of the parasite, in one of which the parasites are crescentic in shape. The examination of a drop of blood from a patient now enables a doctor to recognise which of these three forms of malaria he is dealing with.

Laveran observed that certain forms of the parasite presented "flagella," i.e. filaments exhibiting very active movements. Manson having observed that flagella were not found in blood first drawn, but only appeared after a little time had elapsed, conceived the idea that the function of these must be that of spores. Having previously observed that a microscopic worm, filaria, is drawn with the blood into the stomach of a kind of mosquito, and finds in the latter a secondary host, he concluded that a similar cycle of events might occur in malaria. Ross tested this theory, and by causing mosquitoes bred in bottles from the larva to bite persons affected with the crescent form of malaria, after repeated unsuccessful attempts, was eventually able to find in comparatively rare mosquitoes which had thus bitten a malarious patient, small rounded bodies embedded in the wall of the stomach. These were watched and found to present appearances identical with those of the parasite of malaria. Similar pigmented bodies were subsequently found in other mosquitoes.

The malarial parasite belongs to the Protozoa, of which it is one of the smallest members. Man is its intermediate host, and the anopheles its definitive or final host. In the red blood corpuscle of man it is a unicellar organism, from 1 μ to 8 μ in diameter. It has two methods of reproduction, endogenous by spore formation and exogenous or sexual. The former occurs in man; the latter in the mosquito. Without the latter, the parasite being unable to pass from man to man, would die with its host. In endogenous multiplication spores are formed which separate from the original parasite and gain access to other red blood corpuscles. The large pigmented spheres and the crescent bodies require to enter the stomach of the anopheles to attain full development. In the anopheles the crescents become spherical, flagella are shot out, having a length of 4 to 5 times the diameter of a red blood corpuscle. These represent the male element, while other spheres without flagella are the females. By the fusion of these two a fertilised cell is produced (the travelling vermicule), which now assumes the shape of a spear-head and is actively mobile. The travelling vermicule pierces the stomach wall of the mosquito and develops into a zygote. If an infected mosquito is examined on a succession of days under the microscope, the following stages can be traced. The zygote consists of pigmented spheres 7 to 8 μ in diameter, lying in the muscular fibres of the mosquito. These grow, and become surrounded by a capsule. Smaller spheres form and subdivide, bud-like processes develop on their surfaces; these gradually become sickle-shaped and protrude into the body cavity. They increase in size. until they attain dimensions of from 40, to 60 μ. Eventually they rupture, and the sickle-shaped bodies (sporozooites) escape and are carried in the body fluid of the mosquito to its salivary glands. These sporozooites are about 14 μ long, and human infection is caused by them. They have been traced as far as the end of the proboscis of the mosquito (page 281).

CHAPTER XLIII

INFECTIVE DISEASES

The prevention of disease depends largely on a knowledge of its causes. Disease may be due to a personal life not in accordance with physiological laws; or to some cause or causes acting ab extra. With advance of knowledge the number of diseases which can be proved to be caused by a contagium vivum introduced from without is steadily increasing. We have already discussed the influence of habits, of clothing, exercise, sleep, and food on health, and have shown how errors in these respects may lead to disease. It now remains to consider more particularly the prevention of diseases, due to the introduction into the system of contagia.

In the study of such diseases three chief factors require consideration: (1) the contagium itself; (2) conditions of environment, as climate, soil, season, weather, etc., which may favour or impede its spread; and (3) personal conditions which similarly influence it. Of these age, heredity, fatigue, injury, diet, and race are specially important.

The first two groups of diseases given in the Registrar-General's classification of causes of death are (1) Specific Febrile or Zymotic Diseases, and (2) Parasitic Diseases. The objection to the word "specific" is that, although in most instances diseases in this group are "specific" in the sense that they are caused by a particular microbe, e.g. tetanus, anthrax, tuberculosis, in a few instances the same lesions may be caused by several microbes, e.g. septicaemia (blood-poisoning), pneumonia. "Zymotic" was the name given by Farr, in view of the analogy of the febrile process to that

259

of alcoholic fermentation. In both there is the introduction of a living germ or germs; in both a period of "incubation" in which nothing can be observed; then follows the active disturbance; and in the disease, as well as in the fermenting liquid, the process is stopped, when the microbes have multiplied to a certain extent, a temporary or permanent protection being the result. The best name for the diseases in this group is "Infective." Parasitic diseases, like ringworm, scabies, or trichinosis, are also infective; but for convenience may be described separately as "parasitic."

The relation between the words "infectious" and "contagious" requires explanation. A disease like measles or small-pox, which can be transmitted from person to person, without immediate contact between the two, is termed infectious. In these cases the infection is conveyed by mucus expectorated or by dust blown about, or carried in apparel, etc., from the first patient. Such diseases may also, of course, be communicated by direct contact. If direct contact between the sick and well is indispensable for the transmission of a disease it is called contagious. There is no such hard line in nature, although some diseases can be more easily communicated than others. The term contagious is usually applied to parasitic diseases like ringworm and scabies, but even these can be communicated by means of infected articles as well as persons. The word contagious should be abandoned for all the acute febrile diseases. The word infective is used to include all specific febrile diseases, however spread. This word, therefore, includes not only infectious and contagious diseases, but also diseases spread by inoculation, i.e. injection of the infection under the skin. Thus malaria is not infectious from patient to patient; but can be inoculated by the mosquito.

Infective Diseases are either acute or chronic. Of acute infective diseases small-pox and enteric fever are typical examples; of chronic, tuberculosis and syphilis.

It was formerly supposed that in certain diseases the contagium or infective agent grew in external noxious matter, a miasm being produced; while in other diseases contagion was only produced direct from patient to patient; and others originated in either way. Hence the classification of infective diseases into (a) miasmatic, (b) contagious, and (c) miasmatico-contagious diseases. This classification has now been abandoned. Thus influenza and ague were formerly thought to be miasmatic; but the former is spread by personal infection; the latter by inoculation of the contagium by an infected mosquito.

Bacteriology has thrown an immense light on the causation of infective diseases. A large number of these have been proved to be caused by bacteria, and by analogy we infer the same thing for many others. Koch has laid down the following postulates as necessary before it can be stated that a particular disease is directly caused by a given microbe:—

(1) The microbe shall be demonstrated in the diseased tissues or blood of man or an animal suffering or dead from the disease.

(2) The microbes shall be isolated from these and cultivated in suitable media until obtained in pure culture. That is to say, matter containing the microbe, taken from the infected source, must be cultivated

in artificial media outside the animal body, under conditions excluding the possibility of the introduction of other microbes, until pure cultures of these microbes are obtained, and these microbes must be transplanted from generation to generation, until it is certain that no trace of non-living matter derived from the original animal body remains in the culture.

(3) A pure culture of the microbe, thus obtained, shall, when introduced into the body of a healthy susceptible animal, reproduce the disease in question.

(4) The microbe in question shall be found in the animal so affected. Kanthack adds a further condition, that

(5) The toxins and poisonous substances obtained from the artificial cultivations shall agree chemically and physiologically with those obtained from the diseased animal.

All the preceding conditions have been fulfilled for anthrax, diphtheria, and tetanus; and the first four conditions have been fulfilled in regard to tuberculosis, glanders, gonorrhœa, malignant œdema, and actinomycosis. In enteric fever and influenza the first two conditions have been met; but inoculation experiments (3) have failed. In leprosy and relapsing fever the first condition is met, but (2) has failed.

In the following diseases the specific microbe has not been isolated, though from analogy it is believed that each of them is caused by such a microbe:—

Measles.
Rubella (German measles).
Typhus fever.
Scarlet fever.
Varicella (chicken pox).
Variola (small-pox).
Whooping Cough.
Mumps.
Hydrophobia, etc.

Erysipelas occupies a special position. It is a specific disease due to a microbe, which, when it attacks other parts than the skin, may produce abscesses, boils, or blood-poisoning.

Bacteria are either saprophytes, i.e. they can grow on dead organic or even inorganic matter; or parasites, i.e. they are dependent for their existence on a living plant or animal which they invade. There are two varieties of each of these, obligate and facultative. An obligate parasite can develop only within a living host; while a facultative parasite can, according to circumstances, lead either a parasitic or saprophytic form of existence. The fact that certain contagia are completely, and others only partially, parasitic brings out important differences in their life-history. Thus, so far as we know, the contagia of scarlet fever, measles, small-pox and hydrophobia do not multiply outside the body. Hence there is a reasonable prospect of annihilating them by measures of disinfection and isolation. The position of diphtheria is doubtful. It may have a saprophytic phase of life. The contagium of tuberculosis, as well as of erysipelas, may have a life outside the host, though to what extent is doubtful. Cholera and enteric fever, although generally communicated by infection, appear sometimes to be communicated by contagia grown in saprophytic life, remote from preceding cases.

The infection caused by bacteria may be local or general. Thus in tetanus and in diphtheria the invading bacteria usually remain at their original point of invasion (under the skin in tetanus, in the throat in diphtheria). In anthrax always, and often in enteric fever, they are present in the general circulation. In both instances the symptoms of disease are due chiefly to the toxic products or toxins formed by the bacteria. These toxins are enzymes, ptomaines, tox-albumins, etc. The specific toxins of anthrax, diphtheria, and tetanus have been identified; and by this means the possibility of neutralising them is created.

The channels of infection, i.e. of invasion of contagia, are the skin and the mucous membranes, particularly of the digestive and respiratory tracts.

The Incubation Period of an infectious disease is the interval elapsing between the receipt of infection and the earliest development of symptoms. The period of incubation of the chief infectious diseases is shown in the following table:—

DISEASE.	BEGINS USUALLY ON THE	BUT MAY POSSIBLY BE AT ANY PERIOD BETWEEN
Scarlet fever	4th day.	1 and 7 days.
Diphtheria	2nd day.	2 and 5 days.
Small-pox	12th day.	1 and 14 days.
Chicken pox	14th day.	10 and 18 days.
Typhus fever	12th day.	1 and 21 days.
Enteric fever	14th-21st day.	1 and 28 days.
Cholera	1st-3rd day.	A few hours and 10 days.
Measles	12th-14th day.	10 and 14 days.
Rötheln (German measles)	14th day.	12 and 18 days.
Mumps	19th day.	16 and 24 days.
Whooping cough	14th day.	7 and 14 days.
Influenza	2nd day.	2 and 6 days.

The period of incubation is several weeks in hydrophobia and syphilis, and may be several years in leprosy.

Following the period of incubation, come the premonitory symptoms, which usually are somewhat sudden in onset.

Persons vary in susceptibility to attack by different infective diseases. The intensity of an attack depends on the condition of the patient, and on the number and the virulence of the particular microbes infecting the patient. In certain families attacks of particular diseases are more severe, and attacks are more liable to occur than in others.

It has been shown in certain diseases that the cells and the fluids of the body have a protective effect against infection. This protective action varies in different persons, and in the same person at different times. The cells of the body (phagocytes) swallow up and destroy a certain number of bacteria. This action is called phagocytosis. It is overcome when the dose of contagium is excessive, or when the vitality of the individual is lowered, especially the local vitality at the part attacked. Thus children with "weak throats" are particularly prone to scarlet fever and diphtheria.

The protection afforded by one attack of an infective disease against its recurrence varies greatly. A second attack of small-pox is very rare, of scarlet fever less uncommon, of diphtheria common. In erysipelas, influenza, pneumonia, and rheumatic fever, second or even more numerous attacks are common.

Immunity against an infective disease may be natural, but is more often acquired by an attack of the disease in question. This latter immunity is active, and is due to the formation in the tissues of the immunised person or animal of substances produced by the reaction of these tissues to the stimulus of the contagium. Thus a pig when it has recovered from an attack of swine-plague has produced what are called in German antikörpers, and its tissues are now a medium unfavourable to the growth of the bacillus of swine-plague. If the serum of the protected pig is injected under the skin of another pig, the latter acquires passive immunity against swine-plague, which is not so persistent as active immunity.

Active Immunity can be produced (1) by an attack of an infective disease, or (2) by artificial inoculation (under the skin) of the contagium of the disease, producing a milder attack of the disease. This may be done (a) by inoculating small doses of a virulent contagium, as in the inoculation of small-pox from a previous patient; or (b) by inoculating an attenuated virus, as in vaccination. Inoculation of small-pox virus usually produced a milder attack than infection by ordinary means; but patients thus inoculated were a great source of danger to other persons. In vaccination the virus of small-pox is employed, which has become attenuated by passing through the calf. In its passage, it has lost the power of producing anything beyond a vesicle at the point of inoculation. The principle of protecting by attenuated virus was extended by Pasteur, who was able to render animals resistant against anthrax, swine-fever, and quarter-evil, and hens against fowl-cholera, by inoculating them with attenuated cultures of the contagia of these diseases. Haffkine has applied the same method on a large scale for cholera.

The above are methods of bacterial vaccination. Salmon and Smith have shown that artificial active immunity can be produced also by (3) toxin-injection. They artificially cultivated the hog-cholera bacillus in broth. This broth was then sterilized, the bacilli being killed, but their products remaining. By injecting pigeons with this sterilized broth they made them resistant to subsequent infection by the bacillus itself, thus proving that immunity can be produced by chemical as well as by biological means. The immunity was proportional to the dose of the toxin absorbed. By gradually increasing the dose, it was found practicable to confer immunity, not only against doses of toxin that would otherwise have been fatal, but also against bacterial infection by the particular bacillus used in manufacturing the toxin.

263

Passive Immunity.—Behring and Kitasato found that if the toxin (free from the bacilli) of tetanus be injected into an animal in increasing doses until it becomes immune against infection by the bacilli of tetanus, the blood serum of the animal in question injected into white mice confers the same immunity on them. The protection thus conferred is only temporary. Exactly the same procedure has been adopted for diphtheria, and it is now found that by injecting anti-diphtheritic serum into children who are exposed to the infection of diphtheria, they can for several weeks be prevented from developing the disease. This is of great practical importance, as meanwhile the source of infection can have been removed. Furthermore, the protective serum is also curative, and by its means diphtheria, if early treated, can be reduced from a dangerous to an insignificant disease.

Various theories have been propounded to explain immunity. Pasteur supposed that the special pabulum or food of the bacillus of the given disease became exhausted; but this does not fit in with the immunity that can be produced by toxins and anti-toxins. Chauveau supposed that certain bacterial products are retained in the body, rendering it unsuitable for further growth of the particular bacillus; just as more than 14 per cent. of alcohol in a saccharine solution prevents further fermentation. This does not explain all the facts. Metschnikoff concluded that the fight of the leucocytes and phagocytes of the body against weaker bacilli, gave the power of fighting and overcoming a more virulent bacilli, and that these properties of the cells were transmitted to later generations of body cells. This theory fails to explain the acquired immunity against toxins as well as against bacteria which occurs. The discovery that the blood and other normal tissue fluids possess some power of destroying bacilli has relegated the phagocytal theory to a secondary position.

Natural Immunity varies in different animals. Thus enteric fever, scarlet fever, and measles are not known to occur except in man. Tuberculosis, anthrax, hydrophobia (called rabies in the dog), glanders and tetanus are common to man and certain other animals. Man, cattle and pigs frequently suffer from tuberculosis; goats, sheep, horses, and dogs are practically immune to it.

Epidemic and Endemic Diseases.—Infective diseases may occur sporadically, in epidemics, or in pandemics, i.e. epidemics spread over a number of countries. The word epidemic is used here to mean specially prevalent, and not to apply only to infective diseases. Thus there may be an epidemic of arsenical poisoning from contaminated beer.

Certain infective diseases are endemic or topical, i.e. they have special homes or centres, from which they occasionally spread as epidemics. Yellow fever, cholera, and malaria belong to this group. In a minor degree enteric fever, epidemic diarrhœa, and tuberculosis may be described as endemic.

Each infective disease has a special seasonal incidence. Of these the most important are the autumnal group, viz.

Epidemic
Diarrhœa,   maximum prevalence in July and August.

264

Enteric Fever	„	„	„	November, but excessive, Aug. to Dec.
Erysipelas	„	„	„	Nov. to Dec.
Diphtheria	„	„	„	Nov. and Dec., excessive, Sept. to Dec.
Scarlet Fever	„	„	„	Oct., excessive in Aug. to Dec.
Of other infective diseases				
Small-pox has its	„	„	„	May, but is excessive Jan. to June.
Whooping Cough	„	„	„	Dec. to May.

Measles commonly has two seasonal maxima, in June and December with intervening minima.

Causes of Epidemics.—Measles recurs in the large towns of England every alternate year. Other infective diseases occur at less regular intervals. The recurrence of epidemics is not solely due to personal infection and the accumulation of a population at susceptible ages. There are longer cycles of the causes of which but little is known. Thus scarlet fever has been shown by Longstaff and Gresswell to become epidemic chiefly in dry years; and I have shown that diphtheria and rheumatic fever become widely epidemic under the same conditions, diphtheria becoming so only when a series of dry years occur in immediate succession.

CHAPTER XLIV

ACUTE INFECTIVE DISEASES

Acute Infectious Diseases are characterised by certain definite characters.

1.—They are usually infectious or contagious. It is preferable to use these two terms as interchangeable. The modes in which infection is received vary greatly with different fevers.

(1) Some can only be propagated by inoculation—the introduction through an abraded surface of a minute quantity of the poison; as in glanders and hydrophobia. Others, again, may be introduced in this way, but are usually acquired in another manner, as scarlet fever, small-pox.

(2) Some are carried through the atmosphere. The contagium of small-pox can be carried as far as any, while that of typhus fever only traverses a few feet. The atmosphere acts as a conveyer of infection, and the infectious matter must necessarily, in most instances, be in the condition of dust to enable it to be wafted by currents of air or disturbed by the movements of persons in an infected room.

(3) Clothes, books, and furniture are not uncommonly carriers of infection. An old letter, or a lock of hair, has even after many years' concealment in an enclosed space produced infection on being brought to light. Woollen articles convey infection more easily than calico, and dark clothes better than light coloured. A fever nurse's clothes should never be woollen, but some washable material.

(4) Drinking water and food often form a vehicle for infection. Milk and water are the two usual sources of infection; but uncooked food, especially oysters and mussels, fed in sewage-polluted estuaries, may produce the same effect. Cholera, enteric fever, dysentery, and summer diarrhœa are the chief diseases from this source; but scarlet fever and diphtheria occasionally have a similar origin. Milk may be infected from having been handed by an infectious patient; or it may possibly convey infection of the disease from which the cow at the time is suffering, e.g., tuberculosis. Water may be contaminated with sewage or the excreta of a single infectious patient.

2. They retain their specific character and origin. Small-pox never produces scarlet fever, nor vice versâ; and it is found universally that all the specific fevers "breed true," each one retaining its identity. More than this, a previous case of the same fever can nearly always be detected on careful examination. Overcrowding and other insanitary conditions diminish the resistance to infection, and may increase its virulence.

3. The behaviour of contagia, when received into the system, is characteristic of these diseases. There is first of all a period of latency or incubation, during which no symptoms are manifested. The incubation period is followed by the characteristic symptoms of the particular fever, which disappear in a variable period, leaving the patient, as a rule, more or less insusceptible to a second attack.

Throughout the progress of the disease, except in the period of incubation, the patient is able to communicate his disease to persons about him who have not been rendered safe by a previous attack. The way in which he thus communicates his disease varies in different cases. In scarlet fever, the throat and skin are the chief sources of contagion; in influenza, whooping-cough, and measles, the secretions from the respiratory passages; in hydrophobia, the saliva; in enteric fever and cholera, the vomit and stools.

Prevention of the Spread of the Chief Acute Infectious Diseases.— We may divide these into three classes. (1) Those which are infectious by contact with the patient or by the atmosphere around him. (2) Those in which the intestinal and renal evacuations are almost alone infectious; as enteric fever and cholera. (3) Those in which inoculation through an abraded surface is generally if not always necessary to produce infection.

SMALL-POX OR VARIOLA

The contagium of small-pox is very tenacious of life. All parts of the body, and all secretions and excretions contain it. As in typhus it adheres to every article in the room, but unlike typhus is possessed of great vitality, and if not exposed to the air may be active after many years. There is considerable evidence indicating that the contagion of small-pox may occasionally be conveyed aerially for a considerable distance, for even a quarter or half a mile from hospitals in which small-pox patients are isolated. Whether this is the aerial convection of infection, or in part at least due to carelessness of persons connected with the hospital in their movements to and fro, may remain an open question; but such hospitals in the midst of towns are in practice a mistake; and in London small-pox has been found to be more manageable since its small-pox patients were all conveyed to extra-urban hospitals. The means for the prevention of small-pox are (1) Isolation of infectious patients. (2) Disinfection of all infected articles. They must be carried out most rigidly in this disease. (3) Vaccination and re-vaccination.

Inoculation of small-pox virus was largely practised as a means of ensuring a comparatively mild attack, until it was made illegal in 1840. Sometimes, however, the attack thus produced was fatal, and every case of inoculated small-pox became a new focus of infection, and a source of high mortality, especially among young children.

Vaccination. About the year 1795 Dr. Edward Jenner was informed by a milk-maid that she could not take small-pox, as she had already contracted the natural cow-pox during milking. Many had previously heard this same statement made; but Jenner was the first to put the matter to the test. He took the lymph or virus from a woman who had accidentally acquired cow-pox (vaccinia) from a cow, and inoculated a boy with it. Some months later he inoculated the same boy with small-pox, and a second time five years afterwards, without producing small-pox on either occasion. Many other experiments were made, all confirming these results; and in 1798 Jenner published his results.

The practice of vaccination gradually became more general, and was followed by a progressive decrease in the mortality from small-pox.

Cow-pox or vaccinia is small-pox modified and mitigated by its passage through the system of the cow, and not a spontaneous disease of the cow. By its passage through the cow it has become attenuated and altered. Instead of a general eruption all over the body, there are vesicles only at the point of inoculation; and vaccinia, unlike small-pox, is not communicable from person to person except by inoculation. Furthermore it is in the vast majority of instances an extremely mild ailment, not involving more than a few days discomfort.

Objection is taken to vaccination for small-pox on the ground that serious diseases such as syphilis, erysipelas, and tuberculosis may be inoculated at the same time. With lymph obtained from healthy children this is impossible. Most of the cases of infection described have been in reality hereditary disease, the local irritation of vaccination serving to call into activity the morbid tendencies of the child. The risk of such infection is infinitesimal; it may be reduced to zero by moderate care and attention to detail. With modern antiseptic methods, it is very rare for a vaccination sore to "go wrong." Erysipelas may be inoculated from dirt getting into a vaccination sore, as it may be into any other sore; but with cleanliness this need not occur; and in fact very seldom does occur. The risks are so small as to be negligible; and if the protection afforded is one tithe of what is claimed for it, no parent is justified in withholding this protection from his infant. The law as to vaccination requires that every infant shall be vaccinated within six months of its birth, domiciliary visits for this purpose being made by the public vaccinator. The obligation can only be avoided by a statement on oath before a magistrate by the parent of conscientious objection to vaccination.

Does Vaccination protect against Small-Pox? The registration of deaths for the whole country only began in 1837, and before this period death-rates from small-pox in terms of the population cannot be accurately stated. Since that time there has been less or more vaccination, so that it is difficult to obtain a true comparison between periods with and without vaccination. Some indication of the facts in London prior to 1801, when the first English census was taken, may be obtained from the fact that in 1796 (two years before the date of Jenner's "Inquiry,") small-pox reached its highest point, causing 18½ deaths out of every 100 total deaths from all causes. In the præ-vaccination period small-pox was 9 times as fatal as measles, and 7½ times as fatal as whooping-cough (McVail), while since vaccination has been practised it has sunk to an insignificant position, when compared with these diseases. Dr. Guy found that in London there were in 48 years of the seventeenth century ten epidemics, in the whole of the eighteenth century 19 epidemics, and in the nineteenth century no epidemic during which the deaths from small-pox caused one-tenth or more than one-tenth of the total deaths from all causes in any year. The worst year under obligatory vaccination in London was 1871, in which barely 4½ per cent. of the total deaths was due to small-pox, a proportion which was exceeded in the eighteenth century ninety-three times.

In Sweden, the highest death-rate before vaccination (1774-1800) was 7·23 per 1,000 inhabitants, the lowest 0·31; under permissive vaccination (1801-1815) the highest 2·57 per 1,000 inhabitants, the lowest 0·12; under compulsory vaccination (1816-85) the highest 0·94 per 1,000 inhabitants, the lowest 0·0005. It has been stated that these results, which might be extended by quotations from the statistics of other countries, have been obtained not by vaccination, but by improved sanitation, including in this term not only improved housing and better water and food supply but also increased means of isolating the infectious sick. Improved housing may by diminishing overcrowding aid in diminishing the spread of this disease. Whether in view of the immense increase in the proportion of the population which lives in towns, it can be said that this has occurred is doubtful. Hospital isolation undoubtedly prevents the spread of infection when promptly effected. But a large share of the improvement in small-pox mortality occurred before either hospital or home-isolation of small-pox patients was generally enforced. There is no reason for supposing that impure water or food, or nuisances about houses have any connection with the origin or spread of small-pox, any more than they have with the origin or spread of measles or whooping-cough; which still remain as prevalent as in the past. Further light can be thrown on the

268

subject by an examination of the age-incidence of small-pox, and of its attack-rate and severity in vaccinated and unvaccinated respectively.

The age incidence of deaths from small-pox has, since 1847, when returns classified according to age became available, undergone a remarkable alteration. Prior to 1870 the small-pox deaths in infants nearly always formed 20 per cent. or more of the total mortality from this disease, between 1870 and 1890 they did not greatly exceed 10 per cent. of the total, while since 1890 they have again begun to form an increasing proportion of the total small-pox mortality. At ages 1-5 the change is even more remarkable. Before 1870 deaths at these ages nearly always exceeded 30 per cent. of the total; since 1870 they have varied between 5 and 14 per cent. of the total; and since 1890 they have, like the proportion of deaths under one, again increased. At the higher ages the proportion of deaths has correspondingly increased, so that the curves of age incidence have become curiously inverted.

The lowered birth-rate can only account for a small portion of this transference of the chief mortality due to small-pox from childhood to adult life.

Furthermore it must not be supposed that the only change which has occurred is that the deaths which formerly occurred in childhood now occur in adult life. The death-rate at all ages has greatly declined. The only explanation which in my judgment satisfactorily explains this remarkable change in age-incidence of small-pox mortality is the fact that vaccination protects children from small-pox and that the protection diminishes, though it never entirely disappears, with advancing years. This conclusion is confirmed by the evidence obtained as to the proportion of vaccinated and unvaccinated attacked, and as to the severity of the attacks occurring when a community is invaded by small-pox.

Attack-rate among Vaccinated.—If the protective effect of vaccination, like that of a preceding attack of small-pox, wears off, it will not be expected that no attacks of small-pox will occur among the vaccinated. For evidence of immunity from attacks we must examine the records as to revaccinated persons exposed to infection. During the six years 1890-95, out of a staff in the London small-pox hospitals varying from 64 to 320, the percentage attacked by small-pox was nil, except in 1892 when it was 1·4, and in 1893 when it was 1·9.

Taking the experience of towns in which during recent years epidemics of small-pox have occurred, the following attack-rates have occurred. By attack-rate is meant the percentage number of attacks occurring among persons living in infected houses. By fatality is meant the number dying out of 100 attacked.

	ATTACK RATE UNDER 10 YEARS OF AGE		ATTACK RATE OVER 10 YEARS OF AGE	
	VACCINATED	UNVACCINATED	VACCINATED	UNVACCINATED
Dewsbury	10·2	50·8	27·7	53·4
Leicester	2·5	35·3	22·2	47·6
Gloucester	8·8	46·3	32·2	50·0

Severity (Fatality) among Vaccinated.—The experience of the same three towns comes out as follows:—

	FATALITY RATE UNDER 10 YEARS OF AGE.		FATALITY RATE OVER 10 YEARS OF AGE.	
	VACCINATED	UNVACCINATED	VACCINATED	UNVACCINATED
Dewsbury	2·2	32·1	2·6	18·7
Leicester	0·0	14·0	1·0	7·8
Gloucester	3·8	41·0	10·0	39·7

In view of such results as the above it is not surprising that the Royal Commission, in their majority report, summed up the advantages of vaccination as follows:

"(1) That it diminishes the liability to be attacked by the disease.

"(2) That it modifies the character of the disease, and renders it (a) less fatal, and (b) of a milder or less severe type.

"(3) That the protection it affords against attacks of the disease is greatest during the years immediately succeeding the operation of vaccination. It is impossible to fix with precision the length of this period of highest protection. Though not in all cases the same, if a period is to be fixed, it might, we think, fairly be said to cover in general a period of nine or ten years.

"(4) That after the lapse of the period of highest protective potency, the efficacy of vaccination to protect against attack rapidly diminishes, but that it is still considerable in the next quinquennium, and possibly never altogether ceases.

"(5) That its power to modify the character of the disease is also greatest in the period in which its power to protect from attack is greatest, but that its power thus to modify the disease does not diminish as rapidly as its protective influence against attacks, and its efficacy during the later periods of life to modify the disease is still very considerable.

"(6) That re-vaccination restores the protection which lapse of time has diminished, but the evidence shows that this protection again diminishes, and that, to ensure the highest degree of protection which vaccination can give, the operation should be at intervals repeated.

"(7) That the beneficial effects of vaccination are most experienced by those in whose case it has been most thorough. We think it may fairly be concluded that where the vaccine matter is inserted in three or four places, it is more effectual than when introduced into one or two places only—and that if the vaccination marks are of an area of half a square inch, they indicate a better state of protection than if their area be at all considerably below this."

SCARLET FEVER

Scarlet Fever and Scarlatina are the same disease. It is extremely infectious, the contagium retaining its virulence for protracted periods. It occurs in epidemics at irregular intervals. During recent years the type of scarlet fever has become greatly attenuated, and this constitutes one of the difficulties of prevention, as the mild form of the disease is apt to be overlooked. The fatality per 100 persons attacked varies greatly with age. It is highest in children under four, rapidly declining with increasing age. Hence the importance of protecting children from attack in early life. Two results follow from the wise precautions taken to prevent attack early in life. (a) With each successive year of life the liability to attack, when exposed to infection, diminishes; (b) the danger of the attack if it occurs and its liability to be fatal becomes rapidly less with greater age. The most common mode of infection is by contact with a previous patient. Outbreaks due to milk infected by a scarlatinal patient also occur. Infected cream has also been known to convey infection. In a milk outbreak the patients would be found chiefly among the customers of a special dairyman, the cases occur almost simultaneously, except secondary cases which may be infected from the first. The simultaneous occurrence of two or more attacks in one house, especially if the same thing happens in a number of houses should throw suspicion on the milk supply. It has been suggested that scarlet fever may originate apart from human infection, from a special disease of the cow, but the evidence on this point is inconclusive.

The duration of infection is usually reckoned until the desquamation of the skin is complete, i.e. about six or seven weeks from the onset of the attack. Occasionally it is more protracted even though desquamation is complete, infection appearing to persist in discharges from the nose and ear and in sore places inside the nostril and possibly in other parts. The period of greatest infectivity is in the earlier part of the disease, when the throat is inflamed. The common notion that the disease is most infectious during the later period, that of desquamation, is erroneous. The micro-organism causing scarlet fever has not certainly been identified. The measures of prevention are those common to infectious diseases.

MEASLES

Measles is an extremely infectious disease, before as well as after the rash appears on the fourth day of the disease. The infectivity of the catarrhal stage constitutes one of the main difficulties in preventing its spread, as measles may be unrecognisable at this stage. The common notion that measles and whooping-cough are comparatively harmless infantile complaints will be dissipated by a study of the comparative death-rate for the five years 1891-5 per million persons living in England and Wales:—

England and Wales.—Death Rates per Million of Population.

Small-pox	*20*
Measles	*408*
Scarlet fever	*183*
Typhus fever	*4*
Enteric fever	*174*
Whooping-cough	*398*

271

It is a mistake also to suppose that measles and whooping-cough are only serious when neglected. Such neglect greatly increases the likelihood of death from bronchitis or pneumonia; but the diseases themselves, especially measles, are frequently fatal during the acute early stage. More children are attacked with measles under the age of five than at any other age, and the greatest number between two and four years of age. The greatest fatality is in the second year of life, when it may be 24 per cent. of those attacked, as compared with between two and three per cent. in the fourth year of life, and a trifling amount at higher ages. These facts explain the folly of allowing children to have an infectious complaint when another child in the house is attacked, "to have it over at one trouble." Such action is pregnant with evil results. (1st) Severe cases occur, in which a fatal result ensues; and even where death does not occur, the child may be left weakly and very prone to become tuberculous. (2nd) Every additional case forms a new centre of infection. It is like the old practice of inoculation for small-pox; the individual is protected, but becomes a source of danger to all around him. If there is only one case of measles in a family the risk to neighbouring households is much smaller than where several children are infected. (3rd) Every year that a child's attack can be delayed, increases his chance of recovery if he is subsequently attacked, and diminishes the likelihood of his being attacked.

The duration of infection should be reckoned as at least three weeks. The contagium of measles does not appear to hang about rooms with the persistence of that of scarlet fever, and less stringent disinfection is required.

WHOOPING COUGH

Very few people have reached adult life without having suffered from this disease, as well as measles. This is chiefly due to the carelessness in mixing infected with healthy children. One frequently hears the peculiar and characteristic cough of a child with whooping-cough, in public assemblies, in railway trains, or in the out-patient rooms of hospitals. The contagium of whooping-cough is conveyed chiefly by the expectoration, which becoming dry, may be scattered like that of phthisis, as dust. Clothing conveys infection easily; visits to infected children should, therefore, be prohibited to all who have to mix with susceptible children.

The duration of infection should be reckoned as at least six weeks from the first recognisable symptoms. It may be longer than this.

DIPHTHERIA

This disease has become increasingly prevalent in the last ten years after a period of only slight prevalence for about twenty-five years. I have shown that epidemics of diphtheria occur during a succession of years of protracted ·drought. Diphtheria is more common in girls than boys, possibly owing to their more affectionate habits; and occurs chiefly under ten years of age, the fifth year of life being that of greatest prevalence. Unlike the acute infections hitherto considered, the bacillus causing diphtheria has been identified and cultivated in the laboratory (called the Klebs-Loeffler bacillus or diphtheria bacillus). Direct infection from patient to patient is probably more common than indirect infection by clothes, etc., though the latter occurs. The infection may hang persistently about a house and its belongings, in the absence of complete purification. When diphtheria is prevalent slighter sore throats occur, sometimes before true diphtheria is detected. This led to the theory that under conditions of overcrowding, especially in schools, there occurred in the micro-organisms causing these sore-throats "the progressive development of the property of infectiveness." Possibly these were slight non-typical attacks of diphtheria. Such attacks occur also during epidemics of diphtheria, and unless specimens ("throat swabs") from these sore-throats are examined bacteriologically, are likely to spread diphtheria by attendance at school, etc. Aggregation in schools seems to intensify the contagium of diphtheria. The practices of kissing, of transferring sweetmeats from mouth to mouth, of cleaning slates with saliva, are common means of spreading it. Effluvia from foul drains and sewers have been commonly held to cause diphtheria. If they aid in producing it, it is rather by lowering the vitality and causing ordinary sore throat. Sore throats and catarrhs make the subjects of them much more prone to diphtheria. Damp houses have been stated to favour the development of diphtheria. Probably they do so in the same way as effluvia from drains. It is likely that the diphtheria bacillus has a saprophytic stage of existence in the soil, as indicated by its excessive prevalence in dry warm years. Besides direct infection from patient to patient and indirect infection by fomites (i.e. in clothing, etc.), milk occasionally causes epidemics of diphtheria. The infection has been usually caused by the handling of the milk by an infectious person. In certain outbreaks no human contamination of the milk could be discovered; and it has been surmised that an analogous disease in the cow may cause diphtheria in man. This is still a moot point. Fowls, cats, and other animals are the occasional victims of diphtheria, and may convey it to man.

The duration of infection in diphtheria is usually less than six weeks; but it may be much more protracted. In some instances long after all naked-eye evidences of diphtheria has disappeared, bacteriological examination may still show the presence of the diphtheria bacillus for two or three months; in rare cases even longer. The protection afforded by one attack of diphtheria against a second is slight and only temporary. The means of prevention are isolation and disinfection as for other infectious diseases. Two additional means are available (a) bacteriological diagnosis; (b) prophylactic injection of antitoxic serum. Many sore throats without membrane on the throat are due to the diphtheria bacillus. Even if membrane be present there may be doubt as to whether the case is true diphtheria. Hence the importance of bacteriological examination.

The patient's throat is swabbed with cotton-wool which has been rolled around a metal probe and sterilised. The wool is then smeared over sterilised and solified blood serum in a test tube. It is then incubated over night at a temperature of 37° C. Next morning the minute growth that has occurred on the surface of the blood serum is spread on a microscopic cover-glass, appropriately stained, and examined microscopically. If diphtheria bacilli are present, they can be recognised by their form and arrangement. The same means enable us to ascertain when a patient has recovered, whether he is fit to be released from isolation.

Antitoxic serum has been found to be a valuable prophylactic and curative agent.

The serum is obtained as follows: Sterilised broth is inoculated with virulent diphtheria bacilli, and grown at 37° C. for a week or more. The broth is then filtered through a Pasteur filter. The filtrate contains toxine free from bacilli. Some of this toxine is injected under the skin of a horse. A few days later the dose is repeated, gradually increasing amounts being injected until injection of further quantities of the toxine is found experimentally not to increase the antitoxic value of the horse's blood serum. Next the horse is bled. Its serum is found to have acquired the power of protecting a guinea-pig against doses of the toxine of diphtheria which would otherwise be fatal. Ten times the quantity of the horse's serum which will protect a guinea-pig (of 250 grammes weight) against ten times the minimum fatal dose of the toxine is called an antitoxic unit.

The treatment of diphtheria in man by the antitoxic serum thus obtained has proved to be remarkably successful. Furthermore, if a susceptible person who has been exposed to the infection of diphtheria, is injected with a small dose of antitoxic serum, he becomes temporarily immune, and does not fall a victim to diphtheria. This is a most important point especially for young children, who may already be incubating a disease which but for this prophylactic injection might occur and prove fatal.

TYPHUS FEVER

This disease was formerly known as spotted or jail-fever, and for many ages has been the scourge of prisons and armies, and all collections of people living in overcrowded and insanitary districts. The history of typhus is the history of human misery. It is essentially associated with filth, overcrowding, and destitution; but when once established by these conditions, it can be carried by infection to others who live amidst healthy surroundings. It generally occurs in winter, when overcrowding is greatest. With free ventilation, the disease cannot be carried more than a few feet. It can be transmitted by clothing. The micro-organism causing it has not been discovered. With the clearance of the rookeries of our great towns, it is rapidly decreasing, and appears likely to become extinct. The means of prevention, in addition to the abatement of nuisances, including overcrowding, are isolation and disinfection.

RELAPSING FEVER

This disease was formerly common in this country, but except in some parts of Ireland has entirely died out. It is caused by a micro-organism (Spirillum Obermeieri) which can be detected in the blood. Inoculation of this will produce the disease in man or in monkeys.

Epidemics of relapsing fever commonly follow in the track of typhus fever; overcrowding and filth being especially associated with typhus, and starvation with relapsing fever, hence its name of "famine fever."

ENTERIC OR TYPHOID FEVER

Enteric fever causes its highest death-rate in early adult life, though it is not peculiar to any age. Eberth in 1880 discovered the Bacillus typhosus in the spleen and other organs of enteric fever patients. This is commonly known as Eberth's bacillus, and is the cause of enteric fever. A few years later it was isolated and can now be grown on agar or gelatine in laboratories. It closely resembles other bacilli which are normal inhabitants of the human intestine; but can be distinguished by certain tests. It is a small rod, rounded at its ends, and from 2 to 4 μ long and three times as long as broad. In the living state it is freely motile, and possesses a number of minute cilia or flagella. Apart from other means of distinction between it and other bacilli, Grüber's serum reaction enables its identity to be ascertained. The bacillus suspected to be the Bac.-typhosus is cultivated in broth in the bacteriological laboratory. A small quantity of blood is taken from the finger of a patient known to be suffering from enteric fever. The serum is separated from the blood corpuscles of this blood by a centrifugalising machine. A drop of the blood serum is diluted with 100 drops of broth culture of the suspected bacillus. If the latter is not the Bac.-typhosus, the individual bacilli when a drop of the mixture is examined under the microscope, will continue to move about freely; if it is the Bac.-typhosus, the bacilli will adhere together in "clumps" and become immobile. Conversely a valuable means of ascertaining whether a suspected case is really suffering from enteric fever is secured, as this blood added to 30 times the amount of a pure culture of the Bac.-typhosus in broth will cause the latter to "clump" within half-an-hour (Widal reaction). Higher dilutions are usually unnecessary.

The chief means of spread of enteric fever is by the urine and fæces; and nurses who have to empty bed-pans unless very careful to wash their hands afterwards, using the nail-brush, are very liable to become infected, probably when eating food afterwards. The urine in a considerable proportion of cases, contains the typhoid bacilli, and it is therefore most important that care should be exercised in the cleansing of all chamber utensils, and that the urine as well as the fæces should be rigidly disinfected. The infectivity of enteric fever has been underrated in the past. When patients with this disease are nursed at home by relatives who do not appreciate the full importance of the necessary precautions, it is rather the rule than the exception for them to fall victims to its infection.

Probably, sometimes the infection has been scattered as dust, owing to small particles of fæces or of urine having become dried on bed linen. The most absolute cleanliness is essential in nursing this disease. In hot climates there is reason to believe that infective dust may be blown about from privies.

Insanitary local circumstances are an important means of spreading enteric fever. It is more prevalent where there are privies than where there are pail-closets; and more prevalent where there are pail-closets, than where water-closets are the rule. Defective drains or soil-pipes are frequently found in houses in which enteric fever originates, and there can be little doubt that the former are at least partially responsible for the latter. The exact link is doubtful. Probably infective dust is blown or aspirated into the room and is inhaled.

The most common cause of enteric fever is infected food or water. Of foods milk not infrequently has been the means of spread of enteric fever. Large epidemics have been traced to this source. Usually this has arisen by washing the milk cans with or wilfully adding contaminated water to the milk. Water, whether added to milk or taken independently, must have contained the specific contagium (the Bac.-typhosus) of enteric fever, to enable it to cause enteric fever. Hence water from a contaminated stream is more likely to have produced this effect than well-water, unless a patient has had enteric fever in the house to which the well is attached, and his dejecta have contaminated the water. Surface waters or spring waters may be contaminated with sewage (as at Maidstone) or deep well waters through fissures (as at Worthing) and thus widespread epidemics be produced. After floods, rivers and wells are most likely to contain the specific contagium of enteric fever, as at such times surface impurities from middens, etc., are apt to be washed into the water.

The means of prevention of enteric fever are the discovery and removal of the cause of an outbreak, and the isolation of each patient and disinfection of all discharges. An early means of diagnosis is secured by Widal's reaction. This is especially useful in cases not presenting characteristic clinical symptoms. The recognition of a disease or at least the suspicion of its presence is an indispensable first step for the taking of precautionary measures.

CHOLERA

Cholera, which was formerly so prevalent, now seldom occurs in this country, and at each successive visit to England its inroads have become less serious. At its last visit in 1893 it scarcely obtained a footing in the country. Thus in the epidemic of 1854 in England it caused 1080, in that of 1866 it caused 672, and in that of 1893 only 45 deaths per million of population. In this country at least it is chiefly spread by infected water and foods, especially by infected water; and the preceding figures form an excellent testimony to our improvement in this respect. For particulars of the Hamburg outbreak, see page 86. In its mode of prevalence and propagation it is very similar to enteric fever, being infectious by means of

276

the evacuations. The means of prevention are the same as for enteric fever. Cholera was shown by Koch to be caused by what is known as the comma bacillus or spirillum of Asiatic cholera, so called because of its curved shape. It is from 1·5μ to 2·6μ long and ·5μ broad. For the supposed connection of enteric fever and cholera with movements of the ground-water, see page 206.

SUMMER OR EPIDEMIC DIARRHŒA

Is a most fatal disease among infants in the third quarter of each year. It is chiefly a disease of urban life, and occurs to a preponderant extent among the children of the artisan and still more of the unskilled labouring classes. It is much less abundant in towns which have adopted the water-carriage system of sewage than in those retaining the conservancy methods of removal of excrement. Towns with the most perfect domestic and street scavenging arrangements have the least epidemic diarrhœa. An impervious soil favours a low diarrhœal mortality; while persons living on porous soils usually have much diarrhœa. I have shewn elsewhere that given two towns equally placed so far as social and sanitary conditions are concerned, their relative diarrhœal mortality is proportional to the height of the temperature and the deficiency of rainfall of each town, particularly the temperature and rainfall of the third quarter of each year. In other words there is a general inverse relationship between rainfall and diarrhœa and a direct relationship between temperature and diarrhœa. Thus wet and cool summers are adverse to diarrhœa. Ballard concluded that the summer rise of diarrhœal mortality does not commence until the mean temperature recorded by the 4-foot earth thermometer has attained somewhere about 56° F., no matter what may have been the temperature previously attained by the atmosphere. This is a convenient index, as the summer warmth does not immediately cause diarrhœa. All the above facts point to the conclusion that the fundamental condition favouring epidemic diarrhœa is an unclean soil, the particulate poison from which infects the air, and is swallowed most commonly with food, especially milk. Thus, diarrhœa, like enteric fever, is a "filth-disease." As the contagium appears to gain entrance by food, the following card of precautions which is distributed each year in the poorer districts of Brighton may be reproduced here:

HOW TO PREVENT DIARRHŒA

During the summer a large number of infants die from diarrhœa. Scarcely a single baby who was being suckled dies from this cause. It is evident, therefore, that in the prevention of this very fatal summer disease, precautions as to food are most important.

Attention to the following points would save many infants' lives:—

1. Do not wean your infant during the hot months of July, August and September. To begin artificial feeding during hot weather is very dangerous.

2. If feeding by hand is absolutely necessary, carefully follow these directions:

277

(a) All milk should be boiled before being given to the infant.

(b) The infants' food must be prepared fresh each time. (For particulars see below.) Milk and water, and still more "pap" or patent foods, if left two or three hours, "go bad," and are then very highly dangerous to the infant.

(c) All jugs or other utensils used for storing milk must be scalded out and kept absolutely clean. They should be covered to prevent access of dust.

(d) The feeding bottle must be thoroughly scalded after each meal, and the tube thoroughly cleansed. It is best to use alternately two boat-shaped bottles without tubes. If the bottle smells sour, something is not clean, and the infant will suffer.

3. Decomposing refuse, such as decaying vegetables, bones, fish-heads, &c., is a fertile source of Diarrhœa. It should be burnt, and not placed in the dust-bin.

4. Scrupulous cleanliness of the house, especially of the rooms where food is stored, is most important. Dust in every form is dangerous to health, and for removing it wet cleansing is preferable to dry. Thus washing and scrubbing are safer means of cleansing floors, &c., than sweeping.

5. Report to the Sanitary Office, Town Hall, any smells or choked closet or drain.

DIRECTIONS FOR PREPARATIONS OF INFANTS' FOOD.

For a Child aged	Mix and then boil	For each Meal
Under 6 weeks	1 part fresh milk 2 parts water 1 teaspoonful cream	4 tablespoonsful.
	Mix and then boil	
6 weeks old	1 part fresh milk 1 part water 2 teaspoonsful cream	8 tablespoonsful.
	Mix and then boil	
From 3 to six months old	2 parts fresh milk 1 part water 2 or 3 teaspoonsful cream.	8 tablespoonsful.

The infant should be fed at regular intervals only, at first every two hours, the interval being gradually increased.

The infant should be fed slowly.

If the milk as prepared above disagrees, freshly boiled barley water should be used instead of water.

The addition of cream is necessary because cows' milk is poorer in cream than mothers' milk, and because it is very often made poorer still by mixing with separated milk before sale. Deficiency of cream causes rickets. A little sugar may

278

also be added to the milk, but this must not be regarded as a substitute for the cream.

TETANUS

Tetanus or lockjaw is not infectious, but is conveyed to man by the inoculation of a wound by dirt or earth which contains the tetanus bacillus. For this reason it is more apt to follow injuries to the hands or feet. Extreme cleanliness of wounds is the only practicable preventive means. Little is known of the history of the tetanus bacillus outside the body; and as to what soils contain it most abundantly. Wounds contaminated by horse manure appear to be especially dangerous.

GLANDERS

Glanders is common in horses. It attacks the mucous membrane of the nose, causing ulceration. It is extremely infectious. Farcy is a more chronic form of the same disease, in which the so-called "farcy-buds" are produced. Its prevention can best be ensured by killing both actually diseased and suspected animals, if the latter give a reaction to mallein. Mallein is a product allied to tuberculin, obtained from cultivations of the bacillus of glanders. It sets up febrile reaction in glandered, but not in healthy horses. Further preventive measures are the temporary closing of public drinking fountains for horses, and the thorough cleansing and disinfection of stables. Men, especially grooms, are sometimes infected by the horse, and the disease is commonly fatal.

HYDROPHOBIA

Hydrophobia is the disease in man which is caused by the bite of a dog or other animal suffering from rabies. It is seldom if ever communicated otherwise than by inoculation. The incubation period in the dog varies from three to six weeks, and in man is usually about the same; but occasionally it is much longer, occasionally even more than a year.

At the Pasteur Institute, Paris, patients who have been bitten by rabid dogs are treated by the inoculation of an attenuated virus of rabies derived from rabbits, with promising results.

Dogs only acquire rabies from dogs or other animals already rabid. So far as is known, it does not arise de novo. Hence the necessity for an extensive area of muzzling when cases of rabies occur. The enforcement of this plan has greatly reduced the amount of hydrophobia in this country in recent years. There has been much misplaced sympathy with dogs on this score. In the dog the symptoms of rabies occur in three stages: a premonitory stage, in which the dog's habits change, he becomes morose and quiet, and dribbles; a second stage, in which he has paroxysms of fury, his voice is high-toned and croupy, and he cannot swallow water; and a third or paralytic stage, in which his jaws drop, he drags his hind legs and soon dies.

279

ERYSIPELAS

Erysipelas occurs on various parts of the skin. It is caused by the inoculation through an abraded surface of a virulent form of the same streptococcus that commonly causes suppuration. It occurs chiefly in debilitated subjects. Some persons are specially prone to it, and may have many attacks. Erysipelas, like scarlet fever, occurs most in years in which there is deficient rainfall; and is probably conveyed by dust. It may spread, though exceptionally, from case to case.

YELLOW FEVER

Yellow fever never occurs in England, except when imported from the West Indies or other countries in which it is endemic. It clings to seaport towns in hot countries; and as a permanent disease is only found when the mean winter temperature is at least 68°-72° F. A frost always stops an epidemic of this disease. The germs of this disease are communicated by mosquitoes, which act as an intermediate host. Dr. J. W. Lazear, although isolated from yellow fever cases, died of it seven days after submitting to the puncture of an infected mosquito, thus proving the communicability of this disease, and entitling himself to an honoured position among scientific martyrs.

PLAGUE

Plague is an Eastern disease, which occasionally shows a tendency to become widely epidemic. It is due to a rod-shaped bacterium, averaging ·8 μ to 1·6 μ in length, which does not form spores. In its characteristic form patients suffering from this disease have inflammatary swellings (buboes) of various glands: hence the name Bubonic Plague. In other cases it simulates ordinary pneumonia, typhus or septicaemia; or the patient may be so slightly ill as to be able to walk about. It appears probable that the bacillus enters the body through cracks or other lesions of the skin, possibly also by inhaling infective dust. The rat is an important factor in the spread of plague. Very commonly plague has been widely prevalent and fatal among them before it attacks human beings. Rats also bring it in ships from infected ports. Hence one of the most important preventive measures is to kill all rats on board ship, before the cargo is unloaded. This has been done by sulphurous acid fumigation in the holds. The use of carbonic oxide gas will probably be found practicable for the same purpose. Manson has put the importance of this point tersely as follows: "To prevent cholera the tea-kettle, malaria the mosquito net, and plague the rat-trap." Flies may carry the infection. It has been suggested that the fleas of rats carry the infection.

ANTHRAX

Anthrax is a very fatal disease in cattle and sheep, occasionally in pigs. Butchers may inoculate themselves with it when dressing a diseased

280

carcase; the tanners similarly when handling the hide; and woolsorters may inhale it when sorting wool derived from a diseased animal.

To prevent the latter, suspected wool must be disinfected by steam, and special arrangements made for carrying off the dust produced during sorting.

PUERPERAL FEVER

Occurs after childbirth. It is caused like erysipelas by the inoculation of septic material. This may be conveyed by dirty instruments (syringes, etc.), or by dirty hands. Hence the importance of extreme cleanliness of hands, finger-nails, and all articles used during and after childbirth.

RHEUMATIC FEVER

Has been commonly attributed to a damp condition of the atmosphere and soil. I have elsewhere shown that this is a mistake, probably arising from the fact that these conditions produce what are called "rheumatic" pains, though they have no true relationship with acute rheumatism (rheumatic fever). I have shown that rheumatic fever occurs chiefly in very dry years, the excess of prevalence in such years being sufficient to justify the use of the term "epidemic." There is strong reason to believe that rheumatic fever is an infective disease, derived, not from other patients suffering from the same disease, but from some outside micro-organism which is ordinarily saprophytic. It follows the rule that when the lesion produced by an infective disease is deep seated (in the joints in this instance), no infection can be communicated to other persons. Some families are much more prone to rheumatic fever than others.

INFLUENZA

Is, like diphtheria, a somewhat mysterious infectious disease. Like the latter it almost disappeared for a series of years, and then again became epidemic in 1889. The previous epidemics of influenza in the 19th century had occurred in 1803, 1833, 1837-8, and 1847-8. The causes of this recurrence of influenza are unknown. It is spread from person to person by direct infection, the infection being conveyed by the mucous discharge from the nose, throat, and lungs. Pocket-handkerchiefs probably are largely responsible for conveying the infection as dust. The disease is particularly fatal to the old; and these should not expose themselves to possible sources of infection, as in public places of assembly, during an epidemic. Every patient attacked with the disease should remain indoors for at least ten days. This is in his own interest, as he thus minimises the risk of such dangerous complications as pneumonia; and it is his duty in the interest of the rest of the community. Many lives might have been saved, had not influenzal patients "struggled about" during the early stages of the disease.

281

MALARIA

Malaria, or Ague, is a generic name given to a disease caused by the invasion of the body by the plasmodium malariæ, discovered by Laveran in 1880. It occurs in two chief types, remittent fever and intermittent fever. For many generations it has been regarded as due to a marshy condition of the soil, associated with decaying vegetable matter, and a moderately high temperature. It is now clear that these conditions are necessary, only because they are necessary for the life of the mosquito. The well-known danger of being out of doors at night in a malarious country is explained by the nocturnal habits of the mosquito. The higher salubrity of the upper stories of houses is explained by the fact that the mosquito does not rise high from the ground; and of high-lying localities by their greater dryness. The value of the mosquito net, of smoke, and of fire as protections from malaria are due to their keeping mosquitos at a distance. The mosquito clings to the puddle or swamp where she was born, and where she will deposit her eggs. Hence the special danger of the immediate vicinity of such collections of water. Thus the prevention of malaria resolves itself chiefly into means for preventing the development of certain species of Anopheles. The conditions necessary for the multiplication of these are (1), an atmospheric temperature from 75° to 104° F.; (2) collections of fresh or slightly brackish water; and (3) the presence in these of low forms of animal and vegetable life. We have already described the cycle of life of the plasmodium malariæ. Man is the chief, if not the only source, from which the mosquito derives this parasite. In native communities the young children, even when apparently not ill with malaria, nearly always harbour these parasites in their blood corpuscles. Hence the importance of Europeans having their dwellings as remote as possible from native houses. Mosquitos do not travel far.

Instances of the prevalence of malaria in the absence of mosquitos are not substantiated. The outbreaks of malaria where the soil has been disturbed after long lying uncultivated, probably mean the formation of puddles favourable to the breeding of the larvæ of mosquitos.

The necessary preventive measures are classified by Manson as:

1. *Suppression of mosquitos.*
2. *Prevention of infection of mosquitos.*
3. *Prevention of infection by mosquitos.*

The suppression of mosquitos involves the draining or filling in of swamps and ponds, the cleansing and canalisation of sluggish streams, and the afforestation of hills to prevent floods. Cultivation of rice and other plants entailing the prolonged flooding of land should be restricted to fields remote from dwellings. Subsoil drainage is helpful. The "painting" of stagnant waters with petroleum, which should be renewed every week or two, frees water for a considerable time from the larvæ of mosquitos. Eucalyptus and other balsamic trees may help to dry up pools, &c.

The prevention of infection of mosquitos is secured by insisting on all malarial patients using mosquito nets. This prevents the access of

282

mosquitos. At the same time patients should vigorously and persistently take quinine, which kills the malarial parasites in the blood, and thus diminishes and finally removes the danger to other persons produced by the intermediation of the mosquito.

The prevention of mosquito bites is secured by rendering the house mosquito-proof by filling in all openings by fine wire gauze, and by having mosquito curtains to all beds; also by fumigating the rooms occasionally with the dried flowers of the chrysanthemum, by strict cleanliness of rooms, and by flushing them with sunlight. The proof of the mosquito theory as to the causation of malaria has been recently supplied by two test experiments. (a) In the first, a number of mosquitos which had been fed on the blood of malarious patients were sent to London from Rome. These were allowed to bite Dr. Manson's son, who had never previously had malaria. A few days later he had a characteristic attack of fever. Malarial parasites were found in his blood. He recovered in a week's time after free dosage with quinine, and the parasites disappeared from his blood. He suffered from a slight relapse about a year later. (b) On a fever-haunted spot in the Roman Campagna a wooden hut was built, and Drs. Sambon and Low, and three others took up their abode here during the malarious season, the only precautions taken being the use of mosquito nets and wire screens in doors and windows. They went about the country daily, but were always home before sunset. They all remained at the end of the season free from malaria.

CHAPTER XLV

TUBERCULOSIS

CONSUMPTION AND OTHER TUBERCULAR DISEASES

Consumption (also called phthisis or phthisis pulmonalis) in the year 1899 caused a recorded death-rate of 1,336, and tubercular diseases of other parts of the body a death-rate of 575 per million of the population. In the same year the chief infectious diseases, including small-pox, measles, scarlet fever, whooping cough, typhus, and enteric fever, and diphtheria, were together responsible for a death-rate of 1,248 per million. In the five years, 1861-65, the mean death-rate from consumption was 2,527 per million, so that a reduction of nearly 50 per cent. has apparently occurred. Notwithstanding this great decline, consumption and other consumptive diseases, which may together be classed under the name tuberculosis, still cause more deaths than all the acute infectious diseases put together. Its importance is emphasised by the fact that between the ages of 20 and 45,

283

one-third of all the deaths of males, and between one-third and one-fourth of all the deaths of females occurring at these ages are due to consumption of the lungs.

Formerly great stress was laid on the hereditary character of consumption. It would appear, however, that what is inherited is simply an increased vulnerability of tissues. Judging by the analogy of other animals it may be said that infants are rarely, if ever, born tuberculous. Bang examined 6,000 head of cattle with the tuberculin test, and found that in calves under 6 months old only 10·7 per cent. reacted, i.e. showed evidence of tuberculosis, between 6 and 12 months old 18·7 per cent., 1 to 2 years 23·2 per cent., and over this age 31·3 per cent. reacted; from which it may be inferred that the infection is nearly always received after birth.

The real cause of tuberculosis was shewn by Koch, in 1881, to be the tubercle bacillus. This is a minute bacillus, the length of which is from a quarter to half the size of a blood corpuscle. These bacilli, obtained from tuberculous growths in the body, Koch was able to cultivate on glycerine agar at blood-heat outside the body. By sub-culturing he obtained pure cultures, and after growing the bacilli for as long as fifty-four days, he inoculated various animals, producing tuberculosis in every case, while in similar check experiments in which all the conditions were the same, barring the absence of bacilli, no tuberculosis resulted.

The tubercle bacilli are easily distinguished from most other bacilli by the fact that after being stained by aniline dyes, such as carbol-fuchsin, the colouration is not removed when the preparation is soaked in dilute acid. By this means the presence of tubercle bacilli in the sputum (expectoration) of a phthisical patient is easily discovered, and a valuable means of early recognition of the disease secured. This is most important, as in its early stages consumption is an easily curable disease. Tubercle bacilli are discharged from the lungs in consumption of the lungs, from the bowels in consumption of the bowels, and so on. Hence the essential necessity for disinfecting these discharges. Such discharges while in a moist condition have, unless they are actually swallowed, little or no capacity for evil. It is when they become dry that they become dangerous. Thus the expectoration of a consumptive patient spat on to the floor or deposited in a pocket handkerchief is, so long as it remains moist, perfectly innocuous. What is evaporated from the wet surface is simply steam, harmless as the steam escaping from the domestic tea-kettle. But when it becomes dry, then comes danger. Dust is formed, which contains the living tubercle bacilli, and with the mere shaking of the handkerchief or the disturbance of the dust on the floor these are inhaled, and often cause consumption. The person thus infected may be a new patient. Often also it is the consumptive patient who is thus re-infected. Consumptive patients tend to recover. But if the patient's disease is daily recruited by fresh doses of the tubercle bacilli inhaled with the dust of previous expectoration, fresh centres of disease are produced, and thus the patient is unwittingly helping to cause his own death.

The infectious character of tuberculosis has been long suspected. In the 18th century, in Naples, there were enactments insisting on the

284

isolation of consumptive patients and disinfection of their furniture, books, etc. We now know, however, that these were counsels of panic, and that for practical purposes the infection may be regarded as confined to the sputum. The expired breath is free from infection except during coughing. That the sputum is infectious can be easily proved by feeding guinea-pigs or the domestic fowl on it. These rapidly become affected by generalised tuberculosis. The simple character of the precautions against infection which are required may be gathered from the following copy of a card which is given to consumptive patients in Brighton:—

Precautions for Consumptive Persons.

Consumption is, to a limited extent, an infectious disease. It is spread chiefly by inhaling the expectoration (spit) of patients which has been allowed to become dry and float about the room as dust.

Do not spit except into receptacles, the contents of which are to be destroyed before they become dry. If this simple precaution is taken, there is practically no danger of infection. The breath of consumptive persons is free from infection.

The following detailed rules will be found useful, both to the consumptive and to his friends:—

1.—Expectoration indoors should be received into small paper bags and afterwards burnt.

2.—Expectoration out of doors should be received into a suitable bottle, to be afterwards washed out with boiling water; or into a small paper handkerchief, which is afterwards burnt.

3.—If ordinary handkerchiefs are ever used for expectoration, they should be put into boiling water before they have time to become dry; or into a solution of a disinfectant, as directed by the doctor.

4.—Wet cleansing of rooms, particularly of bedrooms occupied by sick persons, should be substituted for "dusting" and sweeping.

5.—Sunlight and fresh air are the greatest enemies of infection. Every patient should sleep with his bedroom window open top and bottom, a screen being arranged, if necessary, to prevent direct draught; and, if possible, occupy a separate bedroom. The patient need not fear going out of doors in any weather, if warmly clad.

N.B.—The patient himself is the greatest gainer by the above precautions, as his recovery is retarded and frequently prevented by renewed infection derived from his own expectoration.

6.—Persons in good health have little reason to fear the infection of consumption. Over-fatigue, intemperance, bad air, dusty occupations, and dirty rooms favour consumption.

The most common source of infection is undoubtedly the dried expectoration. Infection may, however, probably be derived from infected food, as milk or meat.

The danger from meat is much less than that from milk, because the former is more generally cooked than the latter, and because the diseased portions of the former would be at least partially removed before it was sold. The abolition of private slaughter-houses, the general establishment of public abattoirs, and efficient meat inspection would do much towards aiding in eliminating tuberculous cattle from herds; because it would no longer be found remunerative to keep tuberculous cows until they become seriously diseased.

The danger from infected milk is probably very great. This has been repeatedly proved experimentally for bovine tuberculosis by experimenting on calves and pigs. A cow may suffer from tuberculosis of its udder, and yet go on freely secreting milk. The milk from such an udder readily produces tuberculosis in calves or pigs drinking it; but if another animal be fed during the same period with boiled milk obtained from the same udder, it remains well.

The presence of tuberculosis in cattle can be determined with almost complete certainty by the tuberculin test. A glycerine extract of pure cultivations of tubercle bacilli (filtered so as to be free from bacilli) was found by Koch to contain substances which, when injected into guinea-pigs suffering from tuberculosis, produced a febrile reaction, and appeared likely to cure the disease. So far as man and larger animals are concerned the hope of cure by this means has not been realised; but as a means of diagnosis, i.e. detection of tuberculosis, injection of a small quantity of tuberculin under the skin, has been found most valuable. If the cow thus injected is suffering from the slightest tuberculosis, it becomes feverish for a few days; if it is healthy no "febrile reaction" occurs. By using this test tuberculous cattle can be detected, they can then be kept in separate sheds, the former sheds cleansed and disinfected; the milk of these cattle kept separate from that of the rest of the herd, and boiled before being drunk, or the infected cattle sent to the butcher. If the disease is strictly localised the carcases can be utilised for food, after careful destruction of all diseased portions. If these means were generally adopted, tuberculosis might gradually be eliminated from the cattle of the entire country, and a serious source of loss to farmers, as well as of danger to children drinking the infected milk, removed. The presence of tubercle bacilli in cow's milk is detected by microscopic examination and by injection of small quantities of the suspected milk into guinea-pigs. The proportion of infected samples found when examinations of milk supplies have been made in different towns has varied from 10 to over 50 per cent.

It is probable that tuberculosis is conveyed by cow's milk only when the tuberculous disease affects the udder. But inasmuch as the udder of a tuberculous animal may become tuberculous very rapidly and without being detected for a considerable time, it is evident that no tuberculous animal of any kind should be allowed to remain in any cowshed where milch cows are kept.

Recently (July, 1901) Koch has thrown doubt on the identity of bovine and human tuberculosis, which was previously accepted, because (unlike some other observers) he has been unable to produce in 19 cattle, on which he experimented, tuberculosis by mixing with their food expectoration of consumptive persons, or inoculating under their skins similar material. Even if these negative results should subsequently be confirmed, the converse proposition does not follow, that bovine tuberculosis cannot be communicated to man; and apart from this possibility milk containing the bacilli of bovine tuberculosis cannot be regarded as wholesome.

The boiling of milk destroys tubercle bacilli. So does a temperature considerably below 212° F. In Denmark, where butter and cheese are manufactured on a large scale, and the raw milk is collected in central dairies, a law was passed in 1898, obliging every proprietor of a dairy to heat all skimmed milk, or butter milk, to a temperature of 85° C. (185° F.) before returning it to the farms. Pasteurization, i.e. the heating of milk in a special apparatus to a temperature of 70° C. (158° F.), and keeping it at this temperature for 30 minutes kills tubercle bacilli. If it is rapidly cooled, the nutritive value and taste of the milk are not spoilt. It is safer, however, to go beyond this point, and the use of an apparatus like the Aylmer or Sentinel Sterilizer can be recommended. More recent experiments have made it doubtful whether tubercle bacilli in milk are always killed in milk at a temperature of 70° C., the pellicle formed on milk when it is heated appearing to shield the bacilli from the effect of the heat. Hence it is desirable that "no sterilizer should be looked upon as thoroughly efficient for the purpose in which a temperature of at least 85° C. (185° F.) is not attained."

The following test may be used to determine whether milk has been efficiently pasteurized:—

Natural milk contains a ferment or enzyme, which is destroyed at a temperature of 176° F. This enzyme splits up hydrogen peroxide (H_2O_2) into water and oxygen, but this effect is not produced in milk heated above 176° F. Take one drop of a dilute aqueous solution of hydrogen peroxide, add it to one teaspoonful of the milk. Next add two drops of a watery solution of paraphenyldiamine. A dark indigo colour is produced with uncooked milk, no change of colour if the milk has been pasteurized. The same test can be used for determining whether butter has been made with pasteurized milk.

Infection is not the sole determining cause of tuberculosis. Certain conditions of environment may determine whether the infection will succeed in "taking root" or not. Of these the following are important:

The nutrition of the individual if defective favours infection. Probably one chief reason why consumption has declined nearly 50 per cent. in the last 50 years is the better, more varied and more abundant food of the population.

Improved housing of the population has greatly helped in the same direction. Tubercular diseases increase with density of population, and are most prevalent in overcrowded tenements. Probably overcrowding chiefly acts by favouring direct infection, but it must also lower the health and power of resistance of the individual against infection.

The drying of the subsoil has been regarded as a chief cause of the reduction of consumption. It is probable, however, that the wet soil merely predisposed to consumption, because it was commonly associated with cold and wet houses, which would favour catarrhs, and open the way for the infection of consumption.

The dryness of the house is a most important matter. If a damp soil means also a damp house it must favour consumption and other chest affections. Damp air, like water, rapidly abstracts heat from the body. Compare, for instance, the discomfort of sitting clad in water at a

287

temperature of 65° F. with the comfort of sitting clad in a dry room at the same temperature! The domestic fowl is naturally immune to anthrax; but by being kept for a few hours with its feet in cold water, it can be rendered susceptible to inoculation with this disease.

The effects of breathing foul air are clearly shewn by the varying death-rate from phthisis in different occupations. Thus, if the comparative mortality figures of agriculturists be represented as 100, that of a commercial clerk = 176, of a draper = 200, of a tailor = 211, of a printer = 244, of a bookbinder = 246.

The effects of breathing dust-laden air are even more marked. Thus, if the comparative mortality figures from phthisis of agriculturists = 100, that of a coal-miner = 166, of a mason = 215, of a chimney-sweep = 249, of a file-maker = 373, of a cutler = 407, of a potter = 453. The last figure probably also shows the influence of alcoholism, which greatly favours tuberculosis.

Means for Preventing Tuberculosis.—The means for preventing tuberculosis from infected milk and meat have been already indicated. They comprise—

(a) Means of eradicating tuberculosis from cattle;

(b) Means of preventing harm from tubercle bacilli in milk or meat;

Under the first head improved conditions of housing of cattle, greater air-space, improved ventilation, a larger proportion of out-door life are important. The use of the tuberculin test, the separation of healthy from diseased cattle; the disinfection of sheds occupied by infected cattle are also essential.

Under the second head come efficient sterilization of suspected food (see p. 13), and the rejection of diseased meat. (See p. 24).

The most important measure against tuberculosis is the prevention of infection from patients with consumption. Under this head are comprised the following steps:—

A. Means of ascertaining the existence of the disease—
  1. Bacteriological diagnosis.
  2. Notification of cases, voluntary or compulsory.
B. Direct preventive measures—
  1. Law against expectoration in places of public resort.
  2. Disinfection and cleanliness.
  3. Isolation.
  4. General sanitary improvement.
C. Education of the public and of patients as to the importance of the preceding measures.

The gratuitous examination of suspected sputum is now being undertaken in certain towns. The earlier the infectious condition of expectoration is detected, the sooner can the necessary precautions be taken.

The notification to the medical officer of health of all cases of consumption I have repeatedly advocated. This is already carried out for the chief acute infectious diseases, and although the difficulties of acting on the information received in regard to a chronic disease like consumption are considerable, they can be overcome with tact and discretion. Voluntary notification is already practised in Brighton, Manchester, and a few other towns. Notification gives increased and more exact opportunities of preventing phthisis by—1. Enabling disinfection and cleansing of affected rooms to be effected; 2. Enabling instructions to be given to the patient and his relatives as to the exact precautions required; and by 3. Facilitating the removal of the insanitary conditions of home and work which may have caused the case or favoured its untoward progress.

The following scheme of measures of disinfection was prepared by Drs. Niven and Newman and myself for the National Association for the Prevention of Consumption, and is issued by them in pamphlet form:—

In preventing a consumptive person from spreading the disease, two sets of preventive measures are required:—1st, The removal or destruction of the infective matter already disseminated by the patient's discharges, especially by his phlegm; and, 2nd, the prevention of future dissemination. For the latter purpose the main object is not to permit any discharge to become dry before being destroyed. Before the consumptive person has learned the personal precautions which must be taken, and up to the time when he has been trained to carry them out carefully, he has probably distributed a considerable amount of infective matter. This is especially liable to accumulate in a dangerous form at home, where the space is small, and light and ventilation are defective. Infective particles will be found in greater abundance on and near the floors, on ledges, and in room-hangings. But the personal clothing and bedclothes will also have become infected. Hence it is necessary to disinfect the floor, walls, and ceiling of the rooms occupied by the patient, as well as the furniture, carpet, bedclothes, &c.

When this has been done, if the personal precautions advised are carried out by the consumptive, further disinfection should not be needed.

It is, however, difficult to make sure that personal precautions are fully carried out, and rooms should therefore be subsequently cleaned at least once in six months, the floors being scrubbed with soft soap, the furniture washed, the walls cleaned down with dough, and the ceiling whitewashed.

Confined workshops in which a consumptive has worked for some time should be cleansed, and a notice in reference to spitting should be suspended in all workshops. The latter precaution should also be observed in all public-houses and common lodging houses, both of which require special attention to cleansing.

Disinfection of rooms which have been occupied by consumptive patients may be secured in various ways, but the following are the practical rules which must underlie any methods adopted:—

1. Gaseous Disinfection of Rooms, or "Fumigation," as it is termed, by whatever method it is practised, is inefficient in such cases.

2. In order to remove and destroy the dried infective discharges, the Disinfectant must be applied directly to the infected surfaces of the room.

3. The Disinfectant may be applied by washing, brushing, or spraying.

4. Amongst other chemical solutions used for this purpose a solution of Chloride of Lime (1 to 2 per cent.) has proved satisfactory and efficient.

5. In view of the well-established fact that it is the dust from dried discharges which is chiefly infective, emphasis must be laid upon the importance of thorough and wet cleansing of infected rooms.

6. Bedding, carpets, curtains, wearing apparel, and all similar articles belonging to or used by the patient, which cannot be thoroughly washed, should be disinfected in an efficient steam disinfector.

7. After all necessary measures of Disinfection have been carried out, the essential principle governing the subsequent control of a case of consumption is that all discharges, of whatever kind (especially expectoration from the lungs), should under no circumstances be allowed to become dry.

Besides measures of disinfection and cleanliness, the patient must be placed under the best conditions for overcoming the disease. The same measures tend to prevent infection. Thus abundant food, an open-air life, sleeping with bedroom windows widely open, avoidance of dust, abundance of sunshine, are all important. The importance of sunlight in the prevention of consumption can scarcely be exaggerated. Koch found that tubercle bacilli were killed in from a few minutes to some hours, according to the thickness of the layer in which they were exposed to the sunlight. He found that even ordinary daylight produced the same effect, if it lasted long enough; cultures of tubercle bacilli dying in from five to seven days if exposed at the window in compact masses. These experimental facts emphasise the importance of abundant open space about dwelling-houses (see p. 203), the provision of a large window-area (see pages 202 and 216), of staircase ventilation, and lighting, &c.

Scrofula means a tubercular affection of the lymphatic glands. It occurs most commonly in the neck. The infection is usually received from some neighbouring mucous surface, as from the throat, being derived from dried expectoration or diseased milk. The same indications as for the prevention of phthisis hold good for scrofula.

CHAPTER XLVI

NOTIFICATION AND ISOLATION

We are confident from the actual discovery of the micro-organisms causing certain infective diseases, that the other diseases of an analogous nature are similarly caused by living contagia. On this supposition, action is taken for the prevention of these diseases. This action comes under a number of different heads, which may be classified as follows:—

1. Means for the early recognition of the infectious character of a disease. The bacteriological aids to recognition in diphtheria, enteric fever, and phthisis have been already mentioned. It is important to call in medical aid when any suspicious symptoms arise, even when these symptoms do not appear to be urgent. If an infectious disease is not recognised in its early stage, it may be easily overlooked, and the patient cause a serious epidemic. The following hints for teachers are in Brighton sent with each circular letter as to excluding infected children from school. The list is not exhaustive, but may aid in drawing attention to suspicious symptoms. The only safe rule when in doubt is to act as though a case is infectious until a skilled opinion can be obtained.

HINTS AS TO INFECTIOUS DISEASES

As infection is sometimes spread by means of children attending school while suffering from undetected infectious diseases, the following hints may be useful to the teacher:—

1. Any scholar having a sore throat should be sent home and regarded as infectious until the throat has been examined by a doctor.

If a scholar has enlarged glands in the neck, and especially if he or she is very pallid, the suspicion of possible diphtheria should be entertained. Many slight cases of diphtheria escape detection.

2. Any scholar suffering from a severe cold, with sneezing, redness of the eyes and running at the nose, should be sent home. It may mean an influenza cold or the commencement of measles, and both are infectious. This recommendation is particularly important when measles is known to be prevalent.

3. A child with a violent cough, especially if it is severe enough to cause vomiting or nose-bleeding, should be suspected of whooping-cough, and sent home, even if the characteristic "whoop" is not heard.

4. Slight cases of scarlet fever sometimes escape notice, and the patients are sent to school with the skin on the hands, etc., freely "peeling."

5. In any of the above instances, or any other case of suspicion, the Medical Officer of Health, on receiving a confidential intimation, will be glad to make an investigation.

SYMPTOMS OF ONSET OF SCARLET FEVER

Sudden onset.
Usually vomiting.
Always headache.
Feverish, with dry, hot skin.
Sore throat.
Red rash on chest in a few hours.

MEASLES

Severe "cold in the head" for 72 hours before the blotchy rash appears.
Measles is extremely infectious in this preliminary stage.
Consider every severe influenza cold as possibly measles.

DIPHTHERIA

may be very indistinct.
Languor and sore throat.
Glands under and behind jaw are enlarged.
Patient very pallid.
White or yellow patches seen on examining inside throat.
Whenever doubtful, send the scholar home.

WHOOPING COUGH

In a child under seven, a severe cough should always be regarded as possibly whooping-cough, although no "whoop" has yet been heard.

2. The notification of all cases of infectious diseases to the medical officer of health, is clearly a means to an end, that of securing that the preventive measures to be next named are effectively carried out.

3. Means for the production of an artificial immunity. This is only practicable at present for two diseases of this country, small-pox by means of vaccination, and a temporary immunity against diphtheria by a dose of antitoxic serum. Apart from these means, any measures for improving the health of a child tend in the same direction. Enlarged tonsils, "adenoids" at the back of the nose (causing the child to snore at night and to breathe through his mouth), discharges from nostrils or ear, and similar conditions should receive early medical attention.

4. Isolation: preventing the conveyance of the contagium from the sick to the healthy.

5. Disinfection, i.e. destruction of the contagium of the disease.

The Infectious Disease (Notification) Act, 1889, and the corresponding London Act of 1891, impose a dual duty of notification (a) on every medical practitioner attending on or called in to visit an infectious patient, as soon as he becomes aware of its nature; and (b) on the head of the family to which the patient belongs or the nearest relative. The intimation must be sent by each of these to the local medical officer of health, the practitioner being paid a small fee for his trouble. Usually notification by the householder319 is only enforced when no doctor is in attendance. The diseases to which this Act applies are small-pox, cholera, diphtheria, membranous croup[10], scarlet fever, erysipelas, and the fevers known by any of the following names: typhus, typhoid, enteric, relapsing, continued or puerperal. The list of notifiable diseases may be extended by resolution of the Local Authority.

The enforcement of notification is most important for the public health. (a) It enables the medical officer of health to take immediate steps to prevent the spread of infection, by enforcing proper isolation of the patient, efficient disinfection, and by preventing the attendance of children from infected houses, at school, etc. (b) It enables the links of evidence connecting a series of cases to be identified, e.g. cases due to a common milk supply, or attendance at a particular school. (c) It has a valuable educational effect on all concerned in the cases.

ISOLATION

Both the patient and his attendant need to be isolated in diseases like scarlet fever, diphtheria and small-pox. The rule is less absolute in enteric fever. In the following description the standard of requirements taken is that of the most dangerous infectious disease, small-pox. The first point to decide is whether the patient may be safely isolated at home. For small-pox this ought never to be allowed in a town. For other diseases, this may be permitted, if the following conditions can be fulfilled.

For Isolation at Home a couple of rooms are required, preferably on

---

[10] This is diphtheria attacking the larynx

a higher floor or in a detached wing of the house. The w.c. used for the dejecta of the patient must not be used by any other members of the household. All linen, towels, handkerchiefs, etc., should be immersed in actually boiling water containing some washing soda, before leaving the sick-room. Other articles to be washed, if they will be deteriorated by soaking in boiling water or a chemical disinfectant, must be tightly wrapped in bundles, and covered with a clean wet sheet saturated with a strong disinfectant solution. Solid and liquid excreta, expectoration and other discharges must be treated as described on page 303. The nurse should not eat her meals in the patient's room. She should wear a cotton dress to be changed before going out for a walk. Her hands must be thoroughly washed and brushed after handling or helping the patient, particularly in enteric fever. It is advantageous if the nurse has previously had the patient's complaint. Attention on the part of the nurse to minute detail is essential, especially in view of the possibility of receiving infection from infected articles as well as directly from the patient. The measures required for the subsequent disinfection of the sick-rooms and of clothing, bedding, books, etc., are given on page 304.

The use of hospital isolation has rapidly increased in recent years, thus releasing private families from a serious burden. The number of beds which a Local Authority should supply for their district is usually stated as one for every 1,000 inhabitants, but in poorer districts this does not suffice. The site of the hospital should be well removed from houses. There must be a minimum zone of 40 feet between all infected buildings and the boundary walls, and the same distance between neighbouring buildings. A wall at least 6 ft. 6 in. high should enclose the hospital site. The hospital is divided into separate detached pavilions for the treatment of different infectious diseases. A floor space of 156 square feet should be allowed for each bed. The height of the ward should be about 13 feet, its width from 24 to 26 feet, and the total cubic space for each patient should be 2,000 cubic feet for scarlet fever, 2,500 for diphtheria. The lavatories and water-closets are separated from the main ward by a cross-ventilated lobby. In an isolation hospital every surface should be washable; all corners should be rounded off, and all projections on which dust can lodge avoided. The proportion of window space should be about 1 square foot to every 70 cubic feet. Special isolation pavilions are required for cases of doubtful diagnosis. The ventilation and warming of wards must be carefully regulated. Cross-ventilation by windows open on opposite sides of the ward can be maintained in nearly all weathers. The temperature of the ward should be maintained at 55°-60° F.

Ambulances are usually provided by the Local Authority for the removal of infectious patients. The ambulance should be cleansed and disinfected after each journey. The use of private conveyances for infectious patients is forbidden, except under special limitations.

The hospital isolation of small-pox is beset with special difficulties. There is a considerable body of evidence indicating that small-pox may be aerially carried from patients in hospitals to people living within a zone of half a mile, or possibly further. Without accepting the view that aerial dissemination of small-pox to considerable distances from the patient frequently occurs, it still remains true that, either by this means or by errors in the administration of small-pox hospitals, they do frequently constitute a source of danger to persons living in the vicinity. The Local Government Board recommended that a Local Authority should not contemplate the erection of a small-pox hospital. (a) On any site where it would have within a quarter of a mile of it as a centre either a hospital, whether for infectious diseases or not, or a workhouse, or any similar establishment, or a population of 150-200 persons; (b) on any site where it would have within half a mile of it as a centre a population of 500-600 persons, whether in one or more institutions or in dwelling-houses.

QUARANTINE

This term has been chiefly employed to denote the limitation of the movements of vessels coming from infected ports, for a term which, as the name indicates, was formerly forty days, but is now shorter. It may be conveniently employed, however, to signify the restriction of the movements of all persons who have been apparently exposed to infection, or who continue to live in infected dwellings. In this sense we may speak of:

1. *Domestic Quarantine.*
2. *Scholastic Quarantine.*
3. *National and International Quarantine.*

Domestic Quarantine, to a varying extent, is desirable for the members of a family of which one member has been attacked by an infectious disease. For small-pox every member of a household should be kept under strict watch until sixteen days have elapsed since the last contact with the case of small-pox, or until successful vaccination has been secured. For enteric fever this strict watch would be unnecessary, but the remaining members of the household should be warned to call in a doctor on the first symptom of malaise.

Quarantine is specially indicated for certain occupations. Thus if the child of an out-door labourer had been removed to a hospital with scarlet fever, it would be unnecessary to keep the latter away from work during the following week. If, however, he were a milk-carrier, or a tailor, or an assistant in a sweet-stuff shop this would be a desirable measure.

The Quarantine of School Children is more necessary than that of adults, because the former are more susceptible to infection. Children are kept from school:

(a) Because the infectious patient still remains in the house. In this case the healthy children must be kept from school until the patient has ceased to be infectious and disinfection has been thoroughly carried out; and for a further period longer than the longest known period of incubation of the disease in question, a margin being left for contingencies. It would probably be 8 plus 2 weeks for scarlet fever.

(b) Children are kept from school for a period exceeding the longest period of incubation when the patient has been removed to hospital.

294

The table in this page, modified from the Author's School Hygiene, is introduced as furnishing a convenient summary of the subject.

Objection is sometimes taken to the exclusion of children under the above circumstances from school, on the ground that they continue to mix with others in the street or in neighbouring houses. Clearly, however, in a school-room, a suspected child may communicate infection to children coming from widely scattered streets, while out-of-doors the danger is comparatively slight, and among neighbours the danger is very limited in area.

It is assumed in the following table that all infected articles have been disinfected before the termination of the period of quarantine.

DISEASE	DURATION OF INFECTION	DATE AT WHICH SCHOOL ATTENDANCE MAY BE RESUMED	DURATION OF QUARANTINE OF CHILDREN EXPOSED TO INFECTION
Scarlet fever	From 5 to 8 weeks; ceases when all peeling of the skin has been completed, and when the child is free from discharge from the nose or ear or sore places.	Not less than 8 weeks 14 days. from the beginning of the rash, and then only if no sore throat or sore places.	14 days.
Diphtheria	At least 21 days; often much longer. Absence of infection should be confirmed by bacteriological tests.	Not less than 2 months, and not then if strength not recovered, or if any sore throat or any discharge from nose, eyes, ears, etc.	12 days.
Small-pox and Chicken pox	About 4 to 5 weeks	When every scab has fallen off.	18 days.
Measles	From 3 to 4 weeks; when all cough and branny shedding of skin has ceased.	Not less than 4 weeks from beginning of rash.	21 days.
Rötheln (German measles)	2 to 3 weeks	From 3 to 4 weeks from beginning of rash.	21 days.
Mumps	About 21 days from the beginning.	4 weeks from the beginning.	24 days.
Whooping cough	6 weeks from the beginning of whooping, or when the cough has quite ceased.	In about 8 weeks	21 days.
Typhus and enteric fevers	4 to 5 weeks	When strength sufficient.	28 days.
Influenza	2 to 3 weeks	1 month	10 days.

School Closure is occasionally required to prevent the further spread of an infectious disease. This can be enforced on the order of any two members of the Local Sanitary Authority acting on the advice of the medical officer of health. This ought to be only occasionally necessary if notification of infectious diseases is strictly enforced, and if suspicious individual children are excluded from attendance at school. In diphtheria school closure may occasionally be rendered unnecessary by systematic bacteriological examination of the throats of children who had been exposed to infection. School closure is more useful for country than for town schools, as in the former the homes of children are more remote from each other, but it is occasionally necessary for both. For measles school closure is specially indicated in Infants' Schools. We have already seen that this disease is chiefly fatal when caught at a tender age. The early closure of Infants' Schools, and particularly of the Babies' Class is therefore indicated. It is unfortunate that the attendance at school of children under six years of age is encouraged. Such children have more severe and more frequently fatal attacks of diphtheria, scarlet fever, measles, and whooping-cough; and these are frequently acquired at school.

International Quarantine was originally enforced against plague; but in many countries has been extended to other diseases, as cholera, yellow fever, typhus fever, small-pox and leprosy. In England cholera is the only disease in connection with which it has been in the past enforced. It has now been entirely abandoned. It consists in the compulsory isolation at the port of entry of all persons who have come from an infected district, or have been in contact with a case of the infectious disease against which quarantine is enforced, for a length of time which will enable it to be determined whether the persons detained are or are not incubating the disease. If this measure could be strictly enforced, and if infectious diseases were conveyed only by infectious persons, quarantine would undoubtedly be effective. But in practice quarantine cannot be enforced in Europe; and as it cannot be efficiently enforced it forms an ineffective and irrational derangement of commerce. Thus if plague prevailed in France it would be impracticable to detain for ten or twelve days every person entering England. Furthermore, in this instance, infection is brought by rats as well as persons; and measures effective for the latter do not prevent the former from importing infection. Because of its impracticability and of the disorganization of commerce which would be associated with any attempt to enforce it, England has abandoned quarantine and other countries are gradually following its example. England bases its action on the ground that (a) sanitation is the true chief means of defence, especially against cholera. It does not trust to this alone but to this along with (b) medical inspection at the ports, (c) and subsequent medical supervision of persons landed from suspected vessels. By these means a watch can be kept over persons who have been in contact with infection.

Regulations are issued at intervals by the Local Government Board requiring the disinfection by steam of all rags and similar materials imported from towns in which small-pox, cholera, etc., are prevalent.

CHAPTER XLVII

DISINFECTION

By disinfection is meant the destruction of the active cause of each infectious disease. A disinfectant is therefore synonymous with a germicide. Disinfectants must be distinguished from deodorants or deodorisers, such as charcoal, and from antiseptics, which are antagonistic to the growth of bacteria, without necessarily killing them, e.g. common salt. Disinfection may be effected by chemical or physical means.

CHEMICAL DISINFECTANTS

A chemical disinfectant should fulfil the following conditions: 1. It must be an efficient germicide. 2. Its germicidal power should not be destroyed by the fæcal or other polluting matter, with which the bacteria of infection are associated. 3. For many purposes, it must not be destructive to or liable to stain the skin, or fabrics, or other articles to which it is applied. 4. It should preferably not be a virulent poison; and should be moderately cheap. The search for a completely non-poisonous disinfectant is a chimera.

There are three great classes of chemical disinfectants.

1. Oxidising agents, as the halogens (chlorine, etc.) and permanganates.

2. Deoxidising agents, as sulphurous acid (SO_2) and formic aldehyde (CH_2O).

3. Other disinfectants, which act by coagulating protoplasm or otherwise, as carbolic acid, corrosive sublimate.

The number of disinfectants is legion. Only the chief ones can be mentioned and their chief properties described. It is a good rule to eschew the use of all disinfectants of which the exact composition is not given; and all disinfectants which are described by "fancy" names, which are not descriptive of their composition.

A. OXIDISING AGENTS

Chlorine has been most commonly used as chloride of lime ($CaCl_2$, $Ca(ClO)_2$). This is somewhat unstable in composition. A solution of sodium hypochlorite containing 10 per cent. of available chloride is preferable. Chloride of lime for sprinkling on decomposing matter should contain at least 10 to 15 per cent. of available chlorine. Sulphuretted hydrogen and other offensive gases are decomposed by it. Thus

$SH_2 + Cl_2 = S + 2HCl$. Its chief action is as an oxidising agent.

Thus $H_2O + Cl_2 = 2HCl + O$.

A large excess must be used in disinfecting, otherwise the chlorine may simply oxidise fœcal or other organic matter, and not effectually destroy contagia.

Methods of Use—(a) As a gas, by the action of hydrochloric acid on strong chloride of lime. The molecular density of chlorine is 35·5, of formic aldehyde 15, of sulphurous acid 32; and the rate of diffusion of gases being inversely to the square-root of their densities, clearly chlorine does not compare favourably as a gas with formic aldehyde. The bleaching effect of chlorine on coloured articles of apparel is a disadvantage.

(b) As a liquid: used thus chlorine is very efficient, applied either as a spray or brushed on walls and other surfaces. Delépine found that a solution of one part of chloride of lime in 100 parts of water applied to wall paper impregnated with tubercular matter, disinfected it in a few hours, or in a few minutes if the layer of infected matter was not thick.

Bromine, Iodine, and Euchlorine (a mixture of chlorine and Cl_2O_4) are efficient disinfectants.

Iodine Trichloride (ICl_3) was found by Behring to share with corrosive sublimate ($HgCl_2$) carbolic acid and cresol mixed with acids, the halogens (Cl, Br, and I), and chloride of lime a superiority over other disinfectants in their power of killing anthrax spores in a short time.

Permanganates have been largely used as disinfectants, but their value is small. Impure sodium manganate (Na_2MnO_4) with much common salt (NaCl) containing some permanganate is known as "Condy's Green Fluid." "Condy's Red Fluid" consists of permanganate and sulphate of soda. To be of any use it must be employed in 5 per cent. solution. It stains fabrics brown, and it exhausts its feeble disinfecting power in first oxidising decomposing organic matter.

B. DEOXIDISING AGENTS

Sulphurous Acid (SO_2) acts chiefly as a reducing agent on organic matter. It is used chiefly as a gaseous disinfectant, and for this purpose is generated (a) by burning 1 lb. of sulphur for every 1,000 cubic feet of space in the room (which will equal 1·12 per cent. of SO_2). The windows and chimney of the room are first closed; the sulphur is placed in a saucepan supported over a bucket of water, and its ignition is aided by a small quantity of methylated spirit. The door of the room is then sealed, and the room left until the next morning. (b) Carbon disulphide may be burned in a benzoline lamp. (c) SO_2 liquefied under pressure is supplied in cylinders available for convenient use. The experimental results of the action of SO_2 on various bacteria are somewhat discrepant. It probably is fairly efficient for some diseases, but not in tuberculosis.

Formaldehyde or Formic Aldehyde (CH_2O) is produced by the slow and incomplete oxidation of methyl alcohol (CH_3OH) under access of air. A saturated solution in water containing 40 per cent. of the formaldehyde gas is known as formalin. The simple evaporation or heating of formalin is liable to produce the polymeric paraform which is solid and inert. To prevent the formation of paraform when formalin is evaporated, Trillat adds to it a solution of calcium chloride ($CaCl_2$), the mixture being known as formochloral. It is stated that when the air of a room is charged with less than one per cent. of the vapour, rapid and complete disinfection of surfaces occurs, and that it possesses a certain amount of penetrating power into loose fabrics. No damage is done to textile fabrics; and disinfection by this means possesses the advantage over disinfection by sulphurous acid or chlorine that the room can be entered without serious discomfort soon after the disinfection is carried out. In solution formalin is undoubtedly a powerful disinfectant, and in the gaseous condition it is at least equal in value to SO_2, probably better. Formaldehyde is used as a disinfectant.

(a) By evaporating a 60 per cent. solution of CH_2O in methyl alcohol (trade name holzine) over pieces of glowing coke placed under an asbestos plate (Opperman-Rosenberg apparatus). (b) By subliming tabloids of paraform by the heat of a lamp. A methylated spirit lamp is employed, and the moisture from the combustion in this causes the transformation of a considerable proportion of paraform into CH_2O vapour. It is doubtful if the quantity of the latter evolved is sufficient for efficiency. (c) In Trillat's apparatus formalin (i.e. the 40 per cent. solution in water of CH_2O) with $CaCl_2$ solution is heated in an autoclave worked at a pressure of 40 lbs., provided with a pressure gauge and thermometer. In all these methods the room must be carefully sealed, as the tendency for the disinfectant to escape is greater than with SO_2 or Cl. (d) The best method is to spray a solution of formalin 4 oz. to one gallon of water on all the surfaces of the room. This is equal to a strength of 1 in 40 of formalin, or 1 in 100 of formic aldehyde.

C. OTHER DISINFECTANTS

TAR ACIDS.—When coal tar is treated by acids and alkalies in succession, it becomes separated into (1) hydrocarbons, (2) phenols or tar acids, carbolic, cresylic, etc., (3) aniline and other basic substances. The hydrocarbons are known in commerce as "neutral tar oils." They are brown and syrupy, turning milky with water, and feebly disinfectant. The two most important "tar acids" are phenol or carbolic acid (C_6H_5OH) and methyl-phenol, also called cresol or cresylic acid ($C_6H_4(CH_3)OH$). The higher members of this same group yield milky emulsions with water, and are less poisonous than phenol. Various mixtures of them are used as disinfectants, and sold as creolin, Jeye's and Lawes' fluids. Izal belongs to the same series.

Carbolic Acid (phenol) did not kill anthrax spores until a 3 per cent. strength of its solution was used for 7 days (Koch), but sporeless anthrax bacilli were destroyed in a few minutes by a 1 to 2 per cent. solution. The disinfecting power of carbolic acid is greatly increased by adding mineral acids. Carbolic acid and lysol are superior to creolin for disinfecting stools. A 5 per cent. solution of carbolic acid destroys tubercle bacilli in sputum in 24 hours. Carbolic acid powders are in common use. In my opinion quicklime is more valuable.

Cresol is obtained from "crude carbolic acid" by fractional

299

distillation at a temperature between 185° and 205° C. A one-half per cent. solution has equal disinfecting power to a 2 or 3 or sometimes a 5 per cent. of phenol (carbolic acid).

Creolin consists of cresol emulsified in a solution of hard soap. Behring classifies the comparative germicidal power of phenol, cresol, and creolin on bacteria in broth as 1, 4, and 10 respectively. When albumen is present, creolin loses a part of its disinfectant power.

Lysol contains 50 per cent. of cresol, dissolved by means of neutral potash soap. It is completely soluble in water and does not turn milky as creolin does when water is added. It is more effective than creolin, and still more than $HgCl_2$ in albuminous liquids.

Soap has, owing to its alkalinity, disinfectant as well as cleansing action. A temperature of 55°-75° C. greatly aids its action. Antiseptic soaps possess no special value as germicides, but carbolic soap is a useful insecticide.

Lime in a one-tenth per cent. solution destroys typhoid and cholera microbes.

Mercuric Chloride ($HgCl_2$, corrosive sublimate) was found by Koch to destroy anthrax bacilli in a dilution of 1 in 20,000. Others have obtained less favourable results, but it is certainly a powerful germicide. The germicidal effect is greatly diminished by contact with organic matter, an insoluble albuminate of mercury being produced. For this reason $HgCl_2$ is not the best disinfectant for fæces unless mixed with acid, as in the following solution: $HgCl_2$ ½ oz., HCl 1 oz., aniline blue 5 grains to three gallons of water. This gives a solution of 1 in 960. The colouring is added to avoid accidental poisoning. $HgCl_2$ is not a good disinfectant for linen. Stains are apt to be fixed by it, and if linen soaked in it is subsequently washed with soap, without first carefully washing out the $HgCl_2$, it is darkened in colour. It attacks metals, and must not therefore be placed in metal receptacles.

Chloride of Zinc in a solution containing 25 grains to the fluid drachm is known as "Sir William Burnett's solution." It is a good deodorant, but an inefficient disinfectant.

Chinosol ($C_9H_6NKSO_4$) belongs to the quinoline group. It is an almost inodorous powder, very soluble in water, noncorrosive, and does not stain. A solution of 1 in 1200 forms an efficient germicide.

DISINFECTION BY PHYSICAL MEANS

Natural processes tend to the destruction of pathogenic microbes after their elimination from the patient. Of these desiccation, sunlight, and fresh air are the most potent. Heat and cold have a similar effect. Filtration or mechanical separation deprives a contaminated liquid of its microbes.

Desiccation attenuates the virulence of and finally kills most microbes. In laboratory experiments the vibrio of Asiatic cholera when dried dies in from three hours to two days, according to the degree of desiccation. The bacilli of enteric fever, tuberculosis, and diphtheria only die after drying for a few weeks or even months. The anthrax bacillus may

300

retain its vitality for several years in a desiccated state. Clearly, therefore, desiccation has no administrative value in the prevention of disease, and on the contrary it aids the dissemination of the microbes of tuberculosis, small-pox, scarlet fever, etc.

Direct Sunlight kills a large proportion of the sporeless pathogenic microbes. Diffuse is less energetic in its action than direct sunlight. The bacillus of diphtheria is destroyed by a half to one hour's exposure to sunlight. As to tubercle bacilli, see page 289. Downes and Blunt showed that diffused sunlight retards the putrefaction of organic infusions, and that direct sunlight inhibits putrefaction. Sunlight cannot, however, be trusted as an efficient disinfectant. It only secures surface disinfection, and could not be relied upon for pillows, mattresses, etc. M. Ward's experiments showed that the actinic rays of the sun are germicidal, independent of the heat.

Fresh Air, like sunlight, should be employed as a valuable auxiliary, not as an agent to be depended upon apart from systematic disinfection. The experiments of Downes and Blunt showed that light and oxygen together accomplished what neither alone could do. The presence of air in anthrax increases danger. The anthrax bacillus does not form spores in an animal suffering from this disease, and does not do so post mortem, unless the animal is dissected. Hence the importance of keeping the skin unbroken in this disease, only examining a drop of blood to establish the diagnosis.

Filtration is a means of separating microbes from the gases or liquids containing them. For the filtration of water see page 88. The carbolic sheet outside a sick-room is supposed to filter the air leaving the room from microbes. It is probably useless except as a reminder to the nurse to change her dress and adopt other precautions on leaving the sick-room.

Settlement of dust also acts as an aerial disinfectant. If a room be locked up, its air next day is almost free from particles, and all that is then required is disinfection of the surfaces of the room and of the articles in it. Whatever method of disinfection is employed, it is not disinfection of the air, but of the surfaces of a room which is the end in view.

Washing is the most efficacious means of removing infection. It is a mechanical means of removing the particular matter of which the contagium consists from the person or article to which it adheres into the water, which subsequently enters the drain, in the same way as do urine and fæces. Washing is an absolutely efficient means of purifying articles that can be completely submitted to it. A consideration of the physical laws governing the spread of infection will make this clear. The contagia are passive. When contained in a liquid they cannot escape from it under ordinary circumstances. Thus foul smelling gases may escape from sewage, but bacteria do not escape, except rarely during bubbling, or from dried portions of the invert of the sewer. Barring rare accidents "microbes submerged are imprisoned." Contagia are harmless until they become dust. Hence the danger associated with the use of pocket handkerchiefs in such diseases as influenza and phthisis; and the importance of keeping all infectious discharges wet, until they can be finally disposed of.

301

DISINFECTION BY HEAT

Heat may be applied in various ways: (1) Prolonged boiling in water of materials which are not spoilt by this means. (2) Destruction by fire of infected articles. (3) Dry hot air. (4) Steam.

Boiling kills most pathogenic microbes. The cholera vibrio is killed in four minutes at a temperature of 52° C. (126° F.); the typhoid bacillus at 59°.4 C. (138°.8 F.) in ten minutes. If boiling be continued for five minutes, the spores of pathogenic microbes are killed. The addition of one to two per cent. of washing soda to the water hastens this effect. For infected linen nothing beyond this is required.

Destruction by Fire is to be recommended for comparatively worthless articles, such as toys, straw from beds, rags, old clothing and bedding.

Dry Hot Air has been largely used in the past in ovens, for the disinfection of bulky bedding. It is now entirely superseded by steam. Its disadvantages are that (a) heat penetrates very slowly into the interior of bedding. Disinfection in test experiments was not accomplished in the interior of small bundles of clothes in three or four hours. (b) Scorching of articles often occurs. The sole advantage of this method is that bound books and leather goods are less liable to be damaged by it than by steam. If no other apparatus is available a baker's oven will serve to kill the non-sporiferous microbes of cholera, enteric fever, and diphtheria, as well as animal vermin. If, however, we accept the proper test proposed by Buchanan of the efficacy of disinfection, the "destruction of the most stable known infective matter," dry heat is unsatisfactory.

Steam may be employed as a disinfectant either (a) superheated, or (b) saturated, i.e. close to the temperature at which condensation occurs. This temperature depends upon the pressure under which the water has been boiled. At ordinary atmospheric pressure it is 100° C. (212° F.). The temperature of boiling is raised by subjecting the water to pressure. Consequently boiling water and the steam produced from it may be at any temperature. Thus steam may be

(a) Under pressure, with a temperature above 212° F.

(b) Not under pressure, at a temperature of 212° F.

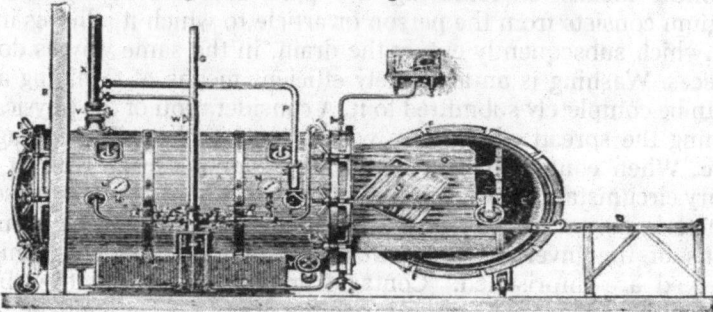

Fig. 57.
Equifex Saturated Steam Disinfector.

302

A—Disinfection chamber. B—Partition wall separating infected from disinfected side. C—Door on disinfected side. D—Door on infected side. EE— Safety-locking bolt for securing door. FF—Stiffening rings on doors. G—Steam inlet from boiler. H—Steam separator for arresting water condensed in G. I— Valve controlling admission of steam to disinfecting chamber. K—Valve controlling admission of steam to coils. LM—Safety valves regulating steam pressure in chamber and coils respectively. NU—Pressure guages indicating steam pressure in chambers and coils respectively. OO—Objects after disinfection. P—Wheeled carriage and cradle for OO. Q—Hinged rails on which P runs. R— Exhaust pipe for steam and air on first admission. S—Thermometer showing rise of temperature (to control complete air evacuation). T—Valve for closing exhaust pipe R when air is completely evacuated. V—Sluice valve to cause sudden escape of steam. W—Cock to admit steam to ejector. X—Exhaust pipe fitted with ejector for escape of steam before and of air during drying. Y—Valve for admission of air for drying under suction of ejector. [In some types of this machine this valve is placed on the lower part of C.]

Steam when admitted into a disinfecting stove comes into contact with cold objects. If the steam is saturated, immediate condensation to 1/1600 part of its original volume occurs. Its latent heat is at the same time evolved. The condensation causes enormous shrinkage in bulk. More steam is thus insucked into the partial vacuum produced, and this is repeated, until in every part of the mattress or other material undergoing disinfection equality of temperature is reached, when condensation of steam will cease, and disinfection is complete. If the steam is superheated and no condensation allowed, disinfection occurs by the relatively slow method occurring with dry heat. In practice at the early stage cooling causes some conversion of superheated into saturated steam, though subsequently the much slower process of disinfection by conduction of heat goes on. Hence superheated steam is a less efficient disinfecting agent than saturated steam.

Superheating is produced in disinfecting stores in two ways: (1) By a jacket around the stove, which is kept at about double the pressure and about 20° to 30° F. hotter than the interior of the stove; as in the older patterns of the Washington Lyon stove. (2) By having a jacket containing a solution of calcium chloride, which is heated by a furnace under the stove. This solution is kept at a constant strength by an automatic supply from a cistern. The temperature of the boiling water is thus raised without pressure to 225° F. This is the principle of Thresh's stove. The object of superheating steam is to assist in rapidly drying materials; but this object can equally well be secured by periodically allowing the sudden escape of the steam confined under pressure, in pressure disinfectors. This last method is the best, as it can not only be utilised at the last stage of the disinfection for drying the articles; but at the earlier stage for sweeping the air out of the stove, and thus removing what, owing to its low conductivity for heat is one of the most serious obstacles to rapid and efficient disinfection.

In the above description it has been assumed that the steam, whether saturated or superheated, is confined, except when the exhaust is employed for drying purposes. Steam may also be employed as current steam. Current steam disinfectors are initially cheap, but more steam, and

303

therefore more fuel, is required in their use; and unless pressure is used by impeding the escape of the steam a temperature of only 212° F. can be secured. Accepting Buchanan's dictum, a stove supplying saturated steam under pressure at a temperature in the interior of the stove of 234° F. is to be preferred. This temperature with saturated steam destroys the spores of the most resistant known microbe (that of symptomatic anthrax). With superheated steam or hot air stoves on the same basis a temperature of 280° F. would be required, which is damaging to most textiles, except horsehair.

THE PRACTICE OF DISINFECTION

The Management of the Sick-room and Patient requires careful and conscientious attention to detail. Certain details are given on page. All unnecessary furniture, carpets, and hangings should be removed as soon as the nature of the illness is known; but unless these articles have been contained in close trunks or drawers, and not opened since before the onset of the illness, they must be disinfected. Food left over from the patient's meals must be burnt, if solid, in the patient's room; if liquid, emptied down the water-closet. Dry sweeping of the floors is to be avoided, only wet brushing or cloths being used. Volatile aerial disinfectants during the sickness are valueless.

The Treatment of Discharges from the Patient is the most important point in the management of infection. The stools should be received into a bed-pan containing a 5 per cent. solution of carbolic acid, a 3 per cent. solution of cresol or lysol, or a 5 per cent. solution of chloride of lime. Milk of lime (20 per cent. strength) is very reliable, when added like the preceding solutions in bulk equal to that of the stool to be disinfected. The urine and vomit, if any, should be treated in exactly the same way. The infection of enteric fever is often spread by undisinfected urine.

Discharges from the throat, nose and mouth of patients should be received into a solution of

lysol 5 oz. to 1 gallon of water, or
carbolic acid 7 oz. to 1 gallon of water,

The efficacy of the carbolic acid solution is increased by adding 2 oz. of NaCl, or 12-14 oz. of NaCl to each gallon. Pocket-handkerchiefs must be avoided, linen rags being employed instead, and placed at once in one of the above solutions or burnt.

The skin may scatter infection, especially in small-pox and scarlet fever. Frequent baths and inunction with vaseline or oil are useful.

The disinfection of hands is most important for all attendants on the infectious sick. A solution of corrosive sublimate 1-1000, or one of the above solutions may be used for this purpose; but this is to be supplemented by the free use of the nail-brush and soap and water. The treatment of linen has been described.

Woollen articles of underclothing, and blankets can be disinfected by steam, which shrinks them less than boiling water. The ordinary

304

laundry processes appear, however, to suffice to rid them of infection, without boiling.

Bedding, curtains, and carpets should be disinfected by steam. Certain precautions are required in removing these to the disinfecting station. Surface disinfection of the room must have been first effected (see below); and the infected bedding should be encased in canvas bags or sheets. When a steam disinfector is inaccessible, the mattress and pillows should be taken to pieces, the covers washed, and their contents disinfected by spraying with formalin solution (1 in 40) or $HgCl_2$ solution (1 in 1,000), and subsequently exposing to sun and air. For disinfection of suits of clothes, current steam may be improvised as follows:—Over two bricks at the bottom of the kitchen "copper" thin floor-boards are placed, above the level of 2 or 3 inches of water previously placed at the bottom of the copper. The cover of the copper is put on, and by means of a brisk fire steam is kept streaming through the clothes. This is continued for an hour, and the clothes then hung out to dry.

Furniture, when wooden, can be washed. If upholstered it can be disinfected by spraying, and then beating and dusting in the open air.

Furs, Boots, and Shoes are spoilt by steam. For the first, spraying freely with formalin (1 in 40), or exposure over a formalin lamp is recommended. Boots and shoes should be filled and washed with a solution of $HgCl_2$, chinosol, or formalin.

The sick-room can only be efficiently disinfected after the patient has left it. The aim is surface disinfection. Aerial disinfection is sufficiently effected by open windows. Four chief methods of surface disinfection are practised. (a) Fumigation by SO_2, formalin, cresol, or other vapours. (b) Spraying the ceiling, walls, floor, and furniture with a disinfectant solution is probably the most convenient method of disinfection. It is more effectual than fumigation, less laborious than rubbing down walls, etc., by bread or wet cloth, and less likely to damage wall-papers than brushing a disinfectant solution on them. Solutions of $HgCl_2$ 1 in 1,000, or chinosol 1 in 1,200, or formalin 1 in 40 are efficient. A special spray apparatus (Fig. 58) is usually employed. A practical point is to spray the wall from below upwards, to prevent the solution running down the wall and producing streaks of discolouration. (c) Washing ceiling and walls with the disinfectant solution may be substituted. A one per cent. solution of hypochlorite of lime is largely used for this purpose, applied by a long-handled whitewash brush. (d) Attrition of walls, etc., by means of bread or dough sterilises them by mechanically removing microbes. The bread is cut into pieces suitable for grasping in the hand, the cut surface being applied to the wall. The crumbs must afterwards be burnt in the room. This is the official method in Germany.

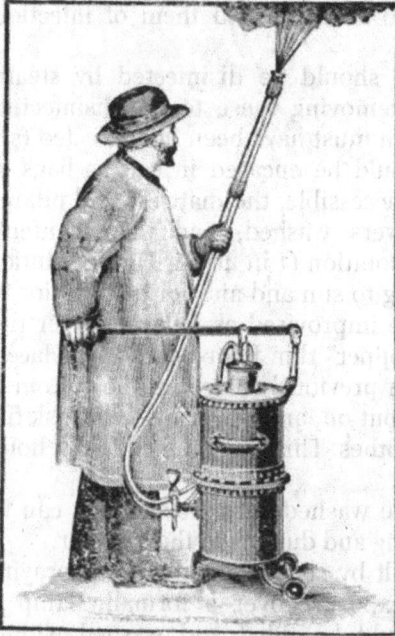

Fig. 58.
Equifex Spray Disinfector in Use.

Floors may be treated like walls and ceiling after the patient has left the room. During his occupancy of the room, tea-leaves or sawdust thoroughly impregnated with lysol or cresol should be sprinkled on the floor before it is swept, or washing substituted for sweeping. Scrubbing with soap and water constitutes the best disinfectant for floors and all other washable surfaces.

Books are difficult of disinfection. Steam damages leather. The penetrating power of dry heat is doubtful. Cheap books should be burnt. Abel discovered virulent diphtheria bacilli on toys six months after the patient, to whom they belonged, had diphtheria. Formalin and phenol vapours have been used to disinfect books in closed chambers, the books being stood on end. Letters can be rendered safe by steam disinfection.

Corpses of infectious patients should be placed in the coffin and buried as early as possible. A thick layer of sawdust saturated with lysol or cresol should be placed at the bottom of the coffin, and the corpse enveloped in cotton wool. Cremation is better than burial.

CHAPTER XLVIII

VITAL STATISTICS

Vital Statistics is the science of numbers applied to the life-history of communities. Its significance is similar to that of the more recently coined word—Demography—though the latter does not necessarily confine itself strictly to study of life by statistical means. Another term has been frequently used in recent years—"Vital and Mortal Statistics." The continued use of the word "mortal" in this connection is undesirable and objectionable. The term "Vital Statistics" is comprehensive and complete, as death is but the last act of life.

Of the problems of life with which the science of Vital Statistics is concerned, population, births, marriages, sickness, and deaths, possess the chief importance; and in the following sketch of the subject I shall concern myself chiefly with these. The subject naturally divides itself into two sections: the sources of information, and the information derived from these sources, and both of these will require consideration.

The importance of numerical standards of comparison in science increases with every increase of knowledge. The value of experience, founded on an accumulation of individual facts, varies greatly according to the character of the observer. As Dr. Guy has put it: "The sometimes of the cautious is the often of the sanguine, the always of the empiric, and the never of the sceptic; while the numbers 1, 10, 100, and 100,000 have but one meaning for all mankind." Hence the importance of an exact numerical statement of facts. The sneering statement that statistics cannot be made to prove anything can only be made by one ignorant of science. In fact, nothing can be proved without their aid, though they may be so ignorantly or unscrupulously manipulated as to appear to prove what is untrue. Instances of fallacious use of figures will be given as we proceed.

An accurate statement of population forms the natural basis of all vital statistics. Thus the comparison of the number of deaths in one with the number of deaths in a second community has no significance unless we know also the number living out of which these deaths occurred. Even then our knowledge would be defective, without further particulars as to the proportion in each population living at different ages, and the number dying at the corresponding ages. For other purposes we should require to know the number married and unmarried, the number engaged in different industries, and so on; in order that the influence of marital conditions, of occupation, etc., on the prospects of life may be calculated. The first desideratum of accurate vital statistics is a census enumeration of the population at such intervals as will not cause the intervening estimates of population to be very wide of the mark. In this country a decennial census is taken, the last occurring in 1901. In the intervals the population of the entire country, and of each town or district is estimated. Various methods of estimating the population have been adopted. (1) If a strict record of emigration and immigration is kept, then in a country in which a complete registration of births and deaths is enforced, the population can be easily ascertained by balancing the natural increase by excess of births over deaths, and the increase or decrease due to migration. This is done in New Zealand, but is impracticable in England, as no complete account of migration can be kept.

(2) The increase of inhabited houses in a district being known year by year, the increase of population may be estimated on the assumption that the number of persons per house is the same as at the last census. This may not be strictly accurate. In 1901 it was found that in England and Wales the average number of persons per house was fractionally less than in 1891.

(3) It may be assumed that the annual increase during the present decennium will be 1/10 of the increase during the last decennium 1891-

1901. If so, the population, e.g. in 1905, is the enumerated population in 1901 plus 4¼; times the annual increase occurring during 1881-91. (The fourth is required because the census is taken early in April, and the population is estimated to the middle of the year). This method is fallacious, because it makes no allowances for the steadily increasing numbers who year by year attain marriageable age and become parents. It assumes, in other words, simple interest, when compound interest is in operation.

(4) The Registrar-General's method, the one generally adopted, assumes that the same rate of increase will hold good as in the preceding intercensal period, i.e. that the population increases in geometrical progression, and not in arithmetical progression as under (3).

The application of this method will be best understood by an example. If the census population of a town is 32,000 in 1891, and 36,000 in 1901, what is the mean population in 1905?

(a) Find the rate of increase in 1891-1901.

If P = population at census 1891,
and if P_1 = population at census 1901,
and if R = rate of increase of population, then
$P_1 = P + Rn$ in the nth year.
$\log P_1 = \log P + 10 \log R.$
$1/10(\log P_1 - \log P) = \log R.$
$(4.556303 - 4.505150)/10 = .0051153 = \log R.$

(b) Apply this to the increase in the next 4¼ years.

Here $P_{1905} = P_{1901} R(17/4)$
$\log P_{1905} = 4.556303 + (17/4)(.0051153)$
$= 4.578043.$

By consulting the table of logs, the population corresponding to this number will be found to be 37,848 = population at the middle of 1905.

Estimates made by the last-named "official" method are liable to error, even for the entire country, and still more when applied to special districts. Thus the decennial rate of increase of the population of England and Wales in the 100 years has varied from 15·8 per cent. in 1821-31 to 11·6 per cent. in 1891-1901. The anomalies are even greater when the official method is applied to great towns. In one decennium such a town may, owing to brisk trade, have a rapid increase of working population with many children, and in the next decennium in consequence of emigration or transmigration there may be little or no increase. The declining birth-rate, which is having a greater effect on the number of population than the declining death-rate, is another cause of disturbance which increases the difficulty in forming a correct estimate of the population in intercensal periods. A quinquennial census is highly desirable, in order to avoid the doubts necessarily associated with estimates of population in the later years of a decennium, and with the birth and death-rates which are based on these estimates.

The Registration of Births and Deaths.—Civil registration of births and deaths began in 1837, but was not compulsory till 1870. It will be going

308

beyond the scope of this chapter to give details of the enactments as to registration. It suffices to state that it is the duty of the practitioner to give a certificate stating the cause of death of his patient to the best of his knowledge and belief. There is no registration of still-births in this country. Many deaths are registered of which the cause of death is not medically certified, and the value of our national vital statistics is considerably diminished on this account. Much improvement is desirable in the medical certification of causes of death. Every medical student ought to receive instruction on this subject before the completion of his studies. Names of symptoms as dropsy, hæmorrhage, convulsions; and obscure names, as abdominal disease, should be avoided. If the patient has recently suffered from injury, or recently passed through childbirth, or had a specific febrile disease, this must not be omitted from the certificate.

The Registration and Notification of Sickness forms another valuable source of information. Various attempts have been made to secure a general registration of disabling sickness, but with only partial success. District and workhouse medical officers appointed since February, 1879, are required to furnish the medical officer of health with returns of pauper sickness and deaths. This source of information might with advantage be more fully utilised by medical officers of health. Sec. 29 of the Factory and Workshops Act, 1895, requires that every medical practitioner attending on or called in to visit a patient whom he believes to be suffering from lead, phosphorus, or arsenical poisoning, or anthrax, contracted in any factory or workshop, shall send to the Chief Inspector of Factories at the Home Office, London, a notice stating the name and full postal address of the patient, and the disease from which he is suffering; a fee of 2s. 6d. being payable for each notification, and a fine not exceeding 40s. being incurred for failure to notify.

The Compulsory Notification of Infectious Diseases is enforced by the Act of 1889, which now applies to the whole country. The list of diseases to be notified is as follows:

"Small-pox, cholera, diphtheria, membranous croup, erysipelas, the disease known as scarlatina or scarlet fever, and the fevers known by any of the following names: typhus, typhoid, enteric, relapsing, continued, or puerperal, and also any infectious disease to which the Act has been applied by the Local Authority in manner provided by the Act."

It is the duty of the medical practitioner to ascertain whether in his own district, such diseases as whooping cough and measles have been added to the schedule of notifiable diseases. It is the duty of (a) the head of the family to which the patient belongs; in his default, of (b), the nearest relatives in the house; in their default, of (c), every person in attendance upon the patient; and in default of any such person, of (d) the occupier of the building, as soon as they become aware that the patient is suffering from an infectious disease to which this Act applies, to send notice thereof to the Medical Officer of the District. (e) The more formal duty of sending to the Medical Officer of Health a certificate stating the name of the patient, the situation of the building, and the infectious disease from which in his opinion the patient is suffering, is imposed on every medical practitioner attending on, or called in, to visit the patient, on becoming aware that the patient is suffering from an infectious disease to which this Act applies. He is entitled to a fee of 2s. 6d. if the case occurs in his private practice, and of 1s. if the case occurs in his practice as medical officer of any public body or institution. He is subject to a fine not exceeding 40s. if convicted of failure to notify. The value of returns of infectious diseases as enabling preventive measures to be taken is increased by interchange of notification returns of different districts. This is now undertaken weekly for a large number of districts by the Local Government Board, and the Registrar-General publishes quarterly summaries of such returns, as well as weekly returns of infectious diseases for the metropolis.

Marriages are usually stated in proportion to the total population, or the number per thousand of population; but a more accurate method would be to base the marriage-rate for comparative purposes on the number of unmarried persons living at marriageable ages. In England the marriage-rate is always higher in large towns than in rural districts. Thus in 1900 the marriage-rate in London was 17·6 as compared with an average marriage-rate in 1891-95 of 15·2 per thousand of the estimated population in England and Wales. The higher marriage-rate in towns is chiefly owing to the fact that higher wages and greater scope for remunerative work attract young country people of marriageable ages to towns.

Births are usually reckoned as a rate per thousand of population. Clearly, however, if one population had a larger proportion than another of women of child-bearing years this method of comparison would not be free from possible error. Even were the proportion of women of child-bearing ages equal, the comparison might be fallacious if in one population the proportion of single women was much higher than in the other. Illegitimate births do not materially vitiate this conclusion, as such births do not constitute more than 4 per cent. of the total births, and this number is not excessive in the districts in which there is the greatest excess of single women, viz. in districts in which a large number of domestic servants are employed. The only strictly accurate method is to subdivide the births into legitimate and illegitimate, stating the former per 1,000 married women of child-bearing years, and the latter per 1,000 unmarried women of child-bearing years. I append an example of the relative accuracy of the three methods above indicated[11]:—

	BIRTH-RATE		
	PER 1,000 INHABITANTS	PER 1,000 WOMEN AGED 15-45	PER 1,000 MARRIED WOMEN AGED 15-45 YEARS
Kensington	21.8	61.6	215.4
Whitechapel	39.9	172.1	328.3
Percentage excess of birth-rate in Whitechapel over that in Kensington	83%	179%	53%

[11] From "Elements of Vital Statistics," by A Newsholme.

Thus, according to the ordinary method (A) of stating the legitimate birth-rate, it is 83% higher in Whitechapel than in Kensington, whereas it is really only 53% higher. Similarly a statement of the illegitimate birth-rate in the two districts "per 1,000 inhabitants," shows an excess of only 6% in Whitechapel, while a statement "per 1,000 unmarried women aged 15-45 years" shows the real excess of 144%. Both in this and other civilised countries there has been in the last 25 years a steady decline in the birth-rate. In England the maximum birth-rate was 36·3 per 1,000 of population in 1876, and the minimum 29·3 in 1899. This diminution is only caused to a minor degree by postponement of marriage to more mature years, and by a larger proportion of celibacy. Nor is there any reasonable ground for the view that a diminished power of either sex to produce children has been produced by alcohol, syphilis, tobacco, or other causes. The main cause of the diminution of the birth-rate is "the deliberate and voluntary avoidance of child-bearing on, the part of a steadily increasing number of married persons."

Deaths are calculated in proportion to every 1,000 of the population, the unit of time being a year. This unit is preserved even when death-rates for shorter periods, e.g. a week, are stated. Thus the death-rates for the 33 great towns published weekly in the chief newspapers are annual death-rates; they represent the number who would die per 1,000 of the population, supposing the same proportion of deaths to population held good throughout the year. The best plan to obtain the weekly annual death-rate is as follows: the correct number of weeks in a year being 52·17747, if the population of a town be 143,956, and the number of deaths in a given week are 35, then the death-rate is 12·687. Thus:—

143,956 / 52·17747 = 2758. 1,000 / 2,758 = 0·3625. This is the factor by which the weekly number of deaths must be multiplied.
35 × 0·3625 = 12·6875 or 12·7.

The above is the crude death-rate. Various corrections are required, which must now be considered. The most important of these are for public institutions, for visitors, and for age and sex. A public institution, e.g. a workhouse, infirmary, or asylum, in a given district may consist almost entirely of persons belonging to another district. The rule is to relegate to the district to which they belong all deaths of inmates of an institution, i.e. subtract all deaths of outsiders occurring in inside institutions, and add all deaths of inhabitants occurring in outside institutions. The population as well as the deaths of these institutions should be excluded, in so far as they are derived from the outside district, in order to make the net death-rate approximately correct.

Theoretically the correction ought to be extended so as to apply to visitors who do not die in public institutions. In practice, however, this cannot be effected, until a central "clearing house" is established. The exclusion of deaths of visitors from the district in which they occur is easy; their inclusion in the returns of the district from which they come is more difficult to secure. For the present, they should be included in the death-rate of the district in which they occur.

311

Death-rate according to Age and Sex.—To obtain a true conception of the death-rate in a community, it is necessary to state the number of deaths in each sex in proportion to the number living at different ages. The importance of this is shown by the following extract from the Registrar-General's report for 1899.

England and Wales.—Deaths to 1,000 living at each of 12 groups of ages.

	ALL AGES	0	5	10	15	20	25	35	45	55	65	75	85 AND UPWARDS
Males	19·5	60·4	3·8	2·2	3·6	5·3	7·1	12·3	20·0	37·2	69·8	1526	300·3
Females	17·3	50·7	3·9	2·3	3·3	4·3	6·1	10·0	15·4	298	61·5	1426	272·0

Thus at ages over 5 and under 45 for males, and under 55 for females, the death-rate is lower than is the total death-rate for all ages. For females at all ages except from 5 to 15, the death-rate is lower than for males. From the above statement it will be clear that a considerable excess of women (as in a residential district with a large number of domestic servants) or a considerable excess of either sex at the ages of 15 to 45 (as in most large towns) in proportion to the number living at other ages, would produce a lower total or crude death-rate, which does not imply any truly more healthy condition than that of another district, which is less favourably constituted so far as the proportion of the sexes and the numbers living at different ages are concerned. By a means of correction now to be described this source of error can be eliminated. The method of obtaining the factor for correction can be best understood by an example. The annual death-rate of England and Wales in 1881-90 was 19.15, and the death-rate at each age-group is given in the following table:

AGES	MEAN ANNUAL DEATH-RATE IN ENGLAND AND WALES 1881-90, PER 1,000 LIVING AT EACH GROUP OF AGES		POPULATION OF HUDDERSFIELD IN 1891		CALCULATED NUMBER OF DEATHS IN HUDDERSFIELD	
	Males	Females	Males	Females	Males	Females
Under 5	61.59	51.95	4,551	4,785	280	249
5	5·35	5·27	4,691	5,081	25	27
10	2·96	3·11	5,113	5,165	15	16
15	4·33	4·42	4,905	5,549	21	25
20	5·73	5·54	4,541	5,461	26	30
25	7·78	7·41	7,466	8,834	58	65
35	12·41	10·61	5,576	6,265	69	66
45	19·36	15·09	3,944	4,649	76	70
55	34·69	28·45	2,393	3,017	83	86
65	70·39	60·36	1,128	1,590	79	96
75 and upwards	162.62	147.98	250	466	41	69
Totals			44,558	50,862	773	799
			|————/		|————/	
			95,420		1,572	

The population of Huddersfield at each of the corresponding periods as given by the census of 1891, is also shown in this table, and in the last column the number of male and female deaths that would occur by applying the death-rates for England and Wales to the population of Huddersfield are shewn. The total number of deaths thus calculated is 1572 in a population of 95,420, and the total death-rate = 16·47 per 1000. This is the standard death-rate, i.e., the death-rate at all ages calculated on the hypothesis that the rates at each of 12 age-periods in Huddersfield were the same as in England and Wales during the ten years of the last intercensal period, viz. 19·15 in 1881-90.[12] But the standard death-rate of Huddersfield would have been 19·15 instead of 16·47, were it not for the fact that the distribution of age and sex in the Huddersfield population is more favourable than in the country as a whole. Hence it must be increased in the ratio of 19·15: 16·47, i.e., multiplied by the factor 19·15/16·47 = 1·1627. When the crude or recorded death-rate for 1900 of 16·78 is multiplied by this factor we obtain the corrected death-rate of 16·78 × 1·1627 = 19·51 per 1000, which is the correct figure to compare with the death-rate of 18.31 for England and Wales in that year. If the death-rate of England and Wales be stated as 1000, then 1000 × 1951/1831 = 1066, is the comparative mortality figure for Huddersfield. Similarly in the year 1900 the comparative mortality figure of London was 1093, of Croydon 831, of Norwich 919, while that of Liverpool was 1539, of Salford 1541. In all the towns except Plymouth and Norwich the corrected death-rate is higher than the crude or recorded death-rate. This implies that, in all except these two towns, the factor of correction is greater than unity.

This is a convenient point for briefly discussing the relationship between the birth-rate and death-rate. The opinion is commonly held that a high birth-rate is a direct cause of a high death-rate, owing to the great mortality amongst infants. The table on page 310 shows that the death-rate at ages under five is three times as high as at all ages together, and it is therefore natural to suppose that a high birth-rate by producing an excessive proportion of persons of tender years will cause a high general death-rate. This might be so, if the birth-rate were to remain high for only five years. But if the high birth-rate continued longer, the proportion of the total population at ages of low mortality would be increased, and the general death-rate would be lowered. We have already seen that in nearly all the great towns, in which the birth-rate is higher than in rural districts, the age distribution of the population is more favourable to a low death-rate than in rural districts; and their higher crude death-rate is made still higher than that of rural districts when the necessary factor of correction is applied.

The Infantile Mortality should be stated in terms of the infantile population. This is more accurately assumed to be equal to the number of births in the given year, than estimated from the number stated to be

---

[12] This was written before the figures for the period 1891-1900 were available; but the method adopted is the same, substituting the death-rates, etc., for the later period.

under one year of age at the last census. The number of deaths under one year of age per 1000 births was for England and Wales in 1899, being lowest in the agricultural counties and highest in manufacturing counties. In the 33 great towns it averaged 172 in the year 1900, ranging from in Croydon, Huddersfield and Halifax to 236 per 1000 births in Preston. Of 1000 male children born in England and Wales in 1881-90, the number surviving at the age of three months was 921, at the age of six months 889, twelve months 839, while the number of female children surviving one year of 1000 born was 869. In towns a smaller number survive. Of the conditions causing this high infantile mortality, ignorance and inexperience on the part of parents bear a considerable part, especially as influencing the food and mode of feeding. The death-rates at other age-groups beyond infancy are given in the table on page 311. Season influences the death-rate. The third quarter of the year has the lowest death-rate, unless the amount of Epidemic Diarrhœa has been excessive. In the first quarter of the year, the highest death-rate usually occurs. Mild winters and cool summers both lower the mortality. The seasonal incidence of infectious diseases need only be mentioned in passing.

Density of Population has important bearings on the death-rate. Thus the urban districts in 1899 had a death-rate of 19·2 and the rural of 16·3 per 1000 of population. Farr found that the death-rate increased with the density of populations, not in direct proportion, but in proportion to the 6th roots of the contrasted populations. This rule does not now hold generally good. It is only after the density has reached a certain degree of intensity that it begins to exert an appreciable effect. Even then it is what is implied in aggregation rather than the aggregation itself that is pernicious. In particular, poverty is usually greater in densely populated districts than elsewhere, with its accompaniments of deficient food and clothing and bad housing. Hence the excess of phthisis in tenemented houses, especially in houses with only three rooms. I have shown that the true density that should be considered is the number of persons to each room, not the number of persons on a given area ("The Vital Statistics of the Peabody Buildings," Roy. Statist. Soc., Feb., 1891).

Occupation and Mortality.—To obtain correct statistics showing the influence of occupation on vitality, one must know the number and age of those engaged in each industry, and the corresponding number of deaths. A statement of the mean age at death of those engaged in different occupations would be most fallacious. The best plan is to restrict the statistics to men aged 25-65, and calculate for these death-rates in a standard population, after the fashion already described. By this means a "comparative mortality figure" can be obtained. For all males it is 1000, for farmers 563, teachers 603, lawyers 821, doctors 966, butchers 1096, plumbers 1120, brewers 1427, innkeepers 1659, potters 1706, file-makers 1810. Speaking generally, the occupations are most unhealthy in which there is most exposure to dust, to the breathing of foul air, and to excessive indulgence in alcoholic drinks.

Deaths from Various Causes.—These may be stated in proportion to total deaths from all causes, or in terms of the population. The first plan

314

must be adopted only when it is desired to ascertain the proportional share of a given cause of death in the total mortality. In 1899, in England and Wales the diseases named in the first column of the table, were the most prolific causes of deaths.

England and Wales, 1899.
Deaths from Various Causes to 10,000 Deaths from all Causes.

Bronchitis	880
Phthisis	729
Pneumonia	685
Old age	541
Diarrhœa, Dysentery	511
Cancer	452
Apoplexy	327
Influenza	213
Whooping cough	174
Measles	172
Diphtheria	160
Enteric fever	108
Scarlet fever	64
Small-pox	3

The diseases in the second column are given in order to indicate their proportional share of the total number of deaths.

The proper plan of stating the death-rate from a given disease is in terms of the population, or better still subdivided into death-rates from the disease for different age-groups as in the table on page 311, if the number of deaths is not too small to admit of this. The importance of stating the death-rate for different age-groups is greatest for such diseases as diarrhœa, whooping cough, and measles, in which most of the deaths occur at ages under five. In the following table are given the death-rates from the causes of death which are most important, either from their magnitude, or because of their preventible character:—

England and Wales, 1899.—Death-rate per 1,000 Persons living.

Small-pox	·005
Measles	·32
Scarlet fever	·12
Influenza	·39
Whooping cough	·32
Diphtheria	·29
Enteric fever	·20
Typhus fever	·001

Cholera	·04
Diarrhœa, Dysentery	·94
Intemperance	·09[13]
Cancer	·83
Phthisis	1·34
Other tubercular diseases	·58
Premature birth	·58
Old age	·99
Apoplexy	·60
Convulsions	·57
Valvular disease of heart	·38
Bronchitis	1·61
Pneumonia	1·26
Gastro-enteritis	·61
Bright's disease	·29
Accidents	·59
Ill defined and not specified causes	·73
————	
All causes	18.33

Determination of Longevity. We have hitherto considered only death-rates, i.e. the number dying each year out of each 1,000 of population. The mean duration of life involves another aspect of the same problem. Although nothing is more uncertain than the duration of individual life, the duration of life for the entire community is subject to so little variation that annuities and life assurance can be made the subject of exact calculations. Of the tests employed to measure the duration of human life the most commonly employed is the mean age at death.

$$\text{Mean age at death} = \frac{\text{sum of ages at death.}}{\text{number of deaths.}}$$

This is a fair method of stating the average longevity of a particular group of persons, if the group is sufficiently large to avoid the possible error caused by paucity of data. But it would be entirely unsafe to assume that by this means a safe standard of comparison between two groups can be formed. Thus in 1890 it was stated that the mean age at death of workmen was 29-30 years, of the well-to-do classes 55-60 years. This statement throws no light on the relative vitality of the two classes under comparison. The well-to-do classes consist largely of those whose working

---

[13] There is no general agreement as to the exact sense in which the words average and mean should be used. They are used here interchangeably.

days are past; and it is as untrustworthy to compare their mean age at death with that of workmen, as it would be to base any conclusion on the fact that mean age at death of bishops is much higher than that of curates. The mean age at death is lowest in countries with a high birth-rate. Hence it would be very fallacious to compare the mean age at death in England and France.

The probable duration of life (vie probable) is a term sometimes employed to denote the age at which any number of children born into the world will be reduced to one half. In practice it can only be ascertained from a life-table.

The true mean duration of life or expectation of life can only be ascertained from a Life Table, and this must therefore be briefly described. This is the true biometer, of equal importance in all inquiries connected with human life with the barometer or thermometer and similar instruments employed in physical research. The Life Table represents "a generation of individuals passing through time." The data required for its construction are the number and ages of the living, and the number and ages of the dying, i.e. the data required for ascertaining the death-rate for each year of life. Theoretically the best plan for forming a Life Table would be to observe a million children, all born on the same day, through life, entering in a column (headed l_x) the number who remain alive at the end of each successive year until all have died; and in a second column (headed d_x) the number dying before the completion of each year of life. This method is impracticable, and were it otherwise, the experience would be obsolete before it could be utilised. The method employed in constructing the national Life Tables for England is, without tracing the history of individuals through life, to assume that the population being given by the census returns and the death-rate for each age for a given decennium being known, that the same death-rate will continue during the remainder of the lives of the population included in the census returns.

The total mean number living and the total number dying for a given age-period are known. The mean chance (p_x) of living one year during this age-period is found by the fraction

$$\frac{Population - \frac{1}{2} Deaths}{Population + \frac{1}{2} Deaths} = p_x$$

It is usual to start with a million or 100,000 children at birth, and to make a separate table for the proportionate number of males and females at birth. Thus in Brighton in 1881-90 these were in the proportion of 51,195 and 48,805. Starting with 51,195 male infants at birth, and multiplying this number by ·84608, the probability of surviving for one year, we obtain 51,195 × ·84608 = 43,315. For the second year of life, the probability of surviving was ·93398; hence the number of survivors is

43,315 × ·93398 = 40,452, and so on.

The general arrangement is shewn in the following example of a Life Table, which only gives the data at or near the two extremes of life, the intermediate figures having been omitted from considerations of space.

317

BRIGHTON LIFE TABLE.—MALES.
(Based on the mortality of the 10 years 1881-90.)

AGE x	DYING IN EACH YEAR OF LIFE d_x	BORN AND SURVIVING AT EACH AGE l_x	SUM OF THE NUMBER LIVING, OR YEARS OF LIFE LIVED AT EACH AGE, $x+1$, AND UPWARDS, TO THE LAST AGE IN THE TABLE $\Sigma l_x + 1$	MEAN AFTER LIFE-TIME (EXPECTATION OF LIFE) AT EACH AGE e_{x^o}
0	7,880	51,195	2,206,174	43·59
1	2,863	43,315	2,162,859	50·43
2	996	40,452	2,122,407	52·96
3	733	39,456	2,082,951	53·29
4	440	38,723	2,044,228	53·29
97	12	29	43	1·60
98	7	17	26	1·53
99	4	10	16	1·48

The 43,315 males surviving to the end of the first year of life out of 51,195 born will each have lived a complete year in the first year, or among them 43,315 years. Similarly the 40,452 males will live among them 40,452 further complete years, and so on, until all the males started with become extinct at the age of 105. Evidently, therefore, the total number of complete years lived by the 51,195 males started with at birth will be

43,315 + 40,452 + 39,456 + 38,723 + ... + 10 + 6 + 4 + 3 + 2 + 1 = 2,206,174 years, this sum being obtained by adding together the numbers living at each age beyond (i.e. below on this table) the age in question right down to its last item. This number of years is lived by 51,195 males. Hence the number of complete years lived by, i.e. the expectation of life of, each male

= 2,206,174 / 51,195 = 43·09 years.

This is the curtate expectation of life. It deals only with the complete years of life, not taking into account that portion of life-time lived by each person in the year of his death, which may be assumed to be on an average half a year. Hence the complete expectation of life according to the above table is 43·59 years.

In the following table the expectation of life (complete) for various towns and for England is given:—

Life Table.—Expectation of Life at Birth.

		Male.	Female.
English Life Table,	1838-54 (*Farr*)	39·91	41·85

„	1871-80 (*Ogle*)	41·35	44·62
„	1881-90 (*Tatham*)	43·66	47·18
London, 1881-90 (*Murphy*)		40·66	44·91
Brighton, 1881-90 (*Newsholme*)		43·59	49·25
Manchester City, 1881-90 (*Tatham*)		34·71	38·44
Glasgow, 1881-90 (*Chambers*)		35·18	37·70

Formulæ of varying degrees of accuracy have been devised for giving in the absence of a Life Table an approximation to the expectation of life.

Willich's Formula is as follows:—If x = expectation of life, and a = present age, then x = 2/3 (80-a). Thus, at the age of 50 years the expectation of life, according to this formula, is 20 years. By the English life-table for 1881-90 it was 18.82 for males, and 20·56 for females. Farr's formula is based on the birth and death-rates. If b = birth-rate and d = death-rate per unit of population, then

Expectation of life = (2 / 3 × 1/d) + (1 / 3 × 1/b).

Thus b for England and Wales, 1889-98 = 30·3 / 1,000 = ·0303.

and d for England and Wales, 1889-98 = 18·4 / 1,000 = ·0184.

(2/3 × 1/·0303) + (1/3 × 1/·0184) = 47.2 years, as compared with the expectation of life for 1881-90 shown in the above table.

In a life-table the number out of which one dies annually ⎫ are
the mean age at death ⎬ identical
and the expectation of life ⎭ in value

when the whole duration of life from birth to death is included in the calculation. This is only true for a stationary or life-table population, in which the number dying is assumed to be regularly replaced by a corresponding number of persons of the same age.

Life Capital.—The life-tables now in use are those based on the experience of 1881-90. The gain in any subsequent year, as in 1900, may be ascertained as follows: the mean population and the death-rate for each age-group as 0-5, 5-10, etc., are calculated. Then the mean death-rate of the same community for 1881-90 is applied to this population. By this means the "calculated number" of deaths in 1900 is obtained. The difference between these numbers and the "actual number" obtained from the death-registers, gives the gain or loss during the year. Next multiply these differences by the mean expectation of life for the corresponding groups of years. By adding the gains thus ascertained and subtracting any losses, we obtain the net gain in "life-capital" (Tatham) during the year 1900.

Tests of the Health of a Community. 1. The general death-rate is the test most commonly applied, and generally trusted. It has its limitations in this respect. It may usually be trusted in comparing a town or district for a single year with preceding years, as the age and sex distribution of a given population only changes slowly. But when comparison with other towns or districts is made, the possibility that erroneous conclusions may be drawn becomes considerable. (a) Before the death-rates of two districts can be compared, either this comparison must be made by means of death-rates for age-groups (0-5, 5-10, ... 65-75, etc.) or the factors of correction, the method of obtaining which is described on page 312, must be applied. (b) It must be ensured that in the two compared districts, an equal amount of correction has been made for deaths occurring in public institutions and among visitors. (c) Even when the above precautions are taken, it is conceivable that a town with a death-rate of 15 per 1,000 may really be as healthy as another with a death-rate of 12 per 1,000, though a statistical justification of this statement is a difficult task.

Social conditions quite irrespective of the sanitary condition or the natural salubrity of a district have an important influence on the death-rate. Poverty and all that it connotes, necessarily involves a higher death-rate than occurs among the well-to-do. Furthermore, the domestic servants employed by the latter frequently die in districts other than those in which they are employed, without any possibility of the requisite correction being made.

2. The zymotic death-rate is frequently quoted as a test of sanitary condition. This is a death-rate based on the deaths from the "seven chief zymotic diseases," small-pox, measles, whooping-cough, diphtheria, scarlet fever, fever (chiefly enteric), and diarrhœa. This death-rate should be entirely discarded, the death-rate from each infectious disease being separately stated. A high death-rate from enteric fever would be a much more serious reflection on the health of a town than a high death-rate for whooping-cough.

The death-rate from each of these diseases in London and in England in 1899 was as follows:—

DEATH-RATE IN 1899 PER 1,000 LIVING.
England and Wales. London.

	England and Wales.	London.
Small-pox	·005	nil
Measles	·32	·47
Scarlet fever	·12	·08
Diphtheria	·29	·43
Typhus	·001	nil
Enteric fever	·20	·18
Whooping cough	·32	·38
Diarrhœa	·94	·92

A statement of the death-rate from each of these diseases for a series of years is a much more trustworthy test than a similar statement for a single year, in which accidental causes may have caused a temporary increase, or than a statement of the average result for a series of years, which tends to conceal the epidemic variations of the disease in question. The danger of such averages has been well exposed by Chadwick in the remark that "a mean between the condition of Dives and Lazarus tends to make it appear that after all Lazarus has not so much to complain of."

3. The infantile mortality is a delicate test of mixed sanitary and

social conditions, and stress may always be laid on it from these standpoints. The importance of comparing death-rates at other age-groups has already been explained.

4. The most delicate and exact method, if all the data are accurate and complete, is to construct a Life Table, and ascertain the expectation of life in comparison with that of other communities.

The preceding statistical tests of the salubrity of a community, and any others that may be available, should all, when practicable, be utilised; and it should always be remembered that these tests, especially the general death-rate, are most trustworthy when contrasting the experience of a community with its past experience, and least trustworthy when contrasting its experience with that of others; owing to the difficulty in the latter case of ensuring the avoidance of error arising from non ceteris paribus.

Statistical Fallacies.—If "fallacies" be regarded as synonymous with "errors," clearly they may occur at every step. They may be classified as errors of data, and errors of methods. The most important errors of data are erroneous estimates of population, and erroneous returns of deaths, especially in the direction of exclusion of certain deaths. Death-rates for short periods are relatively untrustworthy. The erroneous use of the mean age at death as a test of longevity has been mentioned. These are in part also errors of methods, and numerous mixed examples are given below.

Errors from Paucity of Data frequently arise, the "fallacy of small numbers," a too hasty generalization, being the most common fault in medical writings, especially in therapeutics. The degree of approximation to the truth of a varying number of observations is estimated by means of Poisson's formula.

μ = *total number of cases recorded in two groups.*
m = *number in one group.*
n = *number in the other group, so that $\mu = m + n$.*

The extent of variation in the proportion of each group to the whole will vary within the proportions represented by—

$$m/\mu + 2\sqrt{(2mn/\mu3)}, \text{ and } n/\mu - 2\sqrt{(2mn/\mu3)}$$

The larger the number of the total observations (μ), the less will be the value of $2\sqrt{(2mn/\mu3)}$, and the less will be the limits of error in the simple proportion m/μ.

Thus, of 147 cases of enteric fever, 17 died, a fatality of 11·4 per cent. The possible error is determined by the second half of the above formula—

$$= 2\sqrt{(2 \times 17 \times 130 / 1473)} = 2\sqrt{(4,420 / 3,176,523)} = ·0746.$$

i.e. the possibility of error = ·0746 to unity or 7·46 per cent. In other words, in a second series of cases of enteric fever under the same conditions as the above, the fatality may vary from 3·94 to 18·86 per cent., a vague result which indicates that the first series cannot be regarded as establishing more than a primá facie case in favour of any special method of treatment that may have been adopted.

Non ceteris paribus.—The necessity that data to be compared shall be collected on a uniform plan, and be of a strictly comparable nature, is very frequently ignored. The conclusion that the administration of a given antiseptic is a valuable means of treating enteric fever is not demonstrated by the fact that the fatality in the series of cases thus treated is 7 per cent., while in another series treated without antiseptics it is 14 per cent., unless it is shown that the age and other previous conditions of the patients in the two cases were not widely different, and unless the series are sufficiently long to avoid the fallacy due to paucity of data.

Errors from the Composition of Rates.—If the death-rate of A having a population of 10,000 is 10 per 1000, and of B having a population of 20,000 is 15 per 1000, the combined death-rate is not $(10 + 15) / 2 = 12.5$. To obtain the correct combined death-rate, the number of deaths in A (=100) and in B (=300) must first be ascertained, and the death-rate on a population of 30,000 in which 400 deaths occurred will then be found to be 13.3 per 1000.

Errors from Stating Deaths in proportion to Total Deaths.—There is nothing erroneous per se in stating the proportion of deaths at one age as a ratio of the total deaths at all ages, or the deaths from one cause as a ratio of the total deaths from all causes. It is a useful and in fact the only method practicable when it is required to give the proportion of one of these to the other. But beyond this, such a ratio cannot be trusted. For instance, the proportion of fatal accidents among male infants is 12.2, and among female infants 25.1 per cent. of the total fatal accidents in the male and female sex respectively. But it would be erroneous, if it were concluded from these figures that female are more subject to fatal accidents than male infants. The only conclusion that they justify is that at higher ages females are much less subject to fatal accidents than males. In actual facts, for every 1000 infants born, only 2.9 female as against 3.1 males die under one year of age as the result of accident.

Again, suppose the case of two towns, A and B. A with a population of 10,000 has 150 annual deaths, of which 20 are caused by cancer; the general death-rate therefore being 15, and the death-rate from cancer 2.0 per 1000, while the deaths from cancer form 2/15 of the total deaths. B, with the same population as A, has 300 deaths, its death-rate being 30 per 1000, and 40 deaths from cancer, its cancer death-rate being 4.0 per 1000; while the proportion of the deaths from cancer to the total deaths is 2/15 as before. It is useful to know in regard to each of these individual communities that cancer causes 2/15 of its total mortality, but no comparison between the two is practicable on this basis. The only proper comparison is between the death-rate from cancer per 1000 of population in A and B, which shows that it is twice as high in B as in A. A still more accurate method is to ascertain the number of deaths from cancer, and the number living at different age-groups, thus avoiding any errors due to variations in age and sex distribution of population.

Errors as to Averages.—The most common of these results from paucity of data. Note that the results obtained from an average cannot be applied to a particular case. The mean duration or expectation of life, obtained from a life-table, expresses with almost mathematical certainty,

322

the number of years of life of the members of a community taken one with another, but is often not accurate when applied to a single individual.

In Army statistics errors have arisen by failure to comprehend what is meant by the average strength of a force. The statistics must comprise the lives of a given number of persons as well as the deaths occurring among them for an entire year, or allowance must be made in this respect when required.

Hospital statistics for similar reasons are frequently fallacious. Thus death-rates have been frequently given per 100 occupied beds, which are most misleading, as the frequency of succession of patients as well as the nature of the patients' complaints will vary greatly in different hospitals. The only proper method of stating hospital-returns is on the basis of the aggregate annual number of cases treated to a termination. The cases should be further subdivided according to age and sex and disease. Average death-rates for epidemic diseases when used to compare one community with another may give rise to erroneous conclusions. This is inseparable from the nature of such diseases. During the period under comparison, one town may happen to have, say, three epidemics, and the other four; possibly if two or three additional years had been added to the series, the place of the two towns would have been reversed as regards their average death-rate from the disease in question. The proper plan is to give the death-rates from the epidemic disease for every year recorded, to draw a curve of these death-rates for the two towns on the same scale, and to compare the height, the variations of height, and the trend of the curve in each instance.

9 781647 993566